Worldwide Pharmaceutical Regulation Series

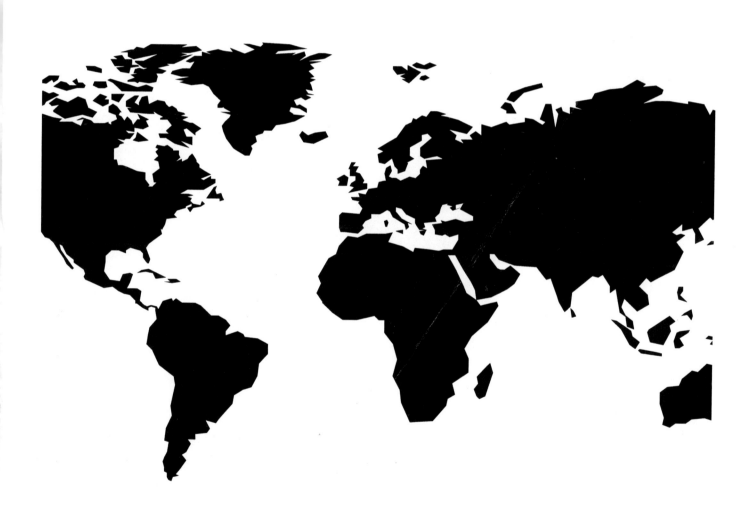

Worldwide Pharmaceutical Regulation Series

New Drug Approval in the United States

Mark Mathieu
with contributions from
Ronald Keeney, M.D.
and
Christopher-Paul Milne

PAREXEL International Corporation
Waltham, MA
Publishers

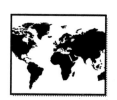

Worldwide Pharmaceutical Regulation Series

New Drug Approval in the United States

by
Mark Mathieu
with contributions from
Ronald Keeney, M.D.
and
Christopher-Paul Milne

Copyright © 2002 by PAREXEL International Corporation, Waltham, MA. All rights reserved. Printed in the United States of America. No part of this work may be reproduced, stored in a retrieval system, or transmitted in any form or by any means, electronic, mechanical, photocopying, recording, or otherwise, without prior written permission of PAREXEL International Corporation.

ISBN Number: 1-882615-57-3

CONTENTS

Chapter 1. An Introduction to the U.S. New Drug Approval Process 1
    The FDA and the Food, Drug and Cosmetic Act 3
    New Drug Development and Approval: The Principal Steps 4
        Preclinical Testing 5
        The Investigational New Drug Application 6
        The FDA's Review of the IND 6
        Clinical Trials 7
        The New Drug Application 8
        The NDA Review Process 9

Chapter 2. Nonclinical Drug Testing 13
    Trends in Nonclinical Testing 14
    FDA Guidance on Nonclinical Testing Requirements. 14
    Types of Nonclinical Studies 16
        Pharmacology Studies 16
            Pharmacological Screening 16
            Pharmacodynamics 16
            Pharmacokinetics 17
        Toxicity Studies 18
            Acute Toxicity Studies 19
            Subacute/Subchronic Studies 20
            Chronic Toxicity Testing 22
            Carcinogenicity Studies 23
            Special Toxicity Studies 25
            Reproductive Toxicity Studies 26
            Genotoxicity Studies 28
            Toxicokinetic Studies 29
    FDA Standards for Nonclinical Testing: Good Laboratory Practice 29
        The Applicability of GLP 30
        Major Provisions of GLP 30
            Organization and Personnel 31
            Testing Facility. 31
            Testing Facility Operation 31
            Test and Control Article Characterization 32
            The Protocol and the Conduct of a Nonclinical Laboratory Study. 32
            Records and Reporting... 32
            Equipment Design... 33
        CDER's GLP Inspections.... 33

Chapter 3. The Investigational New Drug Application.... 35
    Types of INDs 36
    The Applicability of the IND 37
    IND Content and Format Requirements 38

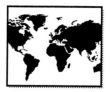

Contents

    Cover Sheet 40
    Table of Contents 41
    Introductory Statement 41
    General Investigational Plan 41
    Investigator's Brochure 44
    Clinical Protocols 45
    Chemistry, Manufacturing, and Control Information 48
    Animal Pharmacology and Toxicology Information 54
    Previous Human Experience with the Investigational Drug 56
    Additional Information 56
Submitting the IND 56
Maintaining/Updating the IND 56
    Protocol Amendments 57
    IND Safety Reports 58
    Annual Reports 61
        Information on Individual Studies 61
        Summary Information 61
        General Investigational Plan 61
        Investigator's Brochure Revisions 61
        Phase 1 Modifications 61
        Foreign Marketing Developments 62
        Request for an FDA Response 62
    Information Amendments 62

Chapter 4. CDER and the IND Review Process 63
    The FDA's Center for Drug Evaluation and Research 64
    CDER's New Drug Review Divisions 67
    Inside the FDA's Drug Review Divisions 74
        Medical/Clinical Discipline 75
        Pharmacology Discipline 75
        Chemistry Discipline 75
        Microbiology Discipline 75
        Project Management Staff 75
    The IND Review Process 76
        Initial Processing of the IND 77
        The IND within the Review Division 77
        The 30-Day Review Clock and IND "Approval" 79
    The Clinical Hold 80
        Clinical Holds and Phase 1 Trials 81
        Clinical Holds and Phase 2 and 3 Trials 81
        How Clinical Holds Work 81
    IND Status 85

Chapter 5. The Clinical Development of New Drugs 87
    The FDA's Role in Clinical Trials 90
    The Structure of Clinical Trials 92
        Phase 1 Clinical Trials 96

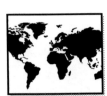

        Pharmacokinetics/Pharmacodynamics and Phase 1 Trials 97
        FDA-Sponsor Communication During Clinical Trials 99
    Phase 2 Clinical Trials 100
    Phase 3 Clinical Trials 104
    Phase 4 Clinical Trials 114

Chapter 6. Good Clinical Practices (GCP) 117
    Responsibilities of the Drug Sponsor 123
    Responsibilities of Investigators 129
    The Institutional Review Board 130
Informed Consent 132

Chapter 7. The New Drug Application 135
  NDA Content and Format Requirements 144
  The Fundamentals of the NDA Submission 145
    The Archival, Review, and Field Copies of the NDA 146
    The Application Form 147
    The Index 148
    Labeling 148
    The NDA Summary 148
    Chemistry Section 152
    Nonclinical Pharmacology and Toxicology Section 159
    Human Pharmacokinetics and Bioavailability Section 160
    Microbiology Section 161
    Clinical Data Section 162
    Safety Update Report Section 165
    Statistical Section 165
    Case Report Tabulations Section 166
    Case Report Forms Section 167
    Patent Information 167
    Patent Certification 167
    Establishment Description 167
    Debarment Certification 167
    Field Copy Certification 168
    User Fee Cover Sheet 168
    Financial Information Section 168
    Other Information 170
  Pre-NDA Meetings 170
  Assembling and Submitting the NDA 172
  Amending the NDA 173

Chapter 8. The NDA Review Process 175
  A Profile of the NDA Review Process 179
  Initial Processing of the NDA 180
  Processing within the Drug Review Division 180
  The FDA's Refuse-to-File Authority 181
  The Preapproval Inspection 182

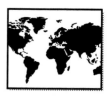

Contents

    The Primary Review Process 185
    Reaching an Institutional Decision on the NDA 189
    Formal Action on an NDA 191
    FDA Action Letters 192
        Approval Letter 192
        Approvable Letter 194
        Not-Approvable Letter 195
    Final Printed Labeling 196
    Draft Package Labeling 197
    The FDA Review of Draft Labeling 200
    Sponsor Rights During the NDA Review Process 200
        The Right to a Timely Review 200
        The Right to Meetings 203
        The Right to Protest and Appeal FDA Actions/Decisions 204
        The Right to Confidentiality 206

Chapter 9. The FDA's Priority Review Policy **209**
    Therapeutic Rating 210
    Chemical Novelty Rating 212
    CDER's Prioritization Policy at Work 214
    The Impact of CDER's Priority Review Policy 214
    Patterns in Priority/Standard Designations for New Drugs 215

Chapter 10. Advisory Committees and the Drug Approval Process **217**
    A Look at Committee Membership 222
    When CDER Uses Advisory Committees 224
    How Advisory Committees Function 226
    How Influential are Advisory Committees? 229
    What Sponsors Should Know About Advisory Committees 230

Chapter 11. Beyond Approval: Drug Manufacturer Regulatory Responsibilities **231**
    General Reporting Requirements 232
    Field Alert Reports 232
    Annual Reports 232
    Other Reports 234
            Advertisements and Promotional Labeling 234
            Special Reports 235
    Adverse Drug Experience Reporting Requirements 235
        Key Definitions Relevant to Adverse Drug Experience Reporting 238
        Adverse Drug Experience Reporting Requirements 239
            15-Day Alert Reports 240
            Periodic Reports 242
        Pending Revisions to the FDA's Postmarketing AE Reporting Requirements 243
    Current Good Manufacturing Practices 244
        The Enforcement of CGMP 249
    Phase 4 Commitments 251

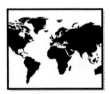

Chapter 12. The Supplemental NDA and Postapproval Changes to Marketed Drugs 255
    When to Submit Supplemental versus Original NDAs 256
    Supplemental NDA Submission Requirements 257
    Postmarketing Manufacturing Changes 258
    FDAMA and Postmarketing Manufacturing Changes 258
    SUPAC and SNDAs for Manufacturing Changes 260
    Labeling Changes 263

Chapter 13. The FDA's Orphan Drug Development Program 267
    The FDA and Orphan Drugs: A Brief History 268
    The Importance of Orphan Drug Designation 268
    A Look at Orphan Drug Incentives 271
    The FDA Approval Process: Advantages for Orphan Drugs? 275

Chapter 14. CDER's Bioresearch Monitoring Program 277
    A Brief History of the Bioresearch Monitoring Program 282
    The Clinical Investigator Compliance Program 283
    Post-Inspectional FDA Actions 288
    The Sponsor/Monitor Compliance Program 289

Chapter 15. Accelerated Drug Approval/Expanded Access Programs 293
    The Treatment IND 296
        Accelerated Drug Development Program (Subpart E) 303
        Accelerated Drug Approval Program (Subpart H) 307
        The Parallel Track Program 308
        Oncology Initiative 310
        "Fast Track" Initiative 312

Chapter 16. The Pediatric Studies Initiative 319
    The Carrot: FDAMA's Pediatric Provision 321
    The Stick: The FDA's 1998 Rule for Assessment of
        Pediatric Safety and Effectiveness 325
    Incorporating FDAMA and the Pediatric Rule into a Drug Development Plan 328
    What Types of Studies Will be Required for FDAMA and the Pediatric Rule? 332
    When to Start Studies 337
    The Present 341
    The Future 343

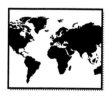

CHAPTER 1

An Introduction to the U.S. New Drug Approval Process

As the gatekeeper to the world's most lucrative pharmaceutical market, the U.S. Food and Drug Administration (FDA) administers what generally is considered to be the world's most demanding drug regulation and approval process. And although studies from the early 1990s suggested that the rigors and inefficiencies of this process resulted in fewer, and the delayed availability of, innovative therapies, much has changed in the intervening years.

Through steadily building momentum under the initial five-year prescription drug user-fee program (PDUFA I), the FDA had improved its drug review performance to the extent that then-FDA Commissioner David Kessler, M.D., proclaimed in December 1996 that the agency had become "a world leader in drug review." In fact, independent studies of global drug reviews suggested that, based on median new drug approval times, the agency had become the fastest among major regulators for perhaps the first time ever.

But CDER's success in approving record numbers of new drugs in record time drew considerable criticism in light of other developments during the late 1990s. After three approved drugs—Redux, Posicor, and Duract—were withdrawn from the market within a nine-month span from late 1997 through mid-1998, agency critics quickly and openly charged that the focus on the speed of drug reviews had come at the expense of drug safety. More recent drug withdrawals, including Rezulin, Lotronex, Raplon, and Baycol, continued to feed these concerns over the safety of new drugs.

Today, international harmonization and an intense focus on risk management and drug safety appear to be the dominant forces driving the next evolutionary phase of new drug regulation in the United States:

- *The Common Technical Document.* By August 2001, the new drug application (NDA) was no longer the sole vehicle through which drug sponsors could formally propose that the FDA approve a new pharmaceutical for marketing in the United States. At that time, the ICH's common technical document (CTD) format became a regulatory option to the NDA for companies seeking FDA approval of a new drug. At the time of its introduction, the CTD was the ICH's most significant achievement: a harmonized core "information package of [clinical, pharmacology/toxicology, and manufacturing] technical data" that could be submitted in the same format and with the same content to obtain marketing authorization in any of the three ICH regions—

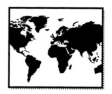

Worldwide Pharmaceutical Regulation Series

the United States, the European Union, and Japan. During a "transition period" that will last until July 2003, companies will have the option of submitting original NDAs and even NDA supplements and amendments in either the CTD or conventional NDA format. Beginning in July 2003, the FDA will "highly recommend" that U.S. marketing dossiers be submitted in the CTD format, although the agency will not be able to implement this as a formal requirement until it undertakes a complete revision of its NDA regulations. It is important to note that the CTD and NDA differ primarily in format and not in content. While it is true that the CTD may provide more information in selected areas than a conventional NDA (see discussion below), the FDA's data and information requirements for drug approval will be unaffected by the CTD. In other words, applications in the CTD format must provide the same data and information as those submitted in the conventional NDA format. In many ways, the CTD simply represents, for now, an alternative format or organizational structure in which data and information that otherwise would be forwarded in the NDA format can be provided to the FDA.

- *Integration of "Risk Management" into New Drug Reviews.* In responding to concerns regarding drug safety, CDER is integrating risk management, or risk intervention, considerations into NDA reviews to control drug risks, center officials first claimed in early 2000. In doing so, the drug center is asking sponsors and its reviewers to consider what additional steps, aside from simply providing risk information on drug labels, can be taken to make newly approved drugs as safe as possible in the marketplace. The use of risk management in drug reviews is, in part, a function of the agency's recognition, through multiple recent product withdrawals, that labeling alone has not been sufficient to ensure the safe use of drugs in a medical system in which drugs are not always prescribed and used according to approved labeling. Risk management alternatives that CDER is evaluating increasingly in new drug reviews include restricted distribution programs, educational programs, patient package inserts, pregnancy registries, special surveillance systems, and safety-related communications. CDER's efforts in this area are now being led by its Review Standards Staff (RSS), which is attempting to create a risk-management framework from early drug development through post-marketing, and which will attempt to develop a systems-based approach for risk communication and risk intervention and for communicating risks to important audiences, including consumers and prescribers.

- *Focus on Postmarketing Surveillance.* While insisting that drug withdrawal rates had not increased, FDA officials openly acknowledged the growing need for a particularly efficient and well-conceived postmarketing drug risk surveillance, assessment, and management program in the face of the speedier and rising numbers of new drug approvals being granted in the United States. Therefore, CDER officials announced a reinvigorated postmarketing drug surveillance program under a newly named Office of Post-Marketing Drug Risk Assessment (OPDRA). In addition, the agency spoke about the need to apply "a new systems framework" to medical product risk management, which would involve a better integration of the efforts of those involved in the prescribing and use of new drugs (patients, practitioners) and better communication of the risks of drug use to both patients and physicians. In 2001, CDER proposed that OPDRA be renamed the Office of Drug Safety, and that it be moved, along with selected other relevant programs, under a new deputy center

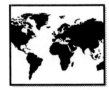

director with special expertise in epidemiology and risk assessment (see Chapter 4). Through either congressional appropriations or industry user fees, the FDA is openly seeking funds to upgrade its postmarketing surveillance efforts. "More rigorous safety monitoring of newly approved drugs in the first few years after a product is on the market could help detect unanticipated problems earlier," the agency claimed in November 2001 statement highlighting the limitations of its current postmarketing surveillance program.

In early 2002, meanwhile, industry and FDA officials were busily discussing the third iteration of the prescription drug user fee program, something that would also have fundamental implications for the drug review process. First on the FDA's agenda, it appeared, was obtaining either higher fees for drug reviews or increased funding from Congress, either of which would better reflect what the agency says is its rising workload and would help shield the resources of other FDA program areas that have suffered as the agency fought to meet its PDUFA goals. The FDA's second goal in negotiating PDUFA III is obtaining additional fees or funding to upgrade the agency's postmarketing surveillance activities. Among the pharmaceutical industry's goals was to obtain more specific performance goals in certain areas (e.g., FDA actions on NDA resubmissions).

Given the number and nature of factors constantly acting upon it, the FDA's new drug approval process can never be characterized as a single, static process. Since new drugs present their own distinct risks and benefits, and because these risks and benefits are evaluated by different FDA reviewers and in the context of a medical knowledge base that is continually evolving, the development and approval paths traveled by two new products are always different, sometimes considerably so. The nature of the drug development and approval process is, in large part, a function of the drug being developed and the condition being studied, and is tailored to ensure that the key questions regarding the compound's safety and effectiveness for this indication are addressed sufficiently before approval.

The FDA and the Food, Drug and Cosmetic Act

Despite the emerging trends outlined above, the foundations of the new drug approval process remain intact within the provisions of the Federal Food, Drug and Cosmetic Act (FD&C Act). Seen by many as the most complex law of its kind, the FD&C Act has at least three basic provisions that continue to shape the new drug development and review process:

1. The FD&C Act defines the term "drug," thereby identifying the universe of products subject to regulation as drugs. The statute defines drugs as "articles intended for use in the diagnosis, cure, mitigation, treatment, or prevention of disease in man..." and "articles (other than food) intended to affect the structure or any function of the body of man...."

2. The FD&C Act defines "new drug," thereby identifying which products are subject to the requirements of the new drug approval process. The law defines "new drug" as: "(1) Any drug (except a new animal drug or an animal feed bearing or containing a new animal drug) the composition of which is such that such drug is not generally recognized, among experts qualified by scientific training and experience to evaluate the safety and effectiveness of drugs, as safe and effective for use under the conditions prescribed, recommended, or suggested in labeling thereof, except that

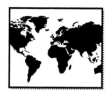

such a drug not so recognized shall not be deemed to be a 'new drug' if at any time prior to the enactment of this Act it was subject to the Food and Drugs Act of June 30, 1906, as amended, and if at such time its labeling contained the same representations concerning the conditions of its use; or (2) Any drug (except a new animal drug or an animal feed bearing or containing a new animal drug) the composition of which is such that such drug, as a result of investigations to determine its safety and effectiveness for use under such conditions, has become so recognized, but which has not, otherwise than in such investigations, been used to a material extent or for a material time under such conditions."

3. The FD&C Act identifies, in the broadest possible terms, the criteria that all new drugs must meet to gain marketing approval. Before a new drug can be marketed in the United States, it must be the subject of an FDA-approved new drug application (NDA), which must contain adequate data and information on the drug's safety and "substantial evidence" of the product's effectiveness.

As similar laws do in other areas, the FD&C Act merely establishes the basic framework and essential principles of new drug approval. The statute must be interpreted, implemented, and enforced. Since the early 1900s, these responsibilities have fallen on the FDA.

It is the interpretive and discretionary powers granted to the FDA under the FD&C Act that give the agency wide-ranging authority. Perhaps the most significant of these powers is the FDA's role in interpreting the legal requirement that a sponsor present substantial evidence of effectiveness prior to a drug's approval. While this is a statutory requirement, it is the FDA that decides what constitutes substantial evidence for each new drug. In deciding, on a case-by-case basis, what constitutes substantial evidence for each new drug, the agency determines the scientific testing and data submissions necessary to obtain marketing approval.

During the late 1990s, CDER made a greater effort to define the concept of substantial evidence and to communicate its expectations to industry. Through a May 1998 guidance entitled, *Providing Clinical Evidence of Effectiveness for Human Drug and Biological Products*, CDER offered what is likely its most detailed discussion ever on the efficacy data necessary to support new drug approval (see Chapter 5). The FDA Modernization Act of 1997 also offered a clarification of the substantial evidence concept by stating that the FDA can accept data from one adequate and well-controlled clinical trial supported by confirmatory evidence as sufficient to establish a drug's effectiveness.

New Drug Development and Approval: The Principal Steps

Despite the changes outlined above, new drugs face a reasonably well-defined development and approval process that has evolved over several decades. In fact, given CDER's commitment to better document and communicate development and approval standards, the drug approval process will likely remain the best understood of the FDA's product approval processes.

The primary stages of the drug development and approval process fall within one of three classes of activities: (1) scientific testing designed to provide data on a product's safety and/or effectiveness; (2) the preparation and submission of these data and other information in regulatory applications; and (3) the FDA's review of regulatory submissions. While all drug development programs involve these core

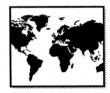

activities, it is important to note how fundamentally different each can be for any two products. Testing and submission requirements, for example, will be shaped by many factors, including the drug's proposed indication, the amount and nature of data already available on the drug and on compounds similar in molecular structure, and the availability of therapeutic alternatives for the target indication.

Preclinical Testing

Clearly, clinical trials represent the ultimate premarketing proving grounds for new pharmaceuticals. Because of the costs and risks inherent in using an untested drug in clinical testing, however, drug sponsors do not leap headlong into a clinical program once they have identified a promising compound. Prior to clinical studies, the sponsor seeks some evidence of the compound's biological activity, and both the sponsor and the FDA seek data indicating that the drug is reasonably safe for initial administration to humans.

Before initiating clinical studies, a drug sponsor must submit an application that provides information showing that the company can manufacture the drug, descriptions of the proposed clinical trials, and data establishing that the drug is reasonably safe for use in initial, small-scale clinical studies. Depending on whether the compound has been studied or marketed previously, the sponsor may have several options for fulfilling the last of these three requirements: (1) compiling existing nonclinical data derived from past *in vitro* laboratory or animal studies on the compound; (2) compiling data from previous clinical testing or marketing of the drug in the United States or another country whose population is relevant to the U.S. population; or (3) undertaking new preclinical studies designed to provide the evidence necessary to support the safety of administering the compound to humans.

For most NMEs and other drugs whose clinical safety and efficacy have not been established previously, preclinical *in vitro* and *in vivo* animal testing represents the first major step toward regulatory approval (see Chapter 2). During preclinical drug development, a sponsor evaluates the drug's toxic and pharmacologic effects. Genotoxicity screening is performed, as well as investigations on drug absorption and metabolism, the toxicity of the drug's metabolites, and the speed with which the drug and its metabolites are excreted from the body. At the preclinical stage, the FDA generally expects that sponsors will: (1) develop a pharmacological profile of the drug; (2) determine the acute toxicity of the drug in at least two species of animals; and (3) conduct short-term toxicity studies, the duration of which is based on the duration of the proposed clinical studies.

Once clinical trials begin, further *in vitro* and *in vivo* animal studies provide information essential to the continued clinical use and, ultimately, the approval of the drug. Long-term and specialized animal tests are needed to support the safety of testing a compound in larger patient populations and over longer periods. These tests also allow researchers to evaluate effects that are impractical or unethical to study in humans, such as drug effects over an entire life span, effects over several generations, and effects on pregnancy and reproduction.

Because preclinical drug development does not involve human exposure to an experimental compound, drug developers have considerable flexibility in manufacturing, shipping, and testing experimental drugs. Virtually the only regulatory limitations facing sponsors are the general animal welfare provisions contained in current federal and state animal protection statutes and regulations, and little more than a single FDA requirement detailed in federal regulations: "A person may ship a drug intended solely for tests in vitro or in animals used only for laboratory research purposes if it is labeled as follows: Caution: Contains a new drug for investigational use only in laboratory research animals, or for tests in vitro. Not for use in humans."

When a sponsor begins to compile safety data for submission to the FDA, however, a set of regulations called Good Laboratory Practice (GLP) apply. Because it will base important regulatory decisions on these data, the FDA uses GLP standards to ensure the quality of animal testing and the resultant data.

The Investigational New Drug Application

When a sponsor believes that it has sufficient data to show that a new drug is adequately safe for initial small-scale clinical studies, the company assembles and submits an investigational new drug application (IND). The IND is the vehicle through which a sponsor seeks an exemption from the statutory requirement that prohibits unapproved drugs from being shipped in interstate commerce. The sponsor seeks this exemption by alerting the FDA of its intent to conduct clinical studies with an investigational new drug.

In the IND, the sponsor submits information in three principal areas: (1) the results of all preclinical testing and an analysis of what implications these results have for human pharmacology; (2) an analysis of the drug's chemical composition and the manufacturing and quality control procedures used in producing the compound; and (3) protocols describing the sponsor's plans for the initial-stage clinical studies proposed in the IND, and information describing the relevant qualifications of the investigators who will carry out these studies.

Among the most significant FDA regulatory reforms implemented in the 1990s were those affecting IND submission requirements. In part an effort to stem the tide of Phase 1 studies moving to European countries, which generally have less demanding submission standards for initial-stage clinical research, the FDA "clarified" its IND content requirements in November 1995. Specifically, the agency established its willingness to accept toxicology data summaries and line listings based upon sponsors' unaudited draft toxicologic reports of completed animal studies in INDs for Phase 1 studies. By accepting the summaries and listings based on unaudited draft reports, and permitting companies to update this information 120 days after trials are initiated, the FDA, in effect, permits sponsors to begin Phase 1 trials months earlier than in the past.

The FDA's Review of the IND

The IND review is unique among the FDA's application review processes. In many respects, this process and the FDA's treatment of INDs reflect the delicate balance between the federal government's responsibility to protect clinical trial subjects from unnecessary risks and its desire to avoid becoming an impediment to the medical research process. Given these dual goals, the FDA must perform a safety review of an IND prior to clinical trials, but has only 30 days in which to reach an initial determination on the filing.

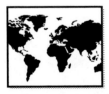

The FDA's review of an IND focuses largely on three areas:

- *Pharmacology/Toxicology Review.* The reviewing pharmacologist examines the results of animal pharmacology and toxicology testing, and attempts to relate these results to human pharmacology.

- *Chemistry Review.* The reviewing chemist evaluates both the sponsor's manufacturing processes and control procedures to ensure that the compound is reproducible and is stable in its pure form. If a drug is either unstable or not reproducible, then the validity of any clinical testing would be undermined and, more importantly, the studies may pose significant risks. The chemistry reviewer also evaluates the drug's characterization and chemical structure, and compares the product's structure and impurity profile to those of other drugs (i.e., drugs known to be toxic).

- *Clinical Review.* The reviewing medical officer, who is generally a physician, evaluates the clinical protocols to ensure: (1) that subjects will not be exposed to unreasonable or unnecessary risks during clinical trials; and (2) that Phase 2 and Phase 3 trials (generally not submitted in the initial IND filing) are adequate in design to provide scientifically valid data.

If the FDA does not contact the applicant within 30 days of the IND submission, the sponsor may initiate clinical trials. In this way, the agency does not approve an IND, but allows clinical testing to proceed through its "administrative silence."

When the FDA decides that a certain clinical trial should be delayed, the agency contacts the sponsor within the 30-day period to initiate what is called a "clinical hold"—the delay of the clinical trial until potential problems or unanswered questions are addressed. Aside from the safety-related reasons mentioned above, the FDA may base a clinical hold on other grounds, including that the IND does not contain sufficient information to assess the risks of using the drug in clinical trials (see Chapter 4).

Clinical Trials

Clinical trials clearly represent the most critical and demanding phase in the drug development process. If a drug survives the rigors of clinical testing, the FDA's ultimate approval decision will be based primarily upon data derived from these studies—the agency estimates that more than 80 percent of the average NDA for an NME consists of clinical data and analyses alone.

If the FDA's new drug review performance was the dominant regulatory controversy of the 1980s and early 1990s, growing clinical development times had clearly supplanted it during the mid-1990s. A seemingly inexorable rise in clinical development times during the past two decades, industry maintained, had made product development costs even more prohibitive, and was offsetting the benefits of the marked improvements in FDA new drug review times.

This reality and changes in the competitive environment for pharmaceuticals helped to accelerate several trends, including industry efforts to streamline its clinical development programs and to leverage its clinical trial efforts internationally. They also may have played a role in a new FDA initiative to better define the clinical trial data necessary to support drug approval. In a May 1998 guidance entitled,

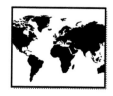

Providing Clinical Evidence of Effectiveness for Human Drug and Biological Products, the agency provided its latest views on the "quantitative and qualitative standards" for establishing drug effectiveness. Further, several new FDA performance goals were established under PDUFA II to help speed the clinical development process.

Although clinical trials for different drugs can vary greatly in design, they are often similar in structure (see Chapter 5). Since researchers may know little about a new compound prior to its use in humans, testing the drug through serially conducted studies permits each phase of clinical development to be carefully designed to use and build upon the information obtained from the research phase preceding it. Clinical programs for most new drugs begin with the cautious use of an investigational compound in small, carefully selected population groups, and proceed into larger, more clinically relevant, and increasingly diverse patient pools.

While there is no statute or regulation that mandates a specific clinical trial structure or design, a clinical development program most often proceeds in three primary stages, or phases:

- Phase 1: The cautious use of a drug in a few patients or normal human volunteers—20 to 80 subjects—to gain basic safety and pharmacological information. Specifically, these studies allow the sponsor to assess a drug's pharmacology and pharmacokinetics, mechanism of action in humans, side effects (of various doses), optimal route of administration, and safe dosage range.

- Phase 2: The use of the compound in a small number of subjects—100 to 200 patients—who suffer from the condition that the drug is intended to treat or diagnose. Phase 2 trials provide additional safety data and the first indication of a drug's clinical effectiveness in its proposed use. Results of Phase 2 studies can establish the foundation for key aspects of Phase 3 study design (e.g., clinical endpoints, target population).

- Phase 3: Use of the drug in a significantly larger group of subjects (i.e., several hundred to several thousand) who suffer from the condition that the drug is proposed to treat or diagnose to gather additional effectiveness and safety information necessary for assessments of the drug's overall risk-benefit relationship. Because certain Phase 3 trials, called "pivotal" trials, will serve as the primary basis for the drug's approval, these studies must meet more rigorous standards (e.g., controls, blinding, randomization, size).

The dire need for therapies for AIDS, cancer, and other life-threatening illnesses compelled the FDA to develop a variety of alternative models for clinical drug development. Some of these programs, which have been implemented by various regulations, were codified into law under the FDA Modernization Act of 1997 (see Chapter 15).

The New Drug Application

Since 1938, the new drug application (NDA) has been the vehicle through which drug sponsors formally propose that the FDA approve a new pharmaceutical for sale and marketing in the United States. To support a drug's approval, an NDA comprises thousands of pages of nonclinical and clinical test data and analyses, drug chemistry information, and descriptions of manufacturing procedures.

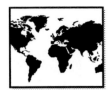

In August 2001, however, the ICH effort produced another option for companies seeking FDA approval to market a new drug in the United States—the common technical document, or CTD. During a "transition period" that will last until July 2003, companies will have the option of submitting U.S. marketing dossiers in either the CTD or conventional NDA format. It is important to note that the CTD differs from the NDA in format but not in content, and that the submission standards necessary to gain FDA approval will not be affected in any way by the transition to the CTD format. Beginning in July 2003, the FDA will "highly recommend" that U.S. marketing dossiers be submitted in the CTD format, although the agency will not be able to implement this as a formal requirement until it undertakes a complete revision of its NDA regulations.

Whether in the NDA or CTD format, the U.S. marketing dossier for a new drug is the largest and most complex premarketing application that the FDA reviews. The application must provide sufficient information, data, and analyses to permit agency reviewers to make several key determinations, including: (1) whether the drug is safe and effective in its proposed use(s), and whether the benefits of the drug outweigh its risks; (2) whether the methods used in manufacturing the drug and the controls used to maintain the product's quality are adequate to preserve its identity, strength, and purity; and (3) whether the drug's proposed labeling is appropriate and, if not, what the drug's labeling should contain.

In recent years, CDER also continued to develop its technical infrastructure to accept electronic NDAs (e-NDAs)—under PDUFA II commitments, the FDA agreed to develop a paperless, electronic application submission system for all applications by fiscal year 2002. Industry appears to be embracing the electronic submission concept: Of the first 61 NDAs filed in fiscal year 2001, for example, 21 (or 35%) were completely electronic submissions.

The NDA Review Process

No other aspect of the U.S. drug development and approval system has evolved as significantly over the past decade as the FDA's NDA review process. So fundamental were these changes—and the improvements in drug review times that resulted from them—that CDER's NDA review performance was transformed from one of the most harshly criticized of FDA activities into what was perhaps the agency's best defense against regulatory reform proposals advanced in the mid-1990s.

The driving forces behind this evolution, of course, were PDUFA I and the changes that CDER implemented to meet the new review timelines associated with this legislation. In the early and mid-1990s, CDER instituted tight controls for managing and tracking drug reviews, and reorganized the center's drug review divisions into smaller, more therapeutically focused units.

But CDER's success in approving record numbers of new drugs in record time drew considerable criticism in light of other developments during the late 1990s. After three approved drugs were withdrawn within a nine-month span from late 1997 through mid-1998, agency critics quickly and openly charged that the FDA's focus on the speed of drug approvals had come at the expense of drug safety, which they claimed was contributing to the estimated 100,000 deaths each year related to adverse drug reactions. CDER officials responded by pointing out that the center's recent record of drug withdrawals compared favorably with its record in earlier years. Several additional drug withdrawals in recent years ensured continuing public attention to the drug safety issue.

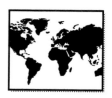

Rising mean and median drug review times and a drop in new drug approvals in 1999 and 2000 ultimately led to industry claims of an FDA drug review "slowdown." Although they conceded that drug reviews may be more conservative in some respects today (e.g., the inability to control prescriber behavior through drug labeling), FDA officials countered that industry's submissions for new drugs had slowed in recent years and that the rise in review times reflected a spate of problematic NDAs submitted years earlier rather than extended reviews for recently submitted applications.

Other CDER initiatives underscored the growing concerns over postmarketing drug safety, and illustrated the center's desire to address such issues during the NDA review process whenever possible. In November 1999, for example, CDER announced that its new drug review divisions and its Office of Post-Marketing Drug Risk Assessment will hold "preapproval safety conferences" on a routine basis prior to approving applications for certain drugs, including new molecular entities, to provide an internal forum for considering the need for any special postmarketing analyses, safety studies, or other special evaluations by the sponsor. Also in response to such concerns, CDER officials promised to integrate the consideration of risk management, or risk intervention, alternatives into NDA reviews by asking sponsors and its own reviewers to consider what additional steps, beyond providing risk information on drug labels, can be taken to make each newly approved drug as safe as possible in the marketplace.

Upon their submission, NDAs are forwarded to one of CDER's 14 new drug review divisions—specifically, the division that handles the therapeutic area relevant to the submission. Within 45 days of the NDA's submission, FDA reviewers—including the lead medical, chemistry, and pharmacology reviewers—will meet to determine if the application is sufficiently complete for a full review. NDAs that meet minimum submission criteria are "filed," or accepted for review, while the FDA issues refuse-to-file (RTF) decisions for deficient applications, which are returned to their sponsors.

Once the review team decides that an NDA is fileable, it begins the "primary" review of the application. During this evaluation, each member of the review team sifts through volumes of research data and information applicable to his or her expertise:

- Clinical Reviewer: Evaluates the data from, and analyses of, clinical studies to determine if the drug is safe and effective in its proposed use(s) and if the product's benefits outweigh its risks.

- Pharmacology/Toxicology Reviewer: Evaluates the entire body of nonclinical data and analyses, with a particular focus on the newly submitted long-term test data, to identify relevant implications for the drug's clinical safety.

- Chemistry Reviewer: Evaluates commercial-stage manufacturing procedures (e.g., method of synthesis or isolation, purification process, and process controls) and the specifications and analytical methods used to assure the identity, strength, purity, and bioavailability of the drug product.

- Statistical Reviewer: Evaluates the pivotal clinical data to determine if there exists statistically significant evidence of the drug's safety and effectiveness, the appropriateness of the sponsor's clinical data analyses and the assumptions under which these analyses were performed, the statistical significance of newly submitted nonclinical data, and the implications of stability data for establishing appropriate expiration dating for the product.

- Biopharmaceutics Reviewer: Evaluates pharmacokinetics and bioavailability data to establish appropriate drug dosing.

- Microbiology Reviewer: For certain drugs (anti-infectives, antivirals, and special pathogens), a CDER microbiologist will evaluate the drug's effects on target viruses or other microorganisms. For sterile drugs and certain non-sterile drug products (e.g., aqueous dosage forms that can support microbial growth), a microbiologist will conduct a product quality assessment.

The filing decision also triggers a division request that the relevant FDA field office undertake what is called a "preapproval inspection" of the sponsor's manufacturing facilities. During such inspections, FDA investigators visit the applicant's production facilities to audit manufacturing-related statements and commitments made in the NDA against actual manufacturing practices employed by the sponsor or contract manufacturer.

When the primary technical reviews are completed, each discipline reviewer must prepare a written evaluation that presents his or her conclusions and recommendations regarding the application. In most cases, the medical reviewer is responsible for evaluating and reconciling the conclusions of reviewers in the other scientific disciplines. This process, and the development of what CDER calls an "institutional decision" on an NDA's approvability, is likely to involve considerable dialogue between the medical reviewer and reviewers in the other disciplines.

During the drug review process, the FDA may seek advice and comment from one of its 15 prescription drug advisory committees (see Chapter 10). When called upon, these expert committees provide the agency with independent, non-binding advice and recommendations.

For NDAs submitted in FY1998 through FY2002, the FDA must meet review performance goals associated with PDUFA II. The new review goals will differ for "priority" drugs (i.e., drugs representing a significant improvement over marketed products) and "standard" drugs (see Chapter 9). A six-month review timeframe will apply to priority applications during PDUFA II, while the agency has agreed to take action on increasing percentages of standard applications within 10 months.

At the completion of its review, CDER must issue an action letter—an approval, approvable, or not-approvable letter. These action letters communicate the results of the review to the applicant and, if necessary, identify what issues or deficiencies must be addressed before the application can be approved. Under its PDUFA II commitments, CDER will develop a regulation establishing that a new type of action letter—a "complete response" letter—will replace both approvable and not-approvable letters.

The center also committed to specific review timeframes for taking action on sponsor resubmissions (i.e., formal company responses to approvable/not-approvable or complete response letters). Applicable review performance goals are based on the type and amount of data provided in these resubmissions.

CHAPTER 2

Nonclinical Drug Testing

For most new molecular entities (NME) and other drugs whose clinical safety and efficacy have not been established previously, preclinical *in vitro* and *in vivo* animal testing represents the first major step toward regulatory approval. According to some estimates, only 1 in every 1,000 compounds studied in preclinical testing progresses beyond this phase. Preclinical screening and testing show that the remaining compounds are unsafe, are poorly absorbed, lack pharmacological activity, or have some other flaw that makes them unworthy of further development.

For those drugs that are researched further, animal studies play several roles in drug development. First, the studies provide the basic toxicological and pharmacological information needed to obtain the FDA's permission to begin clinical trials. While the FDA's decision to approve a new pharmaceutical for marketing is based largely on the results of clinical studies, the agency will not allow an entirely unknown and uncharacterized compound to be administered to human subjects. Before clinical work begins, the agency requires that the drug be administered to, and its short-term effects be studied in, laboratory animals. The FDA uses data from these studies to decide if the drug is sufficiently safe for initial administration to humans.

Once clinical trials begin, further *in vitro* and *in vivo* animal studies provide information essential to the continued clinical use and, ultimately, the approval of the drug. Long-term and specialized animal tests are needed to support the safety of testing a compound in larger patient populations and over longer periods. These tests also allow researchers to evaluate effects that are impractical or unethical to study in humans, such as drug effects over an entire animal life span, effects on pregnancy and reproduction, and effects on development.

Although nonclinical research results are imperfect predictors of clinical responses, laboratory animals remain the best practical experimental models for identifying and measuring a compound's biological activity, and for predicting a drug's clinical effects. (Because animal studies are performed before and during clinical studies, the term "nonclinical" generally is preferable to "preclinical" when discussing the full spectrum of *in vitro* and non-human *in vivo* tests associated with drug development.) By studying a drug's dose-response characteristics, adverse and residual effects, and mechanism, site, degree, and duration of action, drug sponsors and the FDA gain valuable insights on the compound's probable action and effects in humans.

The FDA plays at least four principal roles in the nonclinical testing of drugs:
- the agency determines, sometimes on a case-by-case basis, what nonclinical test

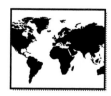

data are needed to show that a drug is sufficiently safe for initial and continued testing in humans;

- the agency, when asked, provides advice to drug sponsors on the adequacy of nonclinical testing programs developed for specific drugs before the animal studies are initiated;
- the agency provides independent analyses of nonclinical test results and conclusions; and
- the agency sets minimum standards for laboratories conducting nonclinical toxicity testing through good laboratory practice (GLP) regulations (see discussion below).

Trends in Nonclinical Testing

Although there are few, if any, studies that measure it directly, nonclinical testing has been affected by industry's need to streamline the drug development process. While most efforts and studies regarding streamlining drug development times have focused on the clinical research process, new benchmarks for preclinical drug development are now emerging. In July 1999, for example, Hoffmann-La Roche reported that it had established "a new benchmark" for preclinical development in taking a new compound from a "proof of concept" study to the start of clinical trials in 18 months.

Early in the new millennium, several emerging initiatives seemed likely to play significant roles in the evolution of nonclinical drug development. These include ongoing government initiatives to develop testing alternatives, the application of genomics and proteomics, efforts to improve nonclinical studies' abilities to predict adverse human effects, and the integration of informatics into toxicity assessments. At its inaugural meeting in December 1999, for example, the Nonclinical Studies Subcommittee of CDER's Pharmaceutical Science Advisory Committee outlined several priorities and areas of focus, including finding new biomarkers to improve the predictive value of nonclinical studies and providing a better interface between nonclinical and clinical studies.

The FDA's August 2001 implementation of a transition period for the "common technical document," a standardized information package of technical data that could be submitted in marketing authorization applications in all three ICH regions, will also have some implications for the presentation of nonclinical data and results (see Chapter 7). From August 2001 until July 2003, industry will have the option of submitting marketing dossiers in the CTD or conventional NDA format. In July 2003, the CTD will become a quasi-requirement, as the FDA states that it will "highly recommend" that the harmonized format be used for all marketing applications.

FDA Guidance on Nonclinical Testing Requirements

Until fairly recently, FDA nonclinical testing requirements were described only in very general terms in two now-outdated guidelines, one published in 1968 by the FDA and the other in 1977 by the U.S. Pharmaceutical Manufacturers Association (PMA). In the late 1980s and early 1990s, FDA toxicologists and pharmacologists were developing several guidance documents to address subjects ranging from animal-testing requirements for specific classes of drugs to the use of computer technology for nonclinical data submissions.

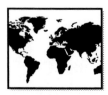

Concurrent with the FDA's efforts to produce updated guidance in this area, the European Community (EC) and Japan were developing testing standards that were often similar in principle but different in detail. In an effort to harmonize these and other testing standards, the regulatory authorities and pharmaceutical industries of these three regions organized the International Conferences on Harmonization (ICH).

The harmonization initiative has had fundamental effects on the FDA's own efforts to develop recommendations for nonclinical testing. Most importantly, the FDA has sought to revise its guidelines to reflect the consensus to which the agency has contributed as part of the ICH process.

The ICH process and its effects on the FDA's efforts will continue for some time. By the late 1990s, the FDA had accepted harmonized recommendations on single dose toxicity testing, the nonclinical safety studies needed to support human clinical trials, and the duration of chronic toxicity testing in rodents. It had also adopted harmonized guidelines on reproductive toxicity studies, toxicokinetics, certain aspects of pharmacokinetics, genotoxicity testing, and carcinogenicity studies. Efforts to finalize guidelines on numerous other nonclinical topics continue, and new topics are destined to enter the process. In addition to outlining the FDA's nonclinical testing requirements, the following discussion analyzes the specific effects that the ICH process has had and is expected to have on these requirements.

FDA officials are always careful to stress the limitations of guidelines, no matter how current. (Note: Under the FDA's 1997 Good Guidance Practices initiative, all new guidelines are being designated as "guidances.") As with any guidances, the agency's nonclinical guidelines are designed only to provide general direction for typical situations; they cannot be applied universally to all drugs and all situations. Therefore, the FDA remains willing to advise sponsors, particularly about unusual cases. FDA staffers will discuss nonclinical testing strategies during the development of these plans, but can usually offer more useful insights if a sponsor develops a nonclinical study program and submits the plan for agency review. Recommendations obtained from such reviews supplement drug sponsors' own expertise and the more general suggestions provided by FDA and ICH guidelines.

Whether or not a sponsor chooses to initiate a dialogue with FDA staff, the types and amount of nonclinical testing ultimately required by the agency will depend on several factors, including:

- a drug's chemical structure, and the similarity of that structure to existing compounds with safety profiles known to the FDA;

- a drug's proposed indication in humans;

- a drug's target patient population (e.g., elderly, infants, women);

- special characteristics of a drug's use pattern (e.g., if a drug is likely to be prescribed as a concomitant medication);

- a drug's proposed route of administration; and

- a drug's proposed duration of administration (i.e., whether for chronic or short-term use).

Types of Nonclinical Studies

When drug sponsors initiate a nonclinical testing program, their first goal is to conduct the studies and collect the data necessary to support the safety of early clinical trials. In the past, these data generally have been limited to short-term animal test results. Today, however, *in vitro* and *in vivo* genotoxicity testing is assuming greater importance during the preclinical phase.

As stated above, preclinical studies represent only part of a drug's nonclinical development. The comprehensive nonclinical testing program needed to support marketing approval for most new drugs involves years of work and several different types of studies.

A final ICH text entitled, M3 *Guidance on Nonclinical Safety Studies for the Conduct of Human Clinical Trials for Pharmaceuticals* (November 1997), hereafter referred to as the M3 guidance, discusses the timing of the various components of nonclinical testing and their relation to the conduct of clinical trials. According to this document, the goals of the nonclinical safety evaluation include "characterization of toxic effects with respect to target organs, dose dependence, relationship to exposure, and potential reversibility. The information is important for the estimation of an initial safe starting dose for the human trials and the identification of parameters for clinical monitoring for potential adverse effects. The nonclinical safety studies, although limited at the beginning of clinical development, should be adequate to characterize potential toxic effects under the conditions of the supported clinical trial."

For the purpose of analysis, nonclinical testing is often divided into two areas: pharmacology and toxicology. Together, pharmacology and toxicology studies are designed to provide an integrated overview of a drug's effects in various animal species.

Pharmacology Studies Because insights gained from pharmacological studies—particularly those regarding adverse effects—can influence the direction of later toxicological testing, pharmacologic work is generally conducted first.

Pharmacological Screening. The pharmacological study of a new drug proceeds in phases. The initial phase, pharmacological screening, is really part of the drug discovery process. It involves the use of *in vitro* and *in vivo* assays designed to determine if a compound has any pharmacological activity. Hundreds of compounds may be subjected to these screenings, with those exhibiting measurable pharmacological effects being selected as "lead chemicals" (i.e., substances to be tested further).

Pharmacodynamics. Once a lead chemical is selected, the sponsor generally begins to compile a more complete qualitative and quantitative pharmacological profile of the compound. This profile consists largely of pharmacodynamic studies, which provide an indication of the drug's action on various receptors or physiological systems in animals.

Some pharmacodynamic studies, called "safety pharmacology studies," should be sufficiently extensive to determine dose-response relationships and the drug's duration and mechanism of action. In these studies, researchers explore the drug's potential adverse effects on major physiological systems and activities (i.e., neurologic, cardiovascular, respiratory, gastrointestinal, genitourinary, endocrine, anti-inflammatory, immunoreactive, chemotherapeutic, and enzymatic) in relation to exposure. The studies are designed to investigate all primary and secondary effects related or unrelated to the desired therapeutic effect, extensions of the therapeutic effect that might produce toxicity at higher

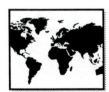

doses, and effects related to interactions with other drugs. According to the ICH's November 1997 M3 guidance, safety pharmacology studies should be performed prior to human exposure. These assessments may be made as part of independent pharmacology studies or incorporated into appropriate toxicology studies. Additional studies may be appropriate following initial clinical studies or toxicology studies.

In July 2000, the ICH parties released a final guidance entitled, S7 *Guideline on Safety Pharmacology Studies for Human Pharmaceuticals*. Although earlier ICH guidances discussed safety pharmacology studies, the S7 guidance is the first to define this phase of development—"those studies that investigate the potential undesirable pharmacodynamic effects of a substance on physiological functions in relationship to exposure in the therapeutic range and above." (Author's note: The S7 guidance states that pharmacology studies also comprise two other categories of studies—primary pharmacodynamic studies ("studies on the mode of action and/or effects of a substance in relation to its desired therapeutic target") and secondary pharmacodynamic studies ("studies on the mode of action and/or effects of a substance not related to its desired therapeutic target...sometimes referred to as part of general pharmacology studies")). The principal objectives of safety pharmacology studies, the guidance notes, are: (1) to identify undesirable pharmacodynamic properties of a substance that may have relevance to its human safety; (2) to evaluate adverse pharmacodynamic and/or pathophysiological effects of a substance observed in toxicology and/or clinical studies; and (3) to investigate the mechanism of the adverse pharmacodynamic effects observed and/or suspected. Among the tests recommended by the guidance is a "safety pharmacology core battery" designed to "investigate the effects of the test substance on vital functions," which are generally the cardiovascular, respiratory and central nervous systems.

Pharmacokinetics. The pharmacology component of preclinical development also includes pharmacokinetic testing, which is designed to obtain information on the extent and duration of systemic exposure to the drug. Generally, these studies are performed both *in vitro* and *in vivo* in multiple species using both radiolabeled and unlabeled test compound. The results are then compared to identify species-to-species drug-response differences that might affect later nonclinical and clinical studies or their interpretation. Today, these studies are considered to be a much more important aspect of preclinical drug development than they were previously, and serve as the basis for subsequent toxicokinetic assessments (see discussion on toxicity studies below). According to the ICH's M3 guidance, exposure data in animals should be evaluated prior to human trials, and additional information on absorption, distribution, metabolism and excretion should become available by the time that early Phase 1 studies (human pharmacology) are complete so that human and animal metabolic pathways can be compared.

It is worth noting that this is one area in which there is little specific international guidance available, and where the ICH regional-specific guidances differ.

Pharmacokinetic studies are designed to yield information about the drug's absorption, distribution, metabolism, and excretion (ADME) pattern. Analytical methodology employed to generate these data may include ultraviolet absorption, fluorescence, high-pressure liquid chromatography, gas chromatography, immunoassay, liquid scintigraphy, autoradiography and mass spectrometry analysis of the parent compound and/or metabolites in tissues or fluids.

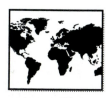

Absorption studies generally involve serial determinations of drug concentration in blood and urine after dosing to indicate the rate and extent of absorption (e.g., following oral administration). Typically, studies using the intravenous route are conducted to serve as a reference. Common pharmacokinetic parameters employed in these assessments include plasma area under the curve (AUC), maximum (peak) plasma concentration (Cmax), and plasma concentration at a specified time after administration of a given dose (C(time)). Bioavailability (i.e., the amount of drug that reaches the systemic circulation) is dependent, in part, on the extent of absorption, but is also influenced by other factors, such as the extent of a drug's metabolism by the liver before it enters the general circulation.

Distribution studies provide information on the extent and time course of tissue accumulation and the elimination of a drug and/or its metabolites. Distribution patterns can be assessed by sacrificing animals at predetermined intervals after dosing, and then measuring the concentration of the drug and/or its metabolites in selected tissues. In general, only single dose studies of distribution are performed. However, in accordance with the adoption of the final ICH guideline entitled, S3B *Pharmacokinetics: Guidance for Repeated Dose Tissue Distribution Studies* (March 1995), repeat dose distribution studies are appropriate for compounds that have: (1) an apparently long half life; (2) incomplete elimination; or (3) unanticipated organ toxicity.

The "volume of distribution" represents another parameter that is useful in assessing drug distribution. The volume of distribution relates the amount of drug in the body to the concentration of drug in the blood or plasma. For drugs that are extensively bound to plasma proteins but not to tissue components, the volume of distribution will approach that of the plasma volume.

The assessment and quantification of a drug's metabolic pattern is essential for a complete understanding of efficacy and toxicity, since species differences in toxicity may be related to differences in metabolism. To assess the metabolic profile of a drug, the concentration of the drug and its major metabolites are measured in plasma, urine, feces, bile, and/or other tissues as a function of time following dose administration. In some cases, toxicological testing of pharmacologically active metabolites may be necessary in addition to testing on the drug itself.

"Clearance" is a measure of an organism's ability to eliminate a drug. The concept represents the rate of a drug's elimination in relation to its concentration (CL = Rate of elimination/C). This excretion parameter can be determined for individual organs and, when added together, will equal total systemic clearance. In general, decreased toxic potential is associated with rapid and complete excretion.

Toxicity Studies *In vitro* and *in vivo* animal toxicity studies are undertaken to identify and measure a drug's short- and long-term functional and morphologic adverse effects. Depending on the nature of a drug, its intended use, and the extent of its proposed study in clinical trials, a toxicity testing program may consist of some or all of the following elements:

- acute toxicity studies;
- subacute or subchronic toxicity studies;
- chronic toxicity studies;
- carcinogenicity studies;
- special toxicity studies;

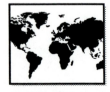

- reproductive toxicity studies;
- genotoxicity studies; and
- toxicokinetic studies.

Because many ongoing FDA and ICH initiatives focus on toxicity testing, drug sponsors are advised to keep abreast of local and international developments and subsequent regulatory changes as they affect these types of studies in particular. In mid-2001, for example, CDER released a spate of new draft guidances in the nonclinical toxicology testing area, including guidances on immunotoxicology and statistical aspects of the design, analysis, and interpretation of animal carcinogenicity studies (see discussions below).

Acute Toxicity Studies. Acute (single dose) toxicity studies are designed to measure the short-term adverse effects of a drug when administered in a single dose, or in multiple doses during a period not exceeding 24 hours. Results from acute toxicity studies should provide information on the following:

- the appropriate dosage for multiple-dose studies;
- the potential target organs of toxicity;
- the time-course of drug-induced clinical observations;
- species-specific differences in toxicity;
- the potential for acute toxicity in humans; and
- an estimate of the safe acute doses for humans.

To determine initial toxicity levels, researchers should evaluate a drug's single dose (acute) toxicity in two mammalian species prior to the first human exposure. These studies should involve dosages that are intended to cause no adverse effects and those intended to cause major (life-threatening) toxicity. The use of vehicle control groups should be considered. According to the ICH's M3 guidance, a dose-escalation study is considered an acceptable alternative to the single-dose design.

The route(s) of administration should include an intravenous route and the route intended for human administration. When intravenous dosing is proposed in humans, use of this route alone in animal testing is sufficient. The animals are then observed for 14 days after drug administration.

The FDA indicates that investigators need to obtain more than just mortality data from acute toxicity studies. At a minimum, researchers should observe and record test animals' clinical signs, and the time of onset, the duration, and the reversibility of toxicity. Gross necropsies should be performed on all animals.

In the past, one type of data derived from acute toxicity studies was the drug's "lethal dose" (LD). LD_{50}, which is calculated using a specific statistical formula, represents the dosage level that kills 50 percent of the test animals. Since 1988, however, the FDA has recommended that classic LD_{50} studies not be conducted (Federal Register 53:39650). In recent years, the value of the "classic" LD_{50} has been seriously questioned internationally for ethical and scientific reasons. Today, in accordance with ICH recommendations for single dose toxicity testing, none of the ICH parties requires or recommends that sponsors determine the "classic" LD_{50}.

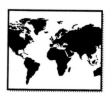

ICH's Duration of Repeated Dose Toxicity Studies to Support Phase I and II Trials in the EU and Phase I, II, and III Trials in the United States and Japan[1]

Duration of Clinical Trials	Minimum Duration of Repeated Dose Toxicity Studies	
	Rodents	Nonrodents
Single Dose	2-4 Weeks[2]	2 Weeks
Up to 2 Weeks	2-4 Weeks[2]	2 Weeks
Up to 1 Month	1 Month	1 Month
Up to 3 Months	3 Months	3 Months
Up to 6 Months	6 Months	6 Months[3]
> 6 Months	6 Months	Chronic[3]

[1] In Japan, if there are no Phase II clinical trials of equivalent duration to the planned Phase III trials, conduct of longer duration toxicity studies should be considered as given in the table below.

[2] In the EU and the United States, 2-week studies are the minimum duration. In Japan, 2-week nonrodent and 4-week rodent studies are needed. In the United States, as an alternative to 2-week studies, single dose toxicity studies with extended examinations can support single dose human trials.

[3] Data from 6 months of administration in nonrodents should be available before the initiation of clinical trials longer than 3 months. Alternatively, if applicable, data from a 9-month nonrodent study should be available before the treatment duration exceeds that which is supported by the available toxicity studies.

Source: ICH M3 Guidance

The LD_{50} has been replaced by single dose administration, increasing dose tolerance studies that measure toxic response as a function of dose. When relevant, major and pharmacologically significant metabolites should be tested in acute toxicity studies. The tests should employ a testing protocol that maximizes the amount of information that can be derived from the smallest number of animals.

In addition to a universal adoption of this approach by the ICH, the FDA has published a revised guidance entitled, *Single Dose Acute Toxicity Testing for Pharmaceuticals* (August 1996). This guidance document indicates that acute toxicity studies, when appropriately designed and conducted, may provide the primary safety data to support single dose pharmacokinetic studies in humans, although nonclinical studies of this nature will require a more comprehensive study design. These toxicity studies should be designed to assess dose-response relationships and pharmacokinetics. Clinical pathology and histopathology should be monitored at an early time and at termination (i.e., ideally, for maximum effect and recovery).

Subacute or Subchronic Studies. Subacute, or subchronic, toxicity testing allows investigators to evaluate a drug's toxic potential and pathologic effects over a longer period. These studies range in length from 14 to 90 days, with the duration generally dependent on the proposed term of clinical use and the duration of proposed clinical trials. According to the ICH's M3 guidance, the duration of the animal toxicity studies conducted in two mammalian species (one non-rodent) should, in principle, equal or exceed the duration of the clinical trial, "up to the maximum recommended duration of the repeated dose toxicity studies" (see exhibit above).

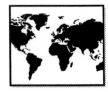

Subacute studies are designed to assess the progression and regression of drug-induced lesions. However, the studies are generally of insufficient duration to identify all secondary effects that may arise during long-term clinical use or during chronic toxicity and carcinogenicity testing.

Independent studies are performed in at least one rodent and one non-rodent species. Typically, the test compound is administered daily at three or more dosage levels. The highest dose used in these studies should be selected to deliberately induce toxic reactions. The lowest dosage should be selected to identify a no-observed adverse (toxic)-effect level (NOAEL)—that is, the dose demonstrating only intended pharmacological effects. When possible, this dose should represent a multiple of the projected average daily clinical dose. Additionally, each study should employ appropriate control groups (i.e., untreated and/or vehicle, positive, comparative).

During such studies, researchers should collect the following data, as appropriate, for the specific test compound:

- observed effects;
- mortality;
- body weight;
- food/water consumption;
- physical examinations;
- hematology/bone marrow/coagulation;
- blood chemistry/urinalysis;
- organ weights;
- gross pathology; and
- histopathology.

The studies in rodents are often used to establish dosing levels for carcinogenicity studies, such as the maximum tolerated dose (MTD). The MTD is the dose just high enough to elicit signs of minimal toxicity without significantly altering the animal's normal life span due to effects other than carinogenicity.

ICH's Duration of Repeated Dose Toxicity Studies to Support Phase III Trials in the EU and Marketing in All Regions[1]

Duration of Clinical Trials	Minimum Duration of Repeated Dose Toxicity Studies	
	Rodents	Nonrodents
Up to 2 Weeks	1 Month	1 Month
Up to 1 Month	3 Months	3 Months
Up to 3 Months	6 Months	3 Months
> 3 Months	6 Months	Chronic

[1] The above table also reflects the marketing recommendations in the three regions, except that a chronic nonrodent study is recommended for clinical use > 1 month.

Source: ICH M3 Guidance

Chronic Toxicity Testing. Chronic toxicity studies, which are tests of 180 days to a year in duration, are designed to determine the following:

- the potential risk in relation to the anticipated dose and period of drug treatment;
- the potential target organs of toxicity;
- the reversibility of any observed toxicities; and
- the no-observed adverse (toxic)-effect level.

The FDA generally requires that sponsors conduct these studies in one rodent (usually rat) and one non-rodent (usually dog) species for both chronic-use drugs and drugs intended for intermittent use to treat chronic or recurrent diseases. Because there is flexibility in this requirement, sponsors should consult the relevant FDA review division for a product-specific assessment.

In accordance with an ICH consensus, the FDA has reduced its recommended maximum duration of chronic toxicity studies in rodents from 12 to 6 months. However, the agency continues to recommend 12-month studies when rodent carcinogenicity bioassays are not performed as part of the drug toxicity profile, but when chronic toxicity testing would otherwise be appropriate.

After considerable discussion and debate, the ICH parties reached consensus on the recommended duration of nonrodent studies through the June 1999 release of a final guidance entitled, S4A *Duration of Chronic Toxicity Testing in Animals (Rodent and Nonrodent Toxicity Testing)*. Although the FDA agreed to reduce the recommended duration of chronic non-rodent studies from 12 months to the ICH-recommended 9 months, the agency included a fairly detailed "note" regarding this consensus: "While FDA considers 9-month studies in nonrodents acceptable for most drug development programs, shorter studies may be equally acceptable in some circumstances and longer studies may be more appropriate in others, as follows:

1. Six-month studies may be acceptable for indications of chronic conditions associated with short-term, intermittent drug exposure, such as bacterial infections, migraine, erectile dysfunction, and herpes.

2. Six-month studies may be acceptable for drugs intended for indications for life-threatening diseases for which substantial long-term human clinical data are available, such as cancer chemotherapy in advanced disease or in adjuvant use.

3. Twelve-month studies may be more appropriate for chronically used drugs to be approved on the basis of short-term clinical trials employing efficacy surrogate markers where safety data from humans are limited to short-term exposure, such as some acquired immunodeficiency syndrome (AIDS) therapies.

4. Twelve-month studies may be more appropriate for new molecular entities acting at new molecular targets where postmarketing experience is not available for the pharmacological class. Thus, the therapeutic is the first in a pharmacological class for which there is limited human or animal experience on its long-term toxic potential."

Dose selection criteria are similar to those described for subacute and subchronic studies, and must reflect the results of these shorter-term studies, as well as structure-activity relationships, pharmacology studies, and pharmacokinetic data. Typically, recovery subgroups and, in some cases, interim

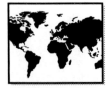

sacrifice subgroups are included. As specified above for subacute and subchronic studies, researchers must collect the data listed, as appropriate, for the drug under investigation.

Chronic studies are often initiated when Phase 2 trials provide indications of a drug's effectiveness, and are conducted concurrently with Phase 3 trials. Data obtained from chronic toxicity tests are used to support the safety of long-term drug administration in clinical trials and, ultimately, the approval of the drug for general marketing.

Carcinogenicity Studies. Multiple aspects of carcinogenicity testing have been discussed as part of the ICH initiative (i.e., need, dose selection, testing approaches). As stated in ICH proceedings, "...a carcinogenicity study is one of the most resource-consuming in terms of animals and time. In the interests of decreased animal use and protection, but without prejudicing safety, such studies should only be performed once... This could be achieved through harmonisation of the requirements of different regulatory systems."

In the past, the FDA has generally required carcinogenicity studies for any drug intended for use for three months or more, and for drugs intended for intermittent use where the total cumulative lifetime exposure may exceed three months. However, in accordance with the adoption of the final ICH guideline entitled, S1A *Guidance on the Need for Long-Term Carcinogenicity Studies of Pharmaceuticals* (March 1996), the agency has revised its requirements and now expects carcinogenicity studies for drugs whose use is continuous for 6 months or is intermittent to treat chronic or recurrent diseases. Consistent with the ICH consensus, completed carcinogenicity studies are not usually needed in advance of clinical trials "unless there is cause for concern." According to the M3 guidance, for drugs designed to treat certain serious diseases, carcinogenicity testing, if needed, may be conducted postapproval.

Today, the FDA generally requires carcinogenicity studies using the mouse and the rat. Carcinogenicity studies in rats are generally two years in duration. If long-term studies are conducted in mice, these are also generally two-year studies.

Ideally, the route of administration selected for carcinogenicity studies should be the intended clinical route. When there is more than one route or there is a change in the proposed clinical route, the carcinogenicity test route should be that which provides the greatest systemic exposure. Similar to chronic toxicity studies, carcinogenicity investigations are not usually initiated until a drug shows some indication of effectiveness in Phase 2 clinical trials.

Also, in accordance with the final ICH guidance entitled, S1C*Dose Selection for Carcinogenicity Studies of Pharmaceuticals* (1994) and a final addendum entitled, S1C(R) *Addendum to 'Dose Selection for Carcinogenicity Studies of Pharmaceuticals': Addition of a Limit Dose and Related Notes* (December 1997), the FDA no longer views dose selection based on the MTD as the only acceptable practice. As stated in the 1994 ICH guidance, the doses selected "should provide an exposure to the agent that (1) allows an adequate margin of safety over the human therapeutic exposure, (2) is tolerated without significant chronic physiological dysfunction and are compatible with good survival, (3) is guided by a comprehensive set of animal and human data that focuses on the properties of the agent and the suitability of the animal, and (4) permits data interpretation in the context of clinical use."

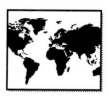

The guidance proposes that any one of several approaches may be appropriate for dose selection in carcinogenicity studies: (1) toxicity-based endpoints; (2) pharmacokinetic endpoints; (3) saturation of absorption; (4) pharmacodynamic endpoints; (5) maximum feasible dose; and (6) additional endpoints. In all cases, appropriate dose-ranging studies are necessary.

Because the approaches for dose selection adopted by ICH offer flexibility and because the factors to be considered in the use of any specific endpoint are complex, it may be prudent for sponsors to ask the agency for an assessment of appropriate dose-selection criteria in individual cases. The prospect of additional revisions to recommended study designs, as well as the expense associated with this aspect of nonclinical testing, should also motivate sponsors to obtain specific FDA guidance before initiating carcinogenicity studies. CDER offers consultation on dose selection and study design issues for carcinogenicity studies through the work of the Carcinogenicity Assessment Committee.

The FDA's most recent guidance on carcinogenicity testing, a May 2001 draft guidance entitled, *Statistical Aspects of the Design, Analysis, and Interpretation of Chronic Rodent Carcinogenicity Studies of Pharmaceuticals*, also emphasizes the "particularly critical" importance of dose selection, and advises companies to consult the S1C guidance. The new draft document provides sponsors with FDA recommendations on the design and interpretation of animal carcinogenicity studies, methods of statistical analysis of tumor data, and the presentation of data and results in reports. "In a carcinogenicity study of a new drug using a series of increasing dosing levels, statistical tests for positive trends in tumor rates are usually of greatest interest, but…, in some situations, pairwise comparisons are considered to be more indicative of drug effects than trend tests," the draft guidance notes.

In July 1997, the ICH parties also agreed to a final guidance entitled, *S1B Testing for Carcinogenicity of Pharmaceuticals*, which the FDA published in February 1998. This guidance outlines experimental approaches that may obviate the need for the routine conduct of two long-term rodent carcinogenicity studies for those pharmaceuticals that currently require such evaluation. A basic scheme comprising one long-term rodent carcinogenicity study (generally, the rat), plus one additional study for carcinogenic activity *in vivo*, is advanced in the guidance. The additional study could be either a short- or medium-term rodent test system or a long-term carcinogenicity study in a second rodent species. Under the final guidance, the additional study must be scientifically justified and must contribute to the overall assessment of carcinogenic potential.

Because of the time and expense associated with carcinogenicity studies, CDER traditionally has been willing to review and comment on proposed carcinogenicity protocols through its Carcinogenicity Assessment Committee and Executive Carcinogenicity Assessment Committee. Some aspects of this process have been formalized by the special protocol question and assessment process outlined in the FDA's PDUFA II commitments. Under this process, CDER must review and respond to specific sponsor questions regarding carcinogenicity, stability, or Phase 3 clinical protocols within 45 days. If CDER's Carcinogenicity Assessment Committee agrees in its response that the protocol data can be used as part of the primary basis for product approval, the PDUFA II commitments state that the center "will not alter its perspective on the issue of design, execution, or analysis unless public health concerns unrecognized at the time of the protocol assessment…are evident." According to CDER data released in early 2001, industry had submitted 128 protocols under the special protocol question and assessment process, most of which were thought to be carcinogenicity protocols.

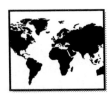

In December 1999, CDER released a draft guidance entitled, *Special Protocol Assessment* to outline the protocol assessment and agreement process for carcinogenicity, stability, and Phase 3 protocols. According to the draft guidance, "a sponsor interested in Agency assessment and agreement on a carcinogenicity protocol should notify the appropriate review division…and discuss planned carcinogenicity testing at an end-of-phase 2 meeting or should notify the director of the appropriate division of an intent to request special protocol assessment by letter at least 30 days prior to submitting the request. With the notice of intent, the sponsor should submit relevant background information so that the Agency may review (or re-review) reference material related to carcinogenicity protocol design prior to receiving the carcinogenicity protocol." In the draft document, CDER noted that it is developing a guidance to describe the type of information that would be appropriate to submit before requesting a carcinogenicity protocol assessment. Protocols submitted for special protocol assessment should be forwarded to the agency at least 90 days before a study's anticipated commencement, the agency recommends.

An October 2000 draft guidance entitled, *Carcinogenicity Study Protocol Submissions* specifies the types of information that CDER considers important in evaluating carcinogenicity protocols. Although that information will vary with the proposed study design and test approach, CDER notes that the following information, in all cases, will facilitate the protocol-review process: the basis for dose selection; a toxicology study report (usually 90-day); metabolic profiles for the drug in humans and in the species employed for assessing carcinogenic potential; toxicokinetic data; exposure data; plasma protein binding data; and a summary of the investigations into genotoxic potential.

In late 1998, CDER published a manual of policies and procedures entitled, *Submission of Preclinical Carcinogencity Protocols and Study Results* (MaPP 7412.3) to provide an administrative mechanism for the submission, and CDER tracking and processing, of proposed carcinogenicity protocols, toxicity data supporting dose selection, and carcinogenicity study results to an existing IND or in advance of a traditional IND submission. This MaPP was to remain in effect until CDER publishes a general MaPP establishing a tracking system for all pre-IND submissions.

In January 2000, CDER released a draft guidance entitled, *Photosafety Testing*, to assist companies in determining whether they should test for photosensitivity and assess the potential human risk for photochemical carcinogenesis and enhancement of UV-induced skin carcinogenesis in the development of topically and systemically administered drug products. According to the draft, the identification of photosensitivity effects before widespread human exposure is preferable to learning of these effects through postmarketing adverse event reports, which CDER claims has been the traditional way that such effects have been discovered.

Special Toxicity Studies. Special toxicity studies include those studies appropriate for a particular formulation or route of administration (e.g., parenteral or local tolerance studies, in vitro hemolysis), and studies conducted in a particular animal model relevant to a human disease or age. At this writing, formal FDA guidance pertaining to special toxicity testing was limited largely to a brief discussion provided in the FDA's *Guideline for the Format and Content of the Nonclinical Pharmacology/Toxicology Section of an Application*. Therefore, sponsors should ask the relevant CDER review division if special toxicity testing is considered applicable. The evaluation of local tolerance should be performed prior to human exposure (and in animals using routes relevant to the proposed clinical administration), although this assessment may be part of other toxicity studies.

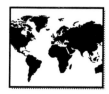

An April 2001 draft guidance entitled, *Immunotoxicology Evaluation of Investigational New Drugs* provides recommendations on when additional, specific immunotoxicology studies should be conducted, the parameters that should be routinely assessed in toxicity studies to determine a drug's effects on immune function, and when additional mechanistic information could help evaluate the significance of a drug's effect on the immune system. While evidence of immunotoxicity can "usually" be observed in standard nonclinical toxicology studies, additional studies are need in some cases, the draft guidance notes. Specific immunotoxicity testing should be conducted (i.e., beyond the standard toxicity studies in two species) when drugs will be administered by the inhalation or topical route, the guidance states. Researchers should also consider specific immunotoxicity studies when a drug has the potential to elicit an antidrug immune response, when use during pregnancy is likely, and when there is an absence of immuntoxicity findings in the toxicity studies but significant accumulation or retention of the drug in immune system tissues or the drug will be used to treat an immune-deficiency disease such as HIV.

Reproductive Toxicity Studies. The FDA requires reproductive testing for any drug to be used in women of childbearing potential, regardless of whether the target population is pregnant women. Generally, these studies have been conducted in a three-segment testing protocol previously recommended by the FDA: (1) Segment I-fertility and general reproductive performance (involving the study of both the male and female rat); (2) Segment II-teratology (conducted in the rat and the rabbit); and (3) Segment III-perinatal and postnatal development (conducted in the rat to evaluate drug effects during the last third of pregnancy and the period of lactation).

In an effort to reduce differences in reproductive toxicity requirements between the EC, Japan, and the United States, the ICH participating parties adopted the final guidance entitled, S5A *Detection of Toxicity to Reproduction for Medicinal Products*, which was released in September 1994. As stated in this guideline, "the aim of reproductive toxicity studies is to reveal any effect of one or more active substances(s) on mammalian reproduction." Therefore, the combination of studies selected should "allow exposure of mature adults and all stages of development from conception to sexual maturity." The integrated sequence of testing has been segregated into the following stages: (A) premating to conception; (B) conception to implantation; (C) implantation to closure of the hard palate; (D) closure of the hard palate to the end of pregnancy; (E) birth to weaning; and (F) weaning to sexual maturity.

The guideline suggests that the "most probable" option for investigating reproductive toxicity is a three-study design:

- Fertility and embryonic development. This study comprises stages A and B, and is conducted in at least one species, preferably the rat. Assessments should include maturation of gametes, mating behavior, fertility, preimplantation stages of the embryo, and implantation. In particular, sponsors should note that, in contrast to the previous Segment I study, this study design uses a histological evaluation of testes, epididymis, and sperm counts to assess drug effects on male fertility.

- Pre- and postnatal development, including maternal development. This phase comprises stages C to F, and is conducted in at least one species, preferably the rat. The study is designed to detect adverse effects on the pregnant/lactating female, and on the development of the conceptus and the offspring following exposure of the female from implantation through weaning. Assessments should include toxicity

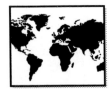

relative to that in nonpregnant females, pre- and postnatal death of offspring, altered growth and development, and functional deficits (e.g., behavior, maturation, and reproduction) in offspring.

- Embryo-fetal development. This study comprises stages C to D, and is usually conducted in two species: a rodent (preferably the rat) and non-rodent (preferably the rabbit). The goal is to detect adverse effects on the pregnant female and the development of the embryo and the fetus consequent to exposure of the female from implantation to closure of the hard palate. Researchers should assess toxicity relative to that in nonpregnant females, embryo-fetal death, and altered growth, including structural changes.

According to the ICH's M3 document, women of childbearing potential may be included in early, carefully monitored studies in the U.S. without the prior conduct of reproduction toxicity studies, provided appropriate precautions are taken (e.g., pregnancy testing, use of highly effective birth control method, and entry after confirmed menstrual period). In the U.S., the assessment of female fertility and embryofetal development should be completed before women of childbearing potential using birth control are enrolled in Phase 3 trials. Women not of childbearing potential (i.e., permanently sterilized, postmenopausal) may be included in clinical trials without reproduction studies, provided the relevant repeated dose toxicity studies, including an evaluation of the female reproduction organs, have been completed.

Subsequent to the acceptance of the above guideline, the ICH parties adopted S5B *Addendum on Toxicity to Male Fertility* (1996). This addendum suggests that the following be taken into account to assess effects on male fertility:

- Provided that no precluding effects have been found in repeated dose toxicity studies, a premating treatment interval of four weeks for males and two weeks for females can be used.

- Histopathology of the testis has been shown to be the most sensitive method for the detection of effects on spermatogenesis. Therefore, good pathological and histopathological examination of the male reproductive organs provides a quick and direct means of detection.

- Sperm analysis can be used as a method to confirm findings by other methods and to characterize effects further.

According to the ICH's M3 guidance, a male fertility study should be completed prior to initiating Phase 3 trials. It adds that men may be included in Phase 1 and 2 trials prior to the male fertility study when an evaluation of the male reproductive organs is performed in the repeated dose toxicity studies.

A November 2001 CDER draft guidance entitled, *Integration of Study Results to Assess Concerns About Human Reproductive and Developmental Toxicities* describes a process for estimating human developmental and reproductive risks as a result of drug exposure when definitive human data are unavailable. The integration process is designed to estimate the likelihood that a drug will increase the risk of adverse human development or reproductive effects. Specifically, the process is based on the evaluation of a complete set of reproductive and general toxicology studies conducted in animals, pharmacokinetics, and the absorption and distribution of metabolic elimination studies conducted in humans and animals. The evaluation also compares animal and human drug-induced pharmacodynamic responses, drug metabolism and disposition, drug-induced pharmacologic and toxic effects, and drug exposures in animal studies against those at the highest recommended dose in humans.

Genotoxicity Studies. Also referred to as "mutagenicity studies," genotoxicity studies (now the preferred term) are used to assess a drug's potential to cause genomic damage that could induce cancer (i.e., somatic cell mutation) and/or heritable defects (i.e., germ cell mutation). These short-term studies include a battery of mammalian and non-mammalian, *in vitro* and *in vivo* tests designed to detect a compound's ability to cause an increase in genetic alterations (e.g., primary DNA damage, chromosomal aberrations). Although genotoxicity tests have not been specified as requirements for pharmaceuticals or described in a CDER guideline, these screening tests have been strongly recommended by the FDA, and are required by both the EC and Japan. (Note: Genotoxicity tests have been described in the FDA's Redbook, or *Toxicological Principles for the Safety Assessment of Direct Food Additives with Color Additives Used in Food.*)

Genotoxicity testing has, however, now been addressed in three final ICH guidances. According to the M3 document, *in vitro* tests for the evaluation of mutations and chromosomal damage "are generally needed" prior to first human exposure. The third test—an *in vivo* test for chromosomal damage—can be conducted during clinical trials. Additional testing should be performed if an equivocal or positive finding is made.

The ICH guidance entitled, S2A *Guidance on Specific Aspects of Regulatory Genotoxicity Tests for Pharmaceuticals*, which was finalized in April 1996, addresses and provides recommendations for the following issues:

- The base set of bacteria strains to be used in bacterial mutation assays;
- Acceptable bone marrow tests for the detection of clastogens *in vivo*;
- Further evaluation of compounds giving positive *in vitro* results;
- Validation of negative *in vivo* tests;
- Definition of the top concentration for *in vitro* tests; and
- Use of male/female rodents in bone marrow micronucleus tests.

Additionally, a companion ICH guidance entitled, S2B *A Standard Battery for Genotoxicity Testing of Pharmaceuticals* was finalized and was published in November 1997. This guidance defines a standard set of genotoxicity tests to be conducted for pharmaceutical registration, and recommends the extent of confirmatory experimentation for *in vitro* genotoxicity tests in the standard battery. The standard test battery calls for the completion of the following tests prior to the initiation of Phase 2 studies:

- a test for gene mutation in bacteria;
- an *in vitro* test with cytogenic evaluation of chromosomal damage with mammalian cells or an *in vivo* mouse lymphoma tK assay; and
- an *in vivo* test for chromosomal damage using rodent hematopoietic cells.

Additional genotoxicity testing may be required if: (1) an equivocal or positive finding is made in the genotoxicity testing battery; or (2) genotoxicity testing is negative, but carcinogenicity testing is positive.

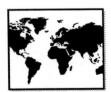

The final ICH guidance also discusses situations in which the standard three-test battery may need modification.

Toxicokinetic Studies. Toxicokinetics is defined "as the generation of pharmacokinetic data, either as an integral component in the conduct of nonclinical toxicity studies or in specially designed supportive studies, in order to assess systemic exposure. These data may be used in the interpretation of toxicological findings and their relevance to clinical safety issues."

A final ICH guideline entitled, SA3 *Toxicokinetics: The Assessment of Systemic Exposure in Toxicity Studies* (1994) has been adopted by the FDA. As stated in this ICH guidance, the primary objective of toxicokinetics is to describe the systemic exposure achieved in animals and its relationship to the dose level and the time course of the toxicity study. Secondary objectives are:

- to relate the exposure achieved in toxicity studies to toxicological findings, and contribute to the assessment of the relevance of these findings to clinical safety;

- to support the choice of species and treatment regimen in nonclinical toxicity studies; and

- to provide information that, in conjunction with the toxicity findings, contributes to the design of subsequent nonclinical toxicity studies.

The objectives may be achieved by the derivation of one or more pharmacokinetic parameters from measurements made at appropriate time points during the course of the individual studies. These measurements usually consist of plasma (or whole blood or serum) concentrations for the parent compound and/or metabolite(s), and should be selected on a case-by-case basis. Plasma (or whole blood or serum) AUC, C_{max}, and C(time) are the most commonly used parameters for assessing exposure in toxicokinetic studies. For some compounds, it may be more appropriate to calculate exposure based on the (plasma protein) unbound concentration. Toxicokinetic studies should be designed to provide information that may be integrated into the full spectrum of nonclinical toxicity testing and then compared to human data.

FDA Standards for Nonclinical Testing: Good Laboratory Practice (GLP)

Manufacturers of drugs and other FDA-regulated products are given considerable freedom during the preclinical screening and testing of new products. Provided that they comply with the U.S. Animal Welfare Act and other applicable animal welfare laws, nonclinical testing laboratories at pharmaceutical companies and private contractors are not limited in the use of animals to screen and measure the activity of drugs.

When the sponsor begins to compile safety data for submission to the FDA, however, standards called Good Laboratory Practice (GLP) apply. To ensure the quality and integrity of data derived from nonclinical testing, the FDA requires that nonclinical laboratory studies designed to provide safety data for an IND, NDA, or other regulatory submission comply with GLP standards. GLP regulations apply to product sponsor laboratories, private toxicology laboratories, academic and government laboratories, and all other facilities involved in animal testing and related analyses whose results will be submitted to the FDA in support of a product's safety.

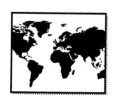

GLP regulations establish basic standards for the conduct and reporting of nonclinical safety testing. Specifically, the regulations set standards in such areas as the organization, personnel, physical structure, maintenance, and operating procedures of nonclinical testing facilities.

GLP regulations, which became effective on June 20, 1979, were the FDA's response to finding, in the mid-1970s, that some nonclinical studies submitted to support the safety of new drugs were not being conducted according to accepted standards. After establishing the initial GLP regulations, the FDA's confidence in the work of nonclinical laboratory facilities increased markedly. As a result, in October 1987, the agency published revised GLP regulations that sought to reduce regulatory and paperwork burdens facing laboratories conducting animal studies.

The Applicability of GLP

On one level, GLP applicability is fairly straightforward. According to FDA regulations, GLP applies to facilities conducting "nonclinical laboratory studies that support or are intended to support applications for research or marketing permits for products regulated by the Food and Drug Administration, including food and color additives, animal food additives, human and animal drugs, medical devices for human use, biological products, and electronic products."

What at times seems more difficult is identifying which nonclinical tests are subject to GLP requirements. The FDA states that GLP applies to "nonclinical laboratory studies," which the regulations define as "*in vivo* or *in vitro* experiments in which test articles are studied prospectively in test systems under laboratory conditions to determine their safety. The term does not include studies utilizing human subjects or clinical studies or field trials in animals. The term does not include basic exploratory studies carried out to determine whether a test article has any potential utility or to determine physical or chemical characteristics of a test article."

As currently interpreted, GLP applies to all "definitive" nonclinical safety studies, including key acute, subacute, chronic, reproductive, and carcinogenicity studies. Preliminary pharmacological screening and metabolism studies are exempt from GLP requirements, as are initial pilot studies such as dose-ranging, absorption, and excretion tests.

The Major Provisions of GLP

The core provisions of GLP establish standards for the nonclinical laboratory's organization, physical structure, equipment, and operating procedures. For purposes of analysis, these standards may be grouped into seven general areas:

- organization and personnel;
- testing facility;
- testing facility operation;
- test and control article characterization;
- the protocol and conduct of the nonclinical laboratory study;
- records and reporting; and
- equipment design.

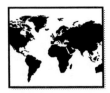

Organization and Personnel GLP regulations regarding a nonclinical laboratory's organization and personnel address four areas: general personnel, testing facility management, study director, and quality assurance unit. Aside from the general qualifications and responsibilities of personnel and management, however, this aspect of GLP focuses primarily on issues regarding the study director and quality assurance unit.

Study Director. GLP requires that the management of the testing facility conducting a nonclinical program designate a scientist or other professional to serve as the study director. This individual has overall responsibility for the "technical conduct of the study, as well as for the interpretation, analysis, documentation, and reporting of results and represents the single point of study control." The FDA does not require that the study director be technically competent in all areas of a study, however.

Quality Assurance Unit. GLP also requires that each testing facility have a quality assurance unit (QAU) comprising one or more persons directly responsible to facility management. The QAU monitors each study to "assure management that the facilities, equipment, personnel, methods, practices, records, and controls" are consistent with GLP. To ensure that such evaluations are made objectively, QAU members may not be involved in any animal study that they monitor.

The GLP regulations specify several major QAU responsibilities in the areas of record maintenance, study inspections, and reports to facility management. At the conclusion of a study, the QAU is required to prepare and sign a statement—to be included with the final report—that specifies the dates on which inspections were made and the findings reported to management and the study director.

Current regulations require that the QAU inspect a nonclinical study at intervals the unit considers adequate to ensure the study's integrity. However, the FDA advises that each study, regardless of its length, be inspected in-process at least once, and that, across a series of studies, all phases be inspected to assure study integrity.

Testing Facility Obviously, the laboratory facility in which the testing program takes place is a primary focus of GLP. Animal care and supply facilities, test substance handling areas, laboratory operation, specimen and data storage, administrative and personnel facilities, methods of dosage preparation, and test substance accountability all must meet detailed requirements. Records indicating compliance must be kept.

In general terms, a testing facility and its equipment must be of suitable size and construction to allow for the proper conduct of the nonclinical study. Animal care areas, for example, must provide for sufficient separation of species/test systems and individual projects, isolation of animals, protection from outside disturbances, and routine or specialized animal housing. Regulated environmental controls for air quality—temperature, humidity, and air changes—and sanitation are needed.

Operation of Testing Facility Each laboratory must base its operations on standard operating procedures (SOPs). SOPs, which are in some respects extensions of nonclinical protocols, are written study methods or directions that laboratory management believes are adequate to ensure the quality and

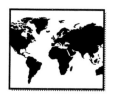

integrity of data obtained from animal tests. The description of research procedures provided by protocols and SOP documents makes possible the verification and reconstruction of studies.

The detailed written procedures specified in the SOPs must be maintained for all aspects of the study, including animal care, laboratory tests, data handling and storage, and equipment maintenance and calibration. Each laboratory area must have accessible laboratory manuals and SOPs relevant to the laboratory procedures being performed. Determining the degree to which SOPs are observed is another QAU responsibility. Any deviations from established SOPs must be authorized by the study director and noted in the raw data. On the other hand, the laboratory's management must approve major changes.

Test and Control Article Characterization Under the 1987 GLP revision, testing facilities are not required to characterize test and control articles before toxicity studies begin. This allows companies to screen out many of the useless compounds before investing resources necessary to characterize them: "FDA has concluded that characterization of test and control articles need not be performed until initial toxicology studies with the test article show reasonable promise of the articles reaching the marketplace. In arriving at this conclusion, the agency considered that prior knowledge of the precise molecular structure is not vital to the conduct of a valid toxicology test. It is important, however, to know the strength, purity, and stability of a test or control article that is used in a nonclinical laboratory study." FDA officials point out that either the sponsor or the testing laboratory may perform the test and control article characterization. The current GLP regulations allow facilities to conduct stability testing of test and control articles either before study initiation or, if this is impossible, through periodic analyses of each batch.

The Protocol and the Conduct of Nonclinical Laboratory Studies A protocol, or testing plan, is a vital element in both clinical and nonclinical studies. GLP regulations state that a nonclinical program must have a written protocol that "clearly indicates the objectives and all methods for the conduct of the study." Included in the 12-item protocol, which the sponsor must approve, should be descriptions of the experimental design and the purpose of the study as well as the type and frequency of tests, analyses, and measurements to be made. Changes made to the protocol during the course of the study must be documented by an official protocol amendment signed by the study director. The study director's approval of protocol amendments assures the FDA of the data's integrity.

Although protocols and SOPs may seem similar, the two have different purposes. The protocol is specific to the study being conducted, while laboratory SOPs are standards used for all research projects at a given facility. For example, SOPs would provide "how to" instructions on a facility's routine procedures for obtaining animal blood samples, caring for animals, and using and maintaining equipment. In contrast, the protocol provides study-specific instructions—for example, how often and from what animals blood samples are to be taken, what tests are to be conducted, and the number, species, sex, age, and weight of the animals to be tested in a particular study.

Records and Reporting A final report must be prepared for each nonclinical laboratory study. Comprehensive reports typically include the summary, testing methods, results, and conclusions of a study, as well as all raw data on each of the test animals. These final reports, as well as all raw data, documentation, protocols, and certain specimens generated during the nonclinical study, must be

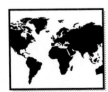

stored in an archive or repository to assure their safety and integrity for specific periods as designated in GLP regulations. Although these regulations state that two to five years is adequate, the FDA sometimes recommends that records be stored indefinitely and that specimens—slides, tissues, and blocks—be stored as long as they can be used to validate data.

Equipment Design GLP regulations specify requirements for the design, maintenance, and calibration of equipment used in nonclinical tests. Equipment used for facility environmental control and automatic, mechanical, or electronic equipment used in the generation, measurement, or assessment of data must be: (1) of appropriate design and adequate capacity to function according to the protocol; (2) suitably located for operation, inspection, cleaning, and maintenance; and (3) adequately tested, calibrated, and/or standardized. SOPs are required to define, in sufficient detail, the methods, materials, and schedules to be used in the routine inspection, cleaning, maintenance, testing, calibration, and standardization of equipment.

CDER's GLP Inspections

To monitor compliance with GLP requirements, the FDA employs a program of on-site laboratory inspections and data audits. According to the agency's Compliance Policy Guide (CPG) 7348.808, the FDA conducts two basic types of GLP compliance inspections: surveillance (or routine) inspections and directed inspections.

Representing the majority of GLP inspections, on-site surveillance inspections are periodic, routine evaluations of a laboratory's GLP compliance. Typically, these evaluations are based on either active or recently completed studies. Routine inspections for monitoring a nonclinical laboratory's GLP compliance are scheduled "approximately every two years" and are unannounced inspections. CDER assigns an estimated 50 to 60 surveillance inspections annually.

Directed inspections are conducted when necessary—when questionable data raise suspicions during an IND or NDA review, for example. The agency may also conduct a directed "data audit" in response to questions or issues that arise during an NDA review (e.g., the NDA review division may request such an inspection when a novel product is under review) or in response to information received from other sources (e.g., complaints). CDER assigns about 15 directed inspections per year. Whenever possible, the FDA will couple directed inspections with routine inspections.

If FDA inspectors find GLP violations within a facility, CDER reviewers will evaluate the violations as described in the establishment inspection report (EIR) and decide on a course of action. When the agency observes noncompliance, it has several options, ranging from the issuance of untitled correspondence, in which CDER would discuss the findings and make recommendations (but not request a formal action or response), to the issuance of a warning letter, in which CDER will generally put a firm on notice regarding noncompliance and establish that specific actions (e.g., action and response) are necessary. In cases involving severe compliance problems, the FDA may disqualify data from an entire nonclinical study.

According to data from GLP inspections conducted in fiscal year 1999, the most common GLP violations were in the areas of equipment maintenance/calibration (62% of laboratories), personnel/management/study director (46%), QAU and operations (38%), and standard operating procedures (38%).

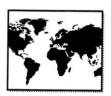

CHAPTER 3

The IND

The investigational new drug application, or IND, is a submission through which a drug sponsor alerts the FDA of its intention to conduct clinical studies with an investigational drug. The IND is a descriptive notification that the sponsor must submit to the FDA, and that the agency has a brief time to review, prior to the initiation of clinical trials.

In legal terms, the IND is a request for an exemption from the federal statute that prohibits an unapproved drug from being shipped in interstate commerce. Current federal law requires that a drug be the subject of an approved new drug application (NDA) before the product is transported or distributed across state lines. Because a sponsor will probably want to ship the investigational drug to clinical sites in other states, it must seek an exemption from this legal requirement.

In many respects, the IND is a product of a successful preclinical development program. During a new drug's early preclinical development, the sponsor's primary goal is to determine if the compound exhibits pharmacological activity that justifies commercial development and if the product is reasonably safe for initial use in humans. When a product is identified as a viable candidate for further development, the sponsor then focuses on collecting the data and information necessary to establish, in the IND, that the product will not expose human subjects to unreasonable risks when used in limited, early-stage clinical studies. Generally, this includes data and information in three broad areas:

Animal Pharmacology and Toxicology Studies. Preclinical data to permit an assessment as to whether the product is reasonably safe for initial testing in humans.

Manufacturing Information. Information pertaining to the composition, manufacture, and stability of, and the controls used for, the drug substance and the drug product to permit an assessment of the company's ability to adequately produce and supply consistent batches of the drug. Further, information on the compound's structure is used to assess whether the compound is similar to drugs known to be toxic.

Clinical Protocols and Investigator Information. Detailed protocols for proposed clinical studies to permit an assessment as to whether the initial-phase trials will expose subjects to unnecessary risks. Also, information on the qualifications of clinical investigators—professionals (generally physicians) who oversee the administration of the experimental compound—to permit an assessment as to whether they are qualified to fulfill their clinical trial duties.

Federal regulations are clear regarding the IND's purpose and the FDA's role in the application's review. As stated in 21 CFR 312.22, "FDA's primary objectives in reviewing an IND are, in all phases of

Worldwide Pharmaceutical Regulation Series

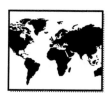

the investigation, to assure the safety and rights of subjects, and, in Phase 2 and 3, to help assure that the quality of scientific evaluation of drugs is adequate to permit an evaluation of the drug's effectiveness and safety."

Unlike NDAs, INDs are never approved by the FDA. Rather, sponsors are permitted to initiate the clinical trials proposed in an IND 30 days after the FDA receives the application, provided that the agency does not contact the applicant during this 30-day period to alert the company otherwise (see Chapter 4). In all cases, however, sponsors are advised to check with a review division before initiating clinical trials to ensure that the IND was received and reviewed.

Types of INDs

This chapter focuses on submissions that are sometimes called "commercial INDs," which are applications filed principally by companies whose ultimate goal is to obtain marketing approval for new products. An October 2000 CDER guidance document defines commercial IND as "an IND for which a sponsor is usually a corporate entity. Other entities may be designated as commercial if it is clear the sponsor intends the product to be commercialized at a later date." In that same guidance, CDER clarified that IND-related user-fee performance goals (e.g., acting on clinical hold responses) are relevant only to commercial INDs and not other categories of submissions (see discussion below).

There are at least a few types of applications that may be grouped within a second class of filings sometimes referred to as "noncommercial" INDs. Interestingly, the vast majority of INDs are noncommercial research submissions. These include the following types of INDs:

Investigator IND (also called research IND). The investigator IND is submitted by a physician who both initiates and conducts an investigation, and under whose immediate direction the investigational drug is administered or dispensed. In most cases, an investigator IND proposes clinical studies on previously studied drugs. A physician might submit a research IND to propose studying an unapproved drug, or an approved product for a new indication or in a new patient population. Generally, however, the physician's motivation is not commercial in nature—in other words, the goal is not to develop data to support marketing approval for an unapproved product or to support new labeling for an approved product. For example, the investigator may simply want to treat patients or obtain data to publish a research paper.

Emergency Use IND. The emergency use IND is a vehicle through which the FDA can authorize the immediate shipment of an experimental drug for a desperate medical situation. According to FDA regulations, "need for an investigational drug may arise in an emergency situation that does not allow time for submission of an IND... In such a case, FDA may authorize shipment of the drug for a specified use in advance of submission of an IND." Emergency use INDs generally are reserved for life-threatening situations in which no standard acceptable treatment is available, and in which there is not sufficient time to obtain institutional review board (IRB) approval. Emergency use INDs are also sometimes called "compassionate use" or "single-patient" INDs. Noting the absence of specific standards for compassionate drug use, FDA officials revealed in mid-2000 that the agency was developing a proposed regulation to outline criteria for a variety of experimental drug access options for patients not enrolled in formal clinical trials.

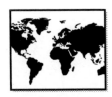

Treatment IND. Although the treatment IND has a history dating back to the 1960s and 1970s, the FDA took steps to formalize the treatment IND concept in a 1987 regulation. Through the FDA's treatment IND program, experimental drugs showing promise in clinical testing for serious or life-threatening conditions are made widely available while the final clinical work is performed and the FDA review takes place (see Chapter 15). The FDA Modernization Act of 1997 codified the treatment IND concept as well as other expanded use programs (e.g., emergency use) into law, and encouraged the FDA to consider changes that might reduce industry reluctance to participate in expanded drug access programs.

A subcategory of commercial IND submissions, called "screening INDs," has gained increasing attention in recent years. After years seemingly on the fringe of regulatory legitimacy, so-called "screening" INDs now have a formal policy statement to support their existence and use. In a May 2001 Manual of Policies and Procedures document (MaPP 6030.4), CDER establishes that a sponsor can, through a screening IND, seek FDA permission to test several closely related chemical entities in initial clinical trials. "In general, CDER policy has been to encourage separate INDs for different molecules and dosage forms," the MaPP notes. "However, in the early phase of drug development, before the developmental path is clear, exploratory studies may be conducted on a number of closely related drugs to choose the preferred compound or formulation. These studies may be best and most efficiently conducted under a single IND.

"Screening INDs are appropriate when single-dose or short-term, repeat-dose clinical trials (≤ 3 days of dosing) are proposed using multiple, closely related compounds. The compounds include different salts or esters and active moieties that are slightly different chemically, but appear to be similar in pharmacodynamic properties. The proposed studies could be a single trial with multiple compounds or similar trials involving only one compound (e.g., several PK studies, one for each compound). The number of compounds tested should usually be ≤ 5. Normally, the intent of the study is to compare the properties of the closely related active moieties to screen for further development." After the early exploratory studies (e.g., Phase 1 tolerance, PK/PD, early pilot efficacy studies) conducted under the screening IND are complete, the application should be withdrawn, MaPP 6030.4 states. When the sponsor plans to conduct further studies for one or more of the moieties or when additional, closely related chemical moieties are to be studied in clinical trials, the sponsor should submit an entirely new IND.

Concurrently with an IND filing (or at any later time), a sponsor can request a "fast track" designation for its drug, provided the therapy addresses unmet medical needs related to a serious and life-threatening condition. This "fast track" designation, which was created under the FDA Modernization Act of 1997, makes a product eligible for accelerated approval and other benefits (see Chapter 15).

The Applicability of the IND

The IND is a requirement for all persons and firms seeking to ship unapproved drugs over state lines for use in clinical investigations. However, the FDA offers exemptions from IND submission requirements for certain types of clinical testing and products, including the following:

- Clinical investigations of a drug product that is lawfully marketed in the United States, provided that all of the following conditions apply: (1) the investigation is

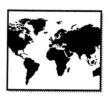

not intended to be reported to the FDA as a well-controlled study in support of a new indication for use, or is not intended to be used to support any other significant change in the drug's labeling; (2) the investigation is not intended to support a significant change in the advertising for a prescription drug; (3) the investigation does not involve a change in the route of administration, dosage level, patient population, or other factor that significantly increases the risks (or decreases the acceptability of the risks) associated with the use of the drug product; (4) the investigation complies with institutional review board (IRB) evaluation and informed consent requirements; and (5) the study's sponsor and investigator do not represent in a promotional context that the drug is safe or effective for the purposes for which it is under investigation, or unduly prolong the study after finding that the results are sufficient to support a marketing application. The FDA has stated that this exemption is intended primarily for practicing physicians.

- Drugs intended solely for testing *in vitro* or in laboratory research animals, provided the drug labels and shipments comply with FDA regulations applicable to investigational drugs.

- Clinical investigations involving the use of a placebo, provided that the investigations do not involve the use of a new drug or otherwise trigger IND submission requirements.

- Certain *in vivo* bioavailability and bioequivalence studies in humans. FDA regulations state, however, that INDs are required for *in vivo* bioavailability or bioequivalence studies in humans if the test product is a radioactively labeled drug product, is a cytotoxic drug product, or contains a new chemical entity. Further, INDs are required for the following types of human bioavailability studies that involve a previously approved drug that is not a new chemical entity: (1) a single-dose study in normal subjects or patients when either the maximum single or total daily dose exceeds that specified in the labeling of the approved product; (2) a multiple-dose study in normal subjects or patients when either the single or total daily dose exceeds that specified in the labeling of the approved product; or (3) a multiple-dose study on a controlled-release product for which no single-dose study has been completed.

In addition to these IND exemptions, FDA regulations provide a mechanism through which individuals and firms can seek an agency waiver from IND requirements. The agency can grant a waiver if certain criteria are met, including that the sponsor's noncompliance will not pose a significant or unreasonable risk to human subjects.

IND Content and Format Requirements

Until the late 1980s, the FDA had less-than-exacting content and format requirements for INDs. A 1987 revision to federal regulations—originally called the "IND Rewrite"—changed this, however, as the FDA sought better organized and more standardized INDs to help expedite reviews.

Another substantive change to IND content requirements came in November 1995, when the FDA clarified its IND data and data presentation requirements in a guidance entitled, *Content and Format of*

Investigational New Drug Applications (IND) *for Phase 1 Studies of Drugs, Including Well-Characterized, Therapeutic, Biotechnology-Derived Products.* Although the FDA characterized the guidance as a "clarification," it really represented a shift in policy, particularly in establishing that the agency would accept toxicology data summaries and line listings based upon sponsors' unaudited draft toxicologic reports of completed animal studies. If industry followed the reduced data requirements outlined in the November 1995 guidance, the FDA claimed that "IND submissions for Phase 1 studies should usually not be larger than two to three, three inch, 3-ring binders." This shift was prompted largely by growing concerns that early-stage clinical research projects were moving to other countries, particularly European countries, which often had less demanding regulatory requirements for initial clinical trials.

In the FDA Modernization Act of 1997, Congress also moved to codify and extend such "clarifications" by adding to the Food, Drug and Cosmetic Act specific language regarding IND submission requirements. The reform legislation states that the IND submission should include: (1) "information on [the] design of the [proposed clinical] investigation and adequate reports of basic information, certified by the applicant to be accurate reports, necessary to assess the safety of the drug for use in clinical investigation;" and (2) "adequate information on the chemistry and manufacturing of the drug, controls available for the drug, and primary data tabulations from animal or human studies."

Within a few years, two initiatives among others are likely to affect the evolution of the IND, at least with respect to its content and format:

The ICH's Common Technical Document (CTD) Initiative. In mid-1997, the ICH parties agreed to embark on their most daunting and significant harmonization initiative—to develop a common technical document, "an information package of technical data, in the same format and with the same content," that could be provided in marketing applications uniformly in all three ICH regions. In mid-2001, the FDA and industry entered a "transition" period during which applicants would have, for the first time, the option of submitting a marketing application in either the conventional NDA format or the harmonized CTD format. Although this effort focuses on marketing, rather than clinical trial authorization, applications, the CTD is expected to have fundamental "trickle down" effects on the types of manufacturing, nonclinical, and clinical data and information submitted in INDs and on the manner in which this information is presented. For a more detailed analysis of the CTD, see Chapter 7.

Submission of eINDs. Although CDER began accepting electronic versions of an IND's pharmacology/toxicology sections in 1994 under its Pharmacology/Toxicology (P/T) Electronic Submission Pilot Project, the center's current plans for eINDs are not based on this effort. Notwithstanding its efforts under this pilot program, CDER has not received or reviewed a completely electronic IND. At this writing, CDER's eIND activities appeared to be advancing on two tracks. First, CDER is party to a CBER effort to develop a formal eIND guidance, which the biologics center hopes to release by early 2002. Once this guidance is published and CDER lists the IND on its e-submissions public docket (92-S-0251), the center will accept eINDs. Meanwhile, however, CDER has proposed an eIND approach and model/prototype that provides a window on how the center wants to approach eNDAs and, ultimately, eCTDs in the future. Specifically, CDER has proposed what it calls an "IND cumulative table of contents" (CTOC), which the center defines as an XML-based "document that would list all the files submitted to an electronic IND, along with information about the type, location, and status of the file and any previously submitted information it references." In part, the

CTOC approach addresses one of the considerable document management-related challenges associated with INDs—that is, that INDs comprise many different files and documents submitted over an extended period (i.e., clinical development). An IND reviewer, says the agency, "would use the CTOC files to access, sort, and search the electronic IND submission's content according to multiple criteria (e.g., amended, replaced, or current documents; submission dates; related documents, etc.)...." Following a January 2001 public meeting to discuss the CTOC approach for the eIND, a few companies submitted examples of INDs employing the CTOC.

According to the current IND application form (Form FDA 1571), an IND will consist of as many as 10 principal sections:

1. Cover Sheet (Form FDA 1571).
2. Table of Contents.
3. Introductory Statement.
4. General Investigational Plan.
5. Investigator's Brochure (IB).
6. Clinical Protocols.
7. Chemistry, Manufacturing, and Control Data.
8. Pharmacology and Toxicology Data.
9. Previous Human Experience (if applicable).
10. Additional Information, including plans for pediatric studies.

The nature of the drug and the available product-related information affect the number of sections included in an IND submission. These and other factors also determine the quantity of information to be included in the application. "Sponsors are expected to exercise considerable discretion...regarding the content of information submitted in each section [of the IND], depending upon the kind of drug being studied and the nature of the available information," FDA regulations state. "The amount of information on a particular drug that must be submitted in an IND depends upon such factors as the novelty of the drug, the extent to which it has been studied previously, the known or suspected risks, and the developmental phase of the drug."

The following sections discuss the content requirements for each component of the IND. Although not included in the listing of IND content requirements above, many INDs include a cover letter that briefly summarizes the purpose and content of the submission. By providing a general introduction to the submission and identifying any previously reached sponsor/FDA agreements, cover letters are often extremely useful to drug reviewers.

Cover Sheet (Form FDA 1571) Form FDA 1571, the first required element of an IND, serves as the cover sheet for the entire IND submission (see sample form below). By completing and signing, or having an authorized representative complete and sign, this form, the sponsor: (1) identifies itself, the investigational drug, the persons responsible for monitoring the clinical trial and safety-related trial information, and the phase(s) of investigation covered by the application; (2) establishes the

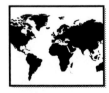

nature of the submission (i.e., initial submission, amendment, etc.); (3) identifies any responsibilities that have been transferred to a contract research organization (CRO); and (4) agrees to comply with applicable regulations, including those requiring the sponsor to refrain from initiating clinical studies until an IND covering the investigations is in effect. A completed copy of Form FDA 1571 is also required with each amendment submitted to the IND.

If the person signing the IND form does not reside or maintain a place of business within the United States, "the IND is required to contain the name and address of, and be countersigned by, an attorney, agent, or other authorized official who resides or maintains a place of business within the United States."

Item 12 of Form 1571 is important because it identifies the various elements that must be addressed in an original IND submission. These elements are discussed below.

Table of Contents FDA regulations offer no guidance on the IND's table of contents. However, the agency does state that sponsors should follow the specified IND format "in the interest of fostering an efficient review of the application." Obviously, the table of contents should be sufficiently detailed to permit FDA reviewers to locate important elements of the application quickly and easily. The table of contents should provide the location of items by volume and page number.

Introductory Statement The IND's introductory statement should provide a description of the drug, the goals of the proposed clinical investigations, and a summary of the previous human experience with the drug. According to FDA regulations, this section should provide "a brief introductory statement giving the name of the drug and all active ingredients, the drug's pharmacological class, the structural formula of the drug (if known), the formulation of the dosage form(s) to be used, the route of administration, and the broad objectives and planned duration of the proposed clinical investigation(s)." The sponsor must also summarize all previous clinical experience with the drug (with reference to other INDs, if applicable), including "investigational or marketing experience in other countries that may be relevant to the safety of the proposed clinical investigation(s)." If a foreign regulatory authority discontinued the drug's testing or marketing for any reason related to safety or effectiveness, the sponsor must identify the country(ies) in which the withdrawal took place and must describe the reason for the withdrawal.

General Investigational Plan The general investigational plan must provide a brief description of the clinical studies planned for the experimental drug. At a minimum, studies planned for the first year should be described. The FDA has stated that the goal of this section is to provide agency reviewers a brief overview of the scale and kind of clinical studies to be conducted during the following year. This general overview should be no more than two to three pages in length, and should provide the necessary context for FDA reviewers to assess the adequacy of technical information to support future studies and to provide advice and assistance to the sponsor.

According to federal regulations, the "plan should include the following: (a) the rationale for the drug or the research study; (b) the indication(s) to be studied; (c) the general approach to be followed in evaluating the drug; (d) the kinds of clinical trials to be conducted in the first year following the submission (if plans are not developed for the entire year, the sponsor should so indicate); (e) the esti-

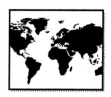

DEPARTMENT OF HEALTH AND HUMAN SERVICES PUBLIC HEALTH SERVICE FOOD AND DRUG ADMINISTRATION **INVESTIGATIONAL NEW DRUG APPLICATION (IND)** **(TITLE 21, CODE OF FEDERAL REGULATIONS (CFR) PART 312)**	Form Approved: OMB No. 0910-0014. Expiration Date: September 30, 2002 See OMB Statement on Reverse. NOTE: No drug may be shipped or clinical investigation begun until an IND for that investigation is in effect (21 CFR 312.40).
1. NAME OF SPONSOR	2. DATE OF SUBMISSION
3. ADDRESS *(Number, Street, City, State and Zip Code)*	4. TELEPHONE NUMBER *(Include Area Code)*
5. NAME(S) OF DRUG *(Include all available names: Trade, Generic, Chemical, Code)*	6. IND NUMBER *(If previously assigned)*

7. INDICATION(S) *(Covered by this submission)*

8. PHASE(S) OF CLINICAL INVESTIGATION TO BE CONDUCTED.   ☐ PHASE 1   ☐ PHASE 2   ☐ PHASE 3   ☐ OTHER _____ *(Specify)*

9. LIST NUMBERS OF ALL INVESTIGATIONAL NEW DRUG APPLICATIONS *(21 CFR Part 312)*, NEW DRUG OR ANTIBIOTIC APPLICATIONS *(21 CFR Part 314)*, DRUG MASTER FILES *(21 CFR 314.420)*, AND PRODUCT LICENSE APPLICATIONS *(21 CFR Part 601)* REFERRED TO IN THIS APPLICATION.

10. IND submissions should be consecutively numbered. The initial IND should be numbered "Serial Number: 000." The next submission (e.g., amendment, report, or correspondence) should be numbered "Serial Number: 001." Subsequent submissions should be numbered consecutively in the order in which they are submitted.	SERIAL NUMBER: ___ ___ ___

11. THIS SUBMISSION CONTAINS THE FOLLOWING: (Check all that apply)

☐ INITIAL INVESTIGATIONAL NEW DRUG APPLICATION (IND)   ☐ RESPONSE TO CLINICAL HOLD

PROTOCOL AMENDMENT(S):   INFORMATION AMENDMENT(S):   IND SAFETY REPORT(S):
☐ NEW PROTOCOL   ☐ CHEMISTRY/MICROBIOLOGY   ☐ INITIAL WRITTEN REPORT
☐ CHANGE IN PROTOCOL   ☐ PHARMACOLOGY/TOXICOLOGY   ☐ FOLLOW-UP TO A WRITTEN REPORT
☐ NEW INVESTIGATOR   ☐ CLINICAL

☐ RESPONSE TO FDA REQUEST FOR INFORMATION   ☐ ANNUAL REPORT   ☐ GENERAL CORRESPONDENCE

☐ REQUEST FOR REINSTATEMENT OF IND THAT IS WITHDRAWN, INACTIVATED, TERMINATED OR DISCONTINUED   ☐ OTHER _____ *(Specify)*

CHECK ONLY IF APPLICABLE

JUSTIFICATION STATEMENT MUST BE SUBMITTED WITH APPLICATION FOR ANY CHECKED BELOW. REFER TO THE CITED CFR SECTION FOR FURTHER INFORMATION.

☐ TREATMENT IND 21 CFR 312.35(b)   ☐ TREATMENT PROTOCOL 21 CFR 312.35(a)   ☐ CHARGE REQUEST/NOTIFICATION 21 CFR 312.7(d)

FOR FDA USE ONLY		
CDR/DBIND/DGD RECEIPT STAMP	DDR RECEIPT STAMP	DIVISION ASSIGNMENT:
		IND NUMBER ASSIGNED:

FORM FDA 1571 (8/01)   PREVIOUS EDITION IS OBSOLETE

12.	**CONTENTS OF APPLICATION**

This application contains the following items: *(check all that apply)*

- ☐ 1. Form FDA 1571 [21 CFR 312.23 (a) (1)]
- ☐ 2. Table of contents [21 CFR 312.23 (a) (2)]
- ☐ 3. Introductory statement [21 CFR 312.23 (a) (3)]
- ☐ 4. General investigational plan [21 CFR 312.23 (a) (3)]
- ☐ 5. Investigator's brochure [21 CFR 312.23 (a) (5)]
- ☐ 6. Protocol(s) [21 CFR 312.23 (a) (6)]
    - ☐ a. Study protocol(s) [21 CFR 312.23 (a) (6)]
    - ☐ b. Investigator data [21 CFR 312.23 (a) (6)(iii)(b)] or completed Form(s) FDA 1572
    - ☐ c. Facilities data [21 CFR 312.23 (a) (6)(iii)(b)] or completed Form(s) FDA 1572
    - ☐ d. Institutional Review Board data [21 CFR 312.23 (a) (6)(iii)(b)] or completed Form(s) FDA 1572
- ☐ 7. Chemistry, manufacturing, and control data [21 CFR 312.23 (a) (7)]
    - ☐ Environmental assessment or claim for exclusion [21 CFR 312.23 (a) (7)(iv)(e)]
- ☐ 8. Pharmacology and toxicology data [21 CFR 312.23 (a) (8)]
- ☐ 9. Previous human experience [21 CFR 312.23 (a) (9)]
- ☐ 10. Additional information [21 CFR 312.23 (a) (10)]

13. IS ANY PART OF THE CLINICAL STUDY TO BE CONDUCTED BY A CONTRACT RESEARCH ORGANIZATION?   ☐ YES   ☐ NO

IF YES, WILL ANY SPONSOR OBLIGATIONS BE TRANSFERRED TO THE CONTRACT RESEARCH ORGANIZATION?   ☐ YES   ☐ NO

IF YES, ATTACH A STATEMENT CONTAINING THE NAME AND ADDRESS OF THE CONTRACT RESEARCH ORGANIZATION, IDENTIFICATION OF THE CLINICAL STUDY, AND A LISTING OF THE OBLIGATIONS TRANSFERRED.

14. NAME AND TITLE OF THE PERSON RESPONSIBLE FOR MONITORING THE CONDUCT AND PROGRESS OF THE CLINICAL INVESTIGATIONS

15. NAME(S) AND TITLE(S) OF THE PERSON(S) RESPONSIBLE FOR REVIEW AND EVALUATION OF INFORMATION RELEVANT TO THE SAFETY OF THE DRUG

I agree not to begin clinical investigations until 30 days after FDA's receipt of the IND unless I receive earlier notification by FDA that the studies may begin. I also agree not to begin or continue clinical investigations covered by the IND if those studies are placed on clinical hold. I agree that an Institutional Review Board (IRB) that complies with the requirements set forth in 21 CFR Part 56 will be responsible for initial and continuing review and approval of each of the studies in the proposed clinical investigation. I agree to conduct the investigation in accordance with all other applicable regulatory requirements.

16. NAME OF SPONSOR OR SPONSOR'S AUTHORIZED REPRESENTATIVE	17. SIGNATURE OF SPONSOR OR SPONSOR'S AUTHORIZED REPRESENTATIVE	
18. ADDRESS (Number, Street, City, State and Zip Code)	19. TELEPHONE NUMBER *(Include Area Code)*	20. DATE

(**WARNING**: A willfully false statement is a criminal offense. U.S.C. Title 18, Sec. 1001.)

Public reporting burden for this collection of information is estimated to average 100 hours per response, including the time for reviewing instructions, searching existing data sources, gathering and maintaining the data needed, and completing and reviewing the collection of information. Send comments regarding this burden estimate or any other aspect of this collection of information, including suggestions for reducing this burden to:

Food and Drug Administration
CBER (HFM-99)
1401 Rockville Pike
Rockville, MD 20852-1448

Food and Drug Administration
CDER (HFD-94)
12229 Wilkins Avenue
Rockville, MD 20852

"An agency may not conduct or sponsor, and a person is not required to respond to a collection of information unless it displays a currently valid OMB control number."

Please DO NOT RETURN this application to this address.

FORM FDA 1571 (8/01)

mated number of patients to be given the drug in those studies; and (f) any risks of particular severity or seriousness anticipated on the basis of the toxicological data in animals or prior studies in humans with the drug or related drugs."

The FDA does not require rigid adherence to the general investigational plan. Provided that it fulfills protocol and information amendment reporting requirements (see discussion below), a sponsor is free to deviate from the plan when necessary.

Investigator's Brochure With the exception of investigator-sponsored applications, all INDs must include a copy of the investigator's brochure (IB)—an information package providing each participating clinical investigator with available information on the drug, including its known and possible risks and benefits. The most recent discussion of the purpose of, and content requirements applicable to, an IB appear in an addendum to the ICH's May 1997 final guideline entitled, *Good Clinical Practice: Consolidated Guideline*:

"The Investigator's Brochure (IB) is a compilation of the clinical and nonclinical data on the investigational product(s) that are relevant to the study of the product(s) in human subjects," the guidance states. "Its purpose is to provide the investigators and others involved in the trial with the information to facilitate their understanding of the rationale for, and their compliance with, many key features of the protocol, such as the dose, dose frequency/interval, methods of administration, and safety monitoring procedures. The IB also provides insight to support the clinical management of the study subjects during the course of the clinical trial. The information should be presented in a concise, simple, objective, balanced, and nonpromotional form that enables a clinician, or potential investigator, to understand it and make his/her own unbiased risk-benefit assessment of the appropriateness of the proposed trial. For this reason, a medically qualified person should generally participate in the editing of an IB, but the contents of the IB should be approved by the disciplines that generated the described data." The ICH consolidated guidance also offers an example of an IB format.

While not as detailed as the ICH guideline's description of investigator's brochure content requirements, FDA regulations call for IBs to include the following principal elements:

- a brief description of the drug substance and formulation, including the structural formula (if known);

- a summary of the pharmacological and toxicological effects of the drug in animals and, to the extent known, in humans;

- a summary of the pharmacokinetics and biological disposition of the drug in animals and, if known, in humans;

- a summary of information relating to the drug's safety and effectiveness in humans obtained from prior clinical studies (reprints of published articles on such studies may be appended when useful); and

- a description of possible risks and side effects anticipated on the basis of prior experience with the drug under investigation or with related drugs, and precautions to be taken or special monitoring to be performed as part of the drug's investigational use.

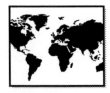

As clinical trials advance, the sponsor must inform investigators "of new observations discovered by or reported to the sponsor of the drug, particularly with respect to adverse effects and safe use." Such information may be distributed to investigators by means of periodically revised IBs, reprints of published studies, reports or letters to clinical investigators, or other appropriate means. Copies of these communications should also be submitted to the IND file. According to the ICH's May 1997 consolidated GCP guideline, the IB should be reviewed at least annually and revised as necessary in compliance with a sponsor's written procedures.

Clinical Protocols FDA regulations state that, along with the general investigational plan, clinical protocols are "the central focus of the initial IND submission." Protocols are descriptions of clinical studies that identify, among other things, a study's objectives, design, and procedures. The FDA reviews clinical protocols to ensure: (1) that subjects will not be exposed to unnecessary risks in any of the clinical trials; and (2) that Phase 2 and Phase 3 clinical study designs are adequate to provide the types and amount of information necessary to show that the drug is safe and/or effective.

In the initial IND submission, the sponsor must provide only protocols for the proposed study or studies that will begin immediately after the IND goes into effect—that is, after the FDA's 30-day review period. Although initial INDs generally include just Phase 1 protocols, some may propose Phase 2 or 3 protocols, particularly if a drug has been studied in clinical trials previously (e.g., in foreign clinical studies).

As stated, the safety of initial Phase 1 studies is the FDA's principal concern in reviewing the original IND submission. Since late-phase clinical studies often are not fully developed until data from Phase 1 studies are obtained, Phase 2 and Phase 3 protocols may be submitted later in the development process.

In its November 1995 IND guidance document, the FDA highlights the regulations' more flexible approach to Phase 1 protocols. "Sponsors are reminded that the regulations were changed in 1987 specifically to allow Phase 1 study protocols to be less detailed and more flexible than protocols for Phase 2 and 3 studies. This change recognized that these protocols are part of an early learning process and should be adaptable as information is obtained, and that the principal concern at this stage of development is that the study be conducted safely. The regulations state that Phase 1 protocols should be directed primarily at providing an outline of the investigation: an estimate of the number of subjects to be included; a description of safety exclusions, and a description of the dosing plan, including duration, dose, or method to be used in determining dose. In addition, such protocols should specify in detail only those elements of the study that are critical to subject safety, such as: 1) necessary monitoring of vital signs and blood chemistries and 2) toxicity-based stopping or dose adjustment rules. In addition, the regulations state that modifications of the experimental design of Phase 1 studies that do not affect critical safety assessments are required to be reported to FDA only in the annual report."

In contrast, the FDA requires that Phase 2 and 3 protocols include detailed descriptions of all aspects of the studies. Federal regulations state that these protocols "should be designed in such a way that, if the sponsor anticipates that some deviation from the study design may become necessary as the investigation progresses, alternatives or contingencies to provide for such deviations are built into

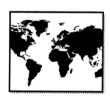

the protocols at the outset. For example, a protocol for a controlled short-term study might include a plan for an early crossover of nonresponders to an alternative therapy." About such contingency plans, which are optional, the FDA has commented that it "strongly encourages the submission of such plans as it believes there is much to be gained in thinking about the planning for possible alternative courses of action early in the protocol development process. Providing in the initial protocol for possible departures from the study design enhances the value or reviewability of study results. Such advance planning also permits both FDA and the sponsor to raise useful questions about study design and supporting information at the earliest possible time."

Agency reviewers report that the language used in the November 1995 guidance and, perhaps to an even greater extent, FDAMA has given some firms the false impression that summary-type protocols are permitted in INDs. Although protocol summaries may be appropriate in some cases and when authorized by a review division, CDER reviewers have been frustrated by the number of summary-type protocols that have been submitted in INDs following FDAMA's passage.

Although the components and level of detail found in a protocol will depend upon the phase covered and other factors, FDA regulations state that a protocol should include seven elements:

1. A statement of the objectives and purpose of the study.

2. The name and address of, and a statement of qualifications (curriculum vitae or other statement of qualifications) for, each investigator; the name of each subinvestigator (i.e., research fellow, resident) working under the supervision of the investigator; the names and addresses of the research facilities to be used; and the name and address of each institutional review board (IRB) responsible for reviewing the protocols (this information may be submitted on Form FDA 1572; see sample below). To address some of the complexities of providing information on foreign investigators, CDER is developing a new guidance entitled, *Submission to an IND of Investigator Information for Non-U.S. Studies*.

3. The criteria for patient selection and exclusion, and an estimate of the number of patients to be studied. Sponsors should be aware of a June 2000 regulation that will allow the FDA to place certain studies under an IND on clinical hold when the agency determines that a sponsor has categorically excluded otherwise eligible men or women with reproductive potential from participating in a study of a drug for a life-threatening disease or condition that affects both genders (see Chapter 4).

4. A description of the study design, including the type of control group to be used, if any, and a description of the methods to be used to minimize bias on the part of subjects, investigators, and analysts.

5. The method for determining the dose(s) to be administered, the planned maximum dosage, and the duration of individual patient exposure to the drug.

6. A description of the observations and measurements to be made to fulfill the objectives of the study.

7. A description of clinical procedures, laboratory tests, or other means to be employed in monitoring the effects of the drug in human subjects and in minimizing risk.

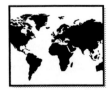

The ICH's May 1997 consolidated GCP guideline also features a discussion of standards for the content of clinical protocols and protocol amendments. According to the GCP guideline, a trial protocol should "generally include the following topics":

> *General Information*: the protocol's title and identifying number, the sponsor and monitor's name and address, the name and title of the investigator responsible for conducting the trial, and the name and address of the person authorized to sign the protocol and any protocol amendments for the sponsor.
>
> *Background Information*: the name and a description of the investigational product, a summary of findings from nonclinical studies, a summary of known and potential risks and benefits to human subjects, and a description of the population to be studied.
>
> *Trial Objectives and Purpose*: a detailed description of the trial's purpose and objectives.
>
> *Trial Design*: a statement of the primary and secondary endpoints (if any) to be measured during the trial, a description of the type/design of the proposed trial (e.g., blinding, controls) and a schematic diagram of trial design, procedures, and stages.
>
> *Selection and Withdrawal of Subjects*: subject inclusion and exclusion criteria and subject withdrawal criteria and procedures.
>
> *Treatment of Subjects*: the treatment(s) to be administered, including the name, dose(s), dosing schedules, route/mode of administration, and treatment and follow-up periods, procedures for monitoring patient compliance, and other treatments permitted and not permitted before and/or during the trial.
>
> *Assessment of Efficacy*: specification of the efficacy parameters, and the methods and timing for assessing, recording, and analyzing these parameters.
>
> *Assessment of Safety*: specification of the safety parameters, a description of the methods and timing for assessing, recording, and analyzing these parameters, a detailing of the procedures for eliciting reports of and for recording and reporting adverse events and intercurrent illnesses, and a description of the type and duration of subject follow-up following adverse events.
>
> *Statistics*: a description of the statistical methods to be employed, including the timing of any planned interim analyses, the planned subject enrollment, the level of significance to be used, criteria for trial termination, procedures for accounting for missing, unused, or spurious data, and methods for the selection of subjects to be included in the analyses.
>
> *Direct Access to Source Documents*: the protocol or other written agreements should specify that the investigators/institutions will permit trial-related monitoring, audits, IRB/IEC review, and regulatory inspections by providing direct access to source data and documents.
>
> *Quality Control and Quality Assurance*.
>
> *Ethics*: a description of the ethical considerations relating to the trial.
>
> *Data Handling and Recordkeeping*.

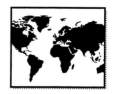

Financing and Insurance: a description of financial- and insurance-related arrangements if not addressed in a separate agreement.

Publication Policy: a description of the publication policy if not addressed in a separate agreement.

Supplements.

The ICH's GCP guideline notes that sponsors may provide site-specific information on separate protocol pages or address these areas in a "separate agreement," and that some of the information may be contained in other documents (e.g., the investigator's brochure) that are referenced in the protocol.

Chemistry, Manufacturing, and Control Information The purpose of the IND's chemistry, manufacturing and control (CMC) section is to establish that the methods used to manufacture and assay the investigational product are adequate to ensure the product's safety. Submission requirements for the IND's CMC section are a function of several factors, including the stage of the clinical trial proposed in the application.

The IND's CMC section was one of two sections affected by the FDA's 1995 IND reform initiative. Specifically, the initiative revised the CMC section in two ways: (1) it suggested that IND sponsors include a new "chemistry and manufacturing introduction;" and (2) it suggested that sponsors provide information on the drug substance and drug product in a pair of "summary reports" (see discussions below).

Based on the FDA's November 1995 guidance document, an IND proposing a Phase 1 clinical study should include CMC information consisting of the following six components:

Chemistry and Manufacturing Introduction. In this introduction, "the sponsor should state whether it believes: 1) the chemistry of either the drug substance or the drug product, or 2) the manufacturing of either the drug substance or the drug product, presents any signals of potential human risk. If so, these signals of potential risks should be discussed, and the steps proposed to monitor for such risk(s) should be described, or the reason(s) why the signal(s) should be dismissed should be discussed. In addition, sponsors should describe any chemistry and manufacturing differences between the drug product proposed for clinical use and the drug product used in the animal toxicology trials that formed the basis for the sponsor's conclusion that it was safe to proceed with the proposed clinical study. How these differences might affect the safety profile of the drug product should be discussed. If there are no differences in the products, that should be stated."

Drug Substance. The FDA states that information on the drug substance should be provided in a "summary report" comprising five elements: (1) a description of the drug substance, including its physical, chemical, or biological characteristics, along with some evidence to support its proposed chemical structure; (2) the name and address of its manufacturer; (3) a description of the general method of preparation of the drug substance (ideally presented as a detailed flow diagram), including a list of the reagents, solvents, and catalysts used; (4) a brief description of the acceptable limits and analytical methods used to assure the identity, strength, quality, and purity of the drug substance; and (5) information sufficient to support the stability of the drug substance during toxicologic studies and the proposed clinical studies (neither detailed stability data nor the stability protocol should be sub-

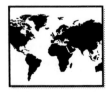

mitted). Reference to the current edition of the U.S. Pharmacopeia or National Formulary may satisfy relevant requirements in the drug substance subsection.

In manufacturing and packaging their products, applicants often utilize components (e.g., drug substances, nonstandard excipients, containers) manufactured by other firms, such as contract manufacturers. In such cases, the contract manufacturer is likely to want to preserve the confidentiality of its manufacturing processes. Since an IND must provide information on these processes, contract manufacturers often submit this information to the FDA in a drug master file (DMF). This allows drug sponsors using the company's products to meet submission requirements by incorporating by reference information provided in the master file. Because the drug sponsor never sees the information in the DMF, the confidentiality of the contract facility's manufacturing processes is maintained. In the IND (or other submission), an incorporation by reference should be made in the section of the application in which the referenced information would normally appear if provided by the applicant.

Traditionally, there have been five different types of DMFs: Type I DMFs, which provide information on manufacturing site, facilities, operating procedures, and personnel information; Type II DMFs, which provide information on drug substances or drug products, drug substance intermediates, and materials use in preparing them; Type III DMFs, which include information on packaging materials; Type IV DMFs, which provide information on excipients, colorants, flavors, essences, or materials used in their preparation; and Type V DMFs, which include FDA-accepted reference information. In a January 2000 final rule, however, CDER eliminated Type I DMFs, and instructed industry to use the other types of DMFs to submit the types of information traditionally provided in Type I DMFs. In 1992, a CDER task force on the DMF system recommended that the agency eliminate Type I DMFs, in part because the information contained in these DMFs was often outdated and was frequently not easily accessible to FDA inspectors, and because more updated information was maintained onsite by manufacturers, where it was more easily available to agency inspectors.

A more detailed discussion of CDER's requirements for, and use of, DMFs can be found in the center's *Guideline for Drug Master Files* (September 1989).

Drug Product. The FDA suggests that the IND provide information on the drug product in a "summary report" comprising as many as six components: (1) a list—usually no more than one or two pages long—of all components, which may include reasonable alternatives for inactive compounds, used in the manufacture of the investigational drug product, including both those components intended to appear in the drug product and those that may not appear, but that are used in the manufacturing process; (2) where applicable, a brief summary of the quantitative composition of the investigational new drug product, including any reasonable variations that may be expected during the investigational stage; (3) the name and address of the drug product manufacturer; (4) a brief, general description of the method of manufacturing and packaging procedures for the product (ideally presented as flow diagrams); (5) a brief description of the proposed acceptable limits and analytical methods used to ensure the identity, strength, quality, and purity of the drug product; and (6) information sufficient to support the stability of the drug substance during the toxicologic studies and the proposed clinical studies (neither detailed stability data nor the stability protocol should be submitted). Reference to the current edition of the U.S. Pharmacopeia or National Formulary may satisfy certain requirements for this section.

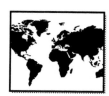

Worldwide Pharmaceutical Regulation Series

DEPARTMENT OF HEALTH AND HUMAN SERVICES
PUBLIC HEALTH SERVICE
FOOD AND DRUG ADMINISTRATION
STATEMENT OF INVESTIGATOR
(TITLE 21, CODE OF FEDERAL REGULATIONS (CFR) PART 312)
(See instructions on reverse side.)

Form Approved: OMB No. 0910-0014
Expiration Date: September 30, 2002
See OMB Statement on Reverse.

NOTE: No investigator may participate in an investigation until he/she provides the sponsor with a completed, signed Statement of Investigator, Form FDA 1572 (21CFR 312.53(c)).

1. NAME AND ADDRESS OF INVESTIGATOR

2. EDUCATION, TRAINING, AND EXPERIENCE THAT QUALIFIES THE INVESTIGATOR AS AN EXPERT IN THE CLINICAL INVESTIGATION OF THE DRUG FOR THE USE UNDER INVESTIGATION. ONE OF THE FOLLOWING IS ATTACHED:

☐ CURRICULUM VITAE   ☐ OTHER STATEMENT OF QUALIFICATIONS

3. NAME AND ADDRESS OF ANY MEDICAL SCHOOL, HOSPITAL, OR OTHER RESEARCH FACILITY WHERE THE CLINICAL INVESTIGATION(S) WILL BE CONDUCTED.

4. NAME AND ADDRESS OF ANY CLINICAL LABORATORY FACILITIES TO BE USED IN THE STUDY.

5. NAME AND ADDRESS OF THE INSTITUTIONAL REVIEW BOARD (IRB) THAT IS RESPONSIBLE FOR REVIEW AND APPROVAL OF THE STUDY(IES).

6. NAMES OF THE SUBINVESTIGATORS (e.g., research fellows, residents, associates) WHO WILL BE ASSISTING THE INVESTIGATOR IN THE CONDUCT OF THE INVESTIGATION(S).

7. NAME AND CODE NUMBER, IF ANY, OF THE PROTOCOL(S) IN THE IND FOR THE STUDY(IES) TO BE CONDUCTED BY THE INVESTIGATOR.

FORM FDA 1572 (8/01)   PREVIOUS EDITION IS OBSOLETE

8. ATTACH THE FOLLOWING CLINICAL PROTOCOL INFORMATION:

☐ FOR PHASE 1 INVESTIGATIONS, A GENERAL OUTLINE OF THE PLANNED INVESTIGATION INCLUDING THE ESTIMATED DURATION OF THE STUDY AND THE MAXIMUM NUMBER OF SUBJECTS THAT WILL BE INVOLVED.

☐ FOR PHASE 2 OR 3 INVESTIGATIONS, AN OUTLINE OF THE STUDY PROTOCOL INCLUDING AN APPROXIMATION OF THE NUMBER OF SUBJECTS TO BE TREATED WITH THE DRUG AND THE NUMBER TO BE EMPLOYED AS CONTROLS, IF ANY; THE CLINICAL USES TO BE INVESTIGATED; CHARACTERISTICS OF SUBJECTS BY AGE, SEX, AND CONDITION; THE KIND OF CLINICAL OBSERVATIONS AND LABORATORY TESTS TO BE CONDUCTED; THE ESTIMATED DURATION OF THE STUDY; AND COPIES OR A DESCRIPTION OF CASE REPORT FORMS TO BE USED.

9. COMMITMENTS:

I agree to conduct the study(ies) in accordance with the relevant, current protocol(s) and will only make changes in a protocol after notifying the sponsor, except when necessary to protect the safety, rights, or welfare of subjects.

I agree to personally conduct or supervise the described investigation(s).

I agree to inform any patients, or any persons used as controls, that the drugs are being used for investigational purposes and I will ensure that the requirements relating to obtaining informed consent in 21 CFR Part 50 and institutional review board (IRB) review and approval in 21 CFR Part 56 are met.

I agree to report to the sponsor adverse experiences that occur in the course of the investigation(s) in accordance with 21 CFR 312.64.

I have read and understand the information in the investigator's brochure, including the potential risks and side effects of the drug.

I agree to ensure that all associates, colleagues, and employees assisting in the conduct of the study(ies) are informed about their obligations in meeting the above commitments.

I agree to maintain adequate and accurate records in accordance with 21 CFR 312.62 and to make those records available for inspection in accordance with 21 CFR 312.68.

I will ensure that an IRB that complies with the requirements of 21 CFR Part 56 will be responsible for the initial and continuing review and approval of the clinical investigation. I also agree to promptly report to the IRB all changes in the research activity and all unanticipated problems involving risks to human subjects or others. Additionally, I will not make any changes in the research without IRB approval, except where necessary to eliminate apparent immediate hazards to human subjects.

I agree to comply with all other requirements regarding the obligations of clinical investigators and all other pertinent requirements in 21 CFR Part 312.

INSTRUCTIONS FOR COMPLETING FORM FDA 1572
STATEMENT OF INVESTIGATOR

1. Complete all sections. Attach a separate page if additional space is needed.
2. Attach curriculum vitae or other statement of qualifications as described in Section 2.
3. Attach protocol outline as described in Section 8.
4. Sign and date below.
5. FORWARD THE COMPLETED FORM AND ATTACHMENTS TO THE SPONSOR. The sponsor will incorporate this information along with other technical data into an Investigational New Drug Application (IND).

10. SIGNATURE OF INVESTIGATOR	11. DATE

(**WARNING**: A willfully false statement is a criminal offense. U.S.C. Title 18, Sec. 1001.)

Public reporting burden for this collection of information is estimated to average 100 hours per response, including the time for reviewing instructions, searching existing data sources, gathering and maintaining the data needed, and completing reviewing the collection of information. Send comments regarding this burden estimate or any other aspect of this collection of information, including suggestions for reducing this burden to:

Food and Drug Administration
CBER (HFM-99)
1401 Rockville Pike
Rockville, MD 20852-1448

Food and Drug Administration
CDER (HFD-94)
12229 Wilkins Avenue
Rockville, MD 20852

"An agency may not conduct or sponsor, and a person is not required to respond to a collection of information unless it displays a currently valid OMB control number."

Please DO NOT RETURN this application to this address.

FORM FDA 1572 (8/01)

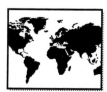

A Brief, General Description of the Composition, Manufacture, and Control of any Placebo Used in the Controlled Clinical Trials. The FDA states that this information should be provided in "diagrammatic, tabular, and brief written" form.

Labeling. The labeling section should comprise "a mock-up or printed representation of the proposed labeling that will be provided to investigator(s) in the proposed clinical trial." Investigational labels must carry a "caution" statement required by federal regulations: "Caution: New Drug-Limited by Federal (or United States) law to investigational use."

Environmental Analysis (EA) Requirements. This section should provide either an environmental assessment, or a claim for a categorical exclusion from the requirement for an environmental assessment. Under a July 1997 final regulation, the FDA established that EAs would be required in INDs (and NDAs) only under "extraordinary circumstances" (e.g., when available data indicate that the expected level of exposure could do serious harm to the environment). Because the use of experimental compounds in clinical trials represents a temporary and low-volume release, however, virtually all INDs traditionally have included only a claim for a categorical exclusion in the past.

To provide further insights regarding the changes brought by the July 1997 regulation, CDER released a final guidance document entitled, *Environmental Assessment of Human Drug and Biologics Applications* (July 1998). This guidance superseded CDER's *Guidance for Industry for the Submission of Environmental Assessments for Human Drug Applications and Supplements* (November 1995).

The FDA emphasizes throughout its regulations and guidelines that the amount and detail of information needed in the IND's CMC section depends on several factors, including the scope and phase of the proposed clinical investigation, the proposed duration of the study, the dosage form, and the quantity of information otherwise available. "Modifications to the method of preparation of the new drug substance and dosage form, and even changes in the dosage form itself, are likely as the investigation progresses," the agency states in its November 1995 IND guidance document. "The emphasis in an initial Phase 1 CMC submission should, therefore, generally be placed on providing information that will allow evaluation of the safety of subjects in the proposed study. The identification of a safety concern or insufficient data to make an evaluation of safety is the only basis for a clinical hold based on the CMC section."

FDA regulations add that "the emphasis in an initial Phase 1 submission should generally be placed on the identification and control of the raw materials and the new drug substance. Final specifications for the drug substance and drug product are not expected until the end of the investigational process." However, when final specifications are not established until just prior to Phase 3 studies, comparability with preceding studies may be necessary. Stability testing should support the duration of use for the proposed clinical studies.

The FDA does require that sponsors comply with Current Good Manufacturing Practices (CGMP) during clinical trials. According to the FDA's *Guideline on the Preparation of Investigational New Drug Products (Human and Animal)* (March 1991), the "FDA recognizes that manufacturing procedures and specifications will change as clinical trials advance. However, as research nears completion, procedures and controls are expected to be more specific because they will have been based upon a growing body of

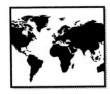

scientific data and documentation.... When drug development reaches a stage where the drugs are produced for clinical trials in humans...then compliance with the CGMP regulations is required. For example, the drug product must be produced in a qualified facility, using laboratory and other equipment that has been qualified, and processes must be validated. There must be written procedures for sanitation, calibration, and maintenance of equipment, and specific instructions for the use of the equipment and procedures used to manufacture the drug. Product contamination and wide variations in potency can produce substantial levels of side effects and toxicity, and even produce wide-sweeping effects on the physiological activity of the drug. Product safety, quality, and uniformity are especially significant in the case of investigational products. Such factors may affect the outcome of a clinical investigation that will, in large part, determine whether or not the product will be approved for wider distribution to the public." A July 2000 draft ICH guidance entitled, *Good Manufacturing Practice Guide for Active Pharmaceutical Ingredients* also includes a brief section on GMP issues for clinical trial-stage drugs.

As the testing and drug development process advances, sponsors must submit IND information amendments to the CMC section of the IND (see discussion below). Most importantly, the amendments must describe the effects of the transition from pilot scale production used for early clinical studies to the larger-scale production methods used for expanded clinical investigations. In February 1998, CDER released a draft guidance entitled, *INDs for Phases 2 and 3 Studies of Drugs, Including Specified Therapeutic Biotechnology-Derived Products: Chemistry, Manufacturing, and Controls Content and Format*. In specifying the chemistry, manufacturing, and controls information that is needed during Phase 2 and 3 clinical trials, the draft guidance claims that it provides IND sponsors with "regulatory relief" in three specific areas. "First, the phase 3 supplementary data and information corroborating the quality and safety criteria established in earlier investigational phases need not be submitted before the initiation of phase 3 studies and can be generated during phase 3 drug development," the draft document states. "This should provide the sponsor with greater flexibility. Second, a sponsor may elect to delay submitting data elements obtained in earlier investigations until phase 3 if they do not affect safety. This allows sponsors to postpone the submission of data and information, even if generated before and during earlier investigational phases. Third, a sponsor may submit summary reports annually and does not need to resubmit data and information already submitted."

In addition to the documents referenced above, the agency has published several guidelines that provide insights regarding the submission of chemistry, manufacturing, and control information in both INDs and NDAs. These include the following: *Guideline for the Format and Content of the Chemistry, Manufacturing, and Controls Section of an Application* (February 1987), *Guideline for Submitting Documentation for the Manufacture of and Controls for Drug Products* (February 1987), *Guideline for Submitting Supporting Documentation in Drug Applications for the Manufacture of Drug Substances* (February 1987), *Guidance for Industry: Container Closure Systems for Packaging Human Drugs and Biologics-Chemistry, Manufacturing, and Controls Documentation* (May 1999), *Documentation for Packaging for Human Drugs and Biologics* (February 1987), *Draft Guidance on the Stability Testing of Drug Substances and Drug Products* (June 1998), *Guideline for Submitting Documentation for the Stability of Human Drugs and Biologics* (February 1987), and *Guidance for Industry for the Submission of Chemistry, Manufacturing, and Controls for Synthetic Peptide Drug Substances* (November 1994).

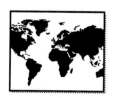

ICH guidelines, such as the 2001 revised final guideline entitled, Q1A(R) *Stability Testing of New Drug Substances and Products* and the final guidance entitled, Q6A *Specifications: Test Procedures and Acceptance Criteria for New Drug Substances and New Drug Products: Chemical Substances*, now provide more updated guidance in certain areas than is available in FDA guidances. While many of the ICH's manufacturing-related guidelines apply more directly to marketing submissions, they may offer insights to IND applicants as well (see Chapter 7).

To assist companies in seeking and participating in productive pre-IND submission meetings on CMC-related issues, CDER issued a February 2000 draft document entitled, *IND Meetings for Human Drugs and Biologics: Chemistry, Manufacturing, and Controls Information*. The meetings, which sponsors must pursue by submitting to the FDA a formal request outlining the specific meeting objectives or desired outcomes, might focus on the drug's physical or chemical characteristics, the source and method of preparation, toxic reagent removal, formulation issues, sterility, or drug stability.

Animal Pharmacology and Toxicology Information The principal focus of the FDA's 1995 IND reform initiative was the application's pharmacology and toxicology section. The agency's "clarification" of its requirements for this section have permitted sponsors to scale back data submissions and to submit INDs months earlier than they could have previously.

In the absence of data derived from previous clinical testing or marketing use, data from animal studies serve as the basis for concluding that a drug is sufficiently safe for initial administration to humans. Therefore, this IND section must include information from the preclinical pharmacology and toxicology studies (animal and *in vitro*) sufficient to establish that the investigational product is reasonably safe for initial use in clinical studies. As is true for the IND's other technical sections, the data and information necessary in the pharmacology and toxicology component depend on several factors, including the nature of the product and the nature and duration of the clinical studies proposed in the IND.

The FDA's November 1995 IND guidance document provides the most detailed and current analysis of content requirements for this section. The guideline suggests that the section comprise four elements:

Pharmacology and Drug Disposition. This section should provide, if known: (1) a description of the pharmacologic effects and mechanism(s) of actions of the drug in animals; and (2) information on the absorption, distribution, metabolism, and excretion of the drug. "A summary report, without individual animal records or individual study results, usually suffices," the agency states in the 1995 IND guidance. "In most circumstances, five pages or less should suffice for this summary. If this information is not known, it should simply be so stated. To the extent that such studies may be important to address safety issues, or to assist in evaluation of toxicology data, they may be necessary; however, lack of this potential effectiveness information should not generally be a reason for a Phase 1 IND to be placed on clinical hold."

Integrated Toxicology Summary. Requirements for the IND's integrated summary of toxicologic effects were the most significantly affected by the FDA's 1995 IND reform initiative. At that time, the agency pointed out that its regulations did not specify whether toxicology data and the study reports should

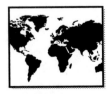

be "final fully quality-assured" individual study reports or earlier, unaudited draft toxicologic reports of completed studies. The agency conceded that most sponsors had concluded that the former were required in INDs.

In clarifying its policy, the FDA stated that, "if final, quality-assured individual study reports are not available at the time of IND submission, an integrated summary report of toxicologic findings based on the unaudited draft toxicologic reports of the completed animal studies may be submitted... Usually, 10 to 15 pages of text with additional tables (as needed) should suffice for the integrated summary."

The FDA guidance document adds that the integrated summary of toxicologic findings should consist of five elements: (1) a brief description of the trial design and any deviations from the design in the conduct of the trials (in addition, the dates of the performance of the trials should be included); (2) a systematic presentation of the findings from the animal toxicology and toxicokinetic studies (i.e., from a systems review perspective); (3) identification and qualifications of the individual(s) who evaluated the animal safety data and concluded that it is reasonably safe to begin the proposed human study; (4) a statement of where the animal studies were conducted and where the records of the studies are available for inspection should an inspection occur; and (5) a declaration that each study subject to good laboratory practice (GLP) regulations was performed in full compliance with GLPs or, if the study was not conducted in compliance with those regulations, a brief statement of the reason for the noncompliance and the sponsor's view on how such noncompliance might affect the interpretations of the findings.

The last three information elements identified above may be supplied as part of the integrated summary or as part of the full data tabulations section.

If an IND includes an integrated summary based on unaudited draft reports, the sponsor should submit an update to the summary within 120 days "after the start of the human study(ies)," the FDA states in an October 2000 guidance entitled, Q&A: *Content and Format of INDs for Phase 1 Studies for Drugs, Including Well-Characterized, Therapeutic Biotechnology-Derived Products*. "The Agency measures the 120-day period based on the Agency's receipt (date receipt stamped on the IND submission) of the *integrated study report* including the toxicology information. If the sponsor does not submit the final, quality-assured report and update at this time, the sponsor should make the final, quality-assured report available upon the request of the Agency and update the Agency on any changes in the findings. In any case, the final, quality-assured report should be submitted with the NDA. The Agency believes that 120 days from submission of an integrated toxicology summary should provide sponsors with adequate time to complete a final, quality-assured document."

Full Toxicology Data Tabulation. For each animal toxicology study that is intended to support the safety of the proposed clinical investigation, the sponsor should submit a full tabulation of data suitable for a detailed review. The agency states that this section should consist of "line listings of the individual data points, including laboratory data points, for each animal in these trials along with summary tabulations of these data points." To facilitate interpretation of the line listings, they should be accompanied by "either: 1) a brief (usually a few pages) description (i.e., a technical report or abstract including a methods description section) of the study or 2) a copy of the study protocol and amendments."

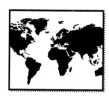

Toxicology GLP Certification. A declaration that each study subject to good laboratory practice (GLP) regulations was performed in full compliance with GLPs or, if the study was not conducted in compliance with those regulations, a brief statement of the reason for the noncompliance.

It is worth noting that CDER began running a pilot program for the electronic submission of the IND's pharmacology and toxicology section in November 1994. Under its Pharmacology/Toxicology (P/T) Electronic Submissions Pilot Project, CDER has accepted computerized preclinical P/T study reports for several INDs. With the release of the agency's March 1997 final rule on electronic signatures and records, however, this program will be incorporated into CDER's larger effort to accept all types of applications in computer format (see Chapter 7).

Previous Human Experience with the Investigational Drug If an investigational drug, or any of its active ingredients, has been marketed or tested in humans previously, the sponsor must provide specific information about any such use that may be relevant to the FDA's evaluation of the safety of either the drug or the proposed investigation. In such cases, the information should be presented in an integrated summary report. If the drug has been marketed outside the United States, the IND must provide a list of the countries in which the drug has been marketed or withdrawn.

Additional Information Any other information that would aid in the evaluation of the proposed clinical study should be included in this section. For example, the section might include information on a drug's dependence and abuse potential (if applicable), or data from special tests on radioactive drugs. Often, the section contains published literature, scientific meeting abstracts, or related materials.

Under a December 1998 final rule, companies developing certain new drugs are required to conduct pediatric studies for the products (see Chapter 16 for a more detailed discussion of the FDA's pediatric rule). Therefore, the agency's IND regulations have been revised to require IND applicants to provide their "plans for assessing pediatric safety and effectiveness" in this section of the application.

Submitting the IND

FDA regulations state that "the sponsor shall submit an original and two copies of all submissions to the IND file, including the original submission and all amendments and reports." In some cases, additional copies may be needed.

The sponsor must provide an accurate and complete English translation for any information originally written in a foreign language. In addition, the applicant must submit the original foreign language document or literature article on which the translation is based.

Maintaining/Updating the IND

Given that clinical development takes place over a multi-year period, a single IND may be "in effect," or "active," for several years or even decades. Because of this, the IND is a "living document" that must be updated continually so that the safety of ongoing and upcoming clinical trials may be periodically reassessed in light of the latest information. Any document submitted to an active IND (i.e., after FDA receipt of an original submission) is referred to as an IND amendment. Each amendment must

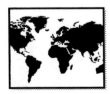

be accompanied by a completed and signed Form 1571, which identifies the purpose and contents of the submission.

Federal regulations require sponsors of active INDs to update their filings through four types of amendments: protocol amendments, information amendments, IND safety reports, and annual reports.

Protocol Amendments Protocol amendments are necessary when a sponsor wants to change a previously submitted protocol or to add a study protocol not submitted in the original IND. New protocols and most protocol changes must have been submitted to the FDA and have received IRB approval before being initiated. However, some sponsors may choose to obtain FDA comments before implementing new protocols or protocol changes.

Protocol amendments that introduce a new protocol should contain the protocol itself along with a brief description of the most clinically significant differences between the new and previous protocols. In explaining this requirement, the FDA writes that "...a detailed and undiscriminating enumeration of the differences would defeat the purpose of this requirement, which is to identify the most important differences between the old and new protocols and to alert FDA reviewers to major changes that may require additional supporting data, such as changes in dose, route of administration, or indication."

Amendments that specify changes to previously submitted protocols are required when a sponsor seeks: (1) to modify a Phase 1 protocol in a manner that significantly affects the safety of clinical subjects; or (2) to modify a Phase 2 or Phase 3 protocol in a manner that significantly affects the safety of the subjects, the scope of the investigation, or the scientific quality of the study. Federal regulations provide the following examples of protocol changes requiring amendments:

- any increase in drug dosage or the duration of individual subject exposure to the drug beyond that in the current protocol, or any significant increase in the number of study subjects;

- any significant change in the design of a protocol, such as the addition or deletion of a control group;

- the addition of a new test or procedure that is intended to improve monitoring for, or reduce the risk of, a side effect or adverse event, or the elimination of a test intended to monitor safety;

- the elimination of an apparent, immediate hazard to subjects (such a change may be implemented prior to an amendment submission, provided that the FDA is subsequently notified through a protocol amendment and that the IRB is properly notified); and

- the addition of a new investigator to carry out a previously submitted protocol (the investigational drug may be shipped to the investigator and the investigator may participate in the study prior to the submission of the amendment, provided the sponsor notifies the FDA within 30 days of the investigator's first participation in the study).

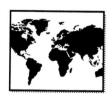

Amendments for changes to existing protocols must provide a "brief description of the change and reference (date and number) to the submission that contained the protocol." Amendments for a new investigator must include "the investigator's name, the qualifications to conduct the investigation, reference to the previously submitted protocol, and all additional information as is required [for other investigators]."

For certain protocol amendments, the FDA requires sponsors to reference the specific technical information that supports the new protocol or protocol change. According to FDA regulations, a protocol amendment must contain a reference, if necessary, to specific technical information in the IND or in a concurrently submitted information amendment to the IND that the sponsor relies on to support any clinically significant change in the new or amended protocol.

Protocol amendments must be prominently identified in one of three ways: "Protocol Amendment: New Protocol," "Protocol Amendment: Change in Protocol," or "Protocol Amendment: New Investigator." Amendments for new protocols or changes in existing protocols must be submitted to the FDA before their implementation. The FDA states, however, that "when several submissions of new protocols or protocol changes are anticipated during a short period, the sponsor is encouraged, to the extent feasible, to include these all in a single submission." Amendments to add new investigators or to provide additional information about investigators may be batched and submitted at 30-day intervals.

IND Safety Reports Sponsors must submit IND safety reports to inform the FDA and all participating investigators of any adverse experience (AE) that is associated with the use of a product and that is both serious and unexpected. The goal of this requirement is to ensure the timely communication of the most important new information about experiences with the investigational drug.

Through a long-awaited October 1997 final rule, the FDA's AE and IND safety reporting requirements were revised in several important ways. Designed to standardize the FDA's pre- and postmarketing AE reporting rules and to harmonize the agency's requirements with international standards, the regulation redefines many of the terms crucial to AE reporting, recasts the reporting timeframes for expedited pre- and postmarketing AE reports, and codifies the use of the MedWatch Form (Form 3500A) for expedited AE reports (i.e., the regulation permits the use of Form 3500A for IND AE reporting, but requires its use for postmarketing AE reporting). Although the regulation did not become effective until April 1998, the FDA allowed companies to implement its provisions immediately upon its publication.

For the purpose of AE reporting, FDA regulations require sponsors to "promptly review all information relevant to the safety of the drug obtained or otherwise received by the sponsor from any source, foreign or domestic, including information derived from any clinical or epidemiological investigations, animal investigations, commercial marketing experience, reports in the scientific literature, and unpublished scientific papers, as well as reports from foreign regulatory authorities that have not already been previously reported to the agency by the sponsor."

Once a sponsor's employee has knowledge of safety-related data, the sponsor is considered to have received that information. Therefore, sponsors must develop efficient mechanisms to ensure that such information is communicated internally (e.g., from subsidiaries, other departments within the company, and CROs).

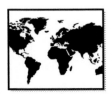

The reporting requirements applicable to adverse experiences are based on factors such as the nature, severity, and probable cause of the experience. The definitions of several terms, some of which were revised by the October 1997 regulation, are critically important in AE reporting:

Serious Adverse Drug Experience. A "serious" AE is "any adverse drug experience occurring at any dose that results in any of the following outcomes: Death, a life-threatening adverse drug experience, inpatient hospitalization or prolongation of existing hospitalization, a persistent or significant disability/incapacity, or a congenital anomaly/birth defect. Important medical events that may not result in death, be life-threatening, or require hospitalization may be considered a serious adverse drug experience when, based upon appropriate medical judgement, they may jeopardize the patient or subject and may require medical or surgical intervention to prevent one of the outcomes listed in this definition. Examples of such medical events include allergic bronchospasm requiring intensive treatment in an emergency room or at home, blood dyscrasias or convulsions that do not result in inpatient hospitalization, or the development of drug dependency or drug abuse."

Unexpected Adverse Drug Experience. An unexpected adverse drug experience is "any adverse drug experience, the specificity or severity of which is not consistent with the current investigator brochure; or if an investigator brochure is not required or available, the specificity or severity of which is not consistent with the risk information described in the general investigational plan or elsewhere in the current application, as amended. For example, under this definition, hepatic necrosis would be unexpected (by virtue of greater severity) if the investigator brochure only referred to elevated hepatic enzymes or hepatitis. Similarly, cerebral thromboembolism and cerebral vasculitis would be unexpected (by virtue of greater specificity) if the investigator brochure only listed cerebral vascular accidents. 'Unexpected,' as used in this definition, refers to an adverse drug experience that has not been previously observed (e.g., included in the investigator brochure) rather than from the perspective of such experience not being anticipated from the pharmacological properties of the pharmaceutical product."

Associated with the Use of the Drug. The phrase "associated with the use of the drug" is interpreted by the regulations to mean "that there is a reasonable possibility that the experience may have been caused by the drug." To harmonize the definition of this phrase with ICH guidances, CDER will be proposing a redefinition as part of a proposed regulation expected in 2000. At the same time, the FDA is expected to propose that the investigator's opinion be given equal weight in the decision on whether or not an AE is reported (i.e., currently, it is the sponsor's final opinion that determines whether an AE is reported).

Life-Threatening Adverse Drug Experience. A "life-threatening" AE is "any adverse drug experience that places the patient or subject, in the view of the investigator, at immediate risk of death from the reaction as it occurred, i.e., it does not include a reaction that, had it occurred in a more severe form, might have caused death."

Disability. A "disability" is "a substantial disruption of a person's ability to conduct normal life functions." The FDA considers only a persistent or significant or incapacitating disability to be serious. Therefore, experiences of relatively minor medical significance, such as a headache, nausea, vomiting, diarrhea, influenza, and accidental trauma (e.g., sprained ankle), would not be considered serious.

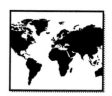

The October 1997 AE final rule revised the reporting timeframes applicable to the two types of IND safety reports that sponsors must make: telephone/facsimile IND safety reports and written IND safety reports.

Telephone/fax reports are required for any unexpected fatal or life-threatening experience associated with the use of the drug. Sponsors must submit these reports within 7 calendar days of their initial receipt of the AE-related information. Companies may make these reports via telephone or facsimile transmission.

Written IND safety reports must be issued to the FDA and participating investigators for any AE that is associated with the use of the drug and that is both serious and unexpected. Such reports must also be made after any finding from animal tests suggesting a significant risk for human subjects. These reports must be issued within 15 calendar days of the sponsor's initial receipt of the information.

The written IND safety reports must identify all safety reports previously filed with the IND concerning a similar adverse experience, and must provide an analysis of the adverse experience's significance in light of the previous, similar reports. Adverse experiences that require telephone/facsimile safety reports must also be the subject of a written IND safety report.

The FDA advises sponsors to submit in written IND safety reports "as much information as possible on a case. In some instances, information for final description and evaluation of a case report may not be available within 15 calendar days. Nevertheless, initial reports should be submitted within this timeframe when the following minimum criteria are met: An identifiable patient; a suspected medicinal product; an identifiable reporter; and an adverse event or outcome that can be identified as serious and unexpected, and for which, in clinical investigation cases, there is a reasonable suspected causal relationship between the investigational product and the adverse event (i.e., the causal relationship cannot be ruled out)."

A safety report to an IND does not necessarily represent the sponsor's concession that there is a relationship between the product and the adverse experience. In fact, the sponsor may state this fact explicitly in the safety report.

The October 1997 final rule also permits the use of the MedWatch Form—FDA Form 3500A—for written IND safety reports. Alternatively, sponsors can submit the reports in a narrative form, or attach a page or pages featuring a narrative description with FDA Form 3500A. Under the regulation, the FDA also permits companies, without agency pre-approval, to make written IND safety reports for foreign AEs on the CIOMS I form.

The agency may request that a sponsor submit IND safety reports in a particular format or at a frequency different than those required by regulations.

In the October 1997 final rule, the FDA stated that it had withdrawn proposed amendments to the IND regulations under which sponsors would have been required to submit a clinical trial "semiannual death and serious adverse experience report," and make a series of other modifications that would reduce investigator and sponsor interpretations in AE reporting, and affect trial protocol devel-

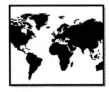

opment, study design, and clinical monitoring. Instead, the agency said that it would develop a guidance document providing recommendations on study design and the monitoring of studies for serious and potentially fatal illnesses, particularly with regard to the detection of AEs similar to those caused by the underlying disease.

Annual Reports Within 60 days of the anniversary date on which the initial IND "went into effect," the sponsor must submit an overview of information collected on the subject product during the previous year. Described by regulations as "a brief report of the progress of the investigation," the annual report should provide the following:

Information on Individual Studies. The FDA requires "a brief summary of the status of each study in progress and each study completed during the previous year. The summary must include the following information on each study: (1) the title of the study (with any appropriate study identifiers such as protocol number), its purpose, a brief statement identifying the patient population and a statement as to whether the study is completed; (2) the total number of subjects initially planned for inclusion in the study, the number entered into the study to date, the number whose participation in the study was completed and planned, and the number who dropped out of the study for any reason; and (3) if the study has been completed or if the interim results are known, a brief description of any available study results."

Summary Information. This section should include all additional product-related information collected during the previous year, as well as summary data from all clinical studies: (1) a narrative or tabular summary showing the most frequent and most serious adverse experiences by body system; (2) a summary of all IND safety reports submitted during the past year; (3) a list of subjects who died while participating in the investigation, with the cause of death for each subject (this list must identify all deaths, including those persons whose cause of death is not believed to be product related); (4) a list of subjects who dropped out during the study due to an adverse experience, regardless of whether the experience is thought to be drug related; (5) a brief description of any information that is pertinent to an understanding of the drug's actions (e.g., information from controlled trials and information about bioavailability); (6) a list of the preclinical studies (including animal studies) completed or in progress during the past year, and a summary of the major preclinical findings; and (7) a summary of any significant manufacturing or microbiological changes made during the past year.

General Investigational Plan. A brief description of the general investigational plan for the coming year must be provided. This plan should be as descriptive as the earlier plans submitted in the original IND and subsequent annual reports. If the plans are not yet formulated, the sponsor must indicate this fact in the report.

Investigator's Brochure Revisions. When the investigator's brochure has been revised, the sponsor must include a description of the revision and a copy of the new brochure.

Phase 1 Modifications. The sponsor must describe any significant Phase 1 protocol modifications that were implemented during the previous year and that were not reported previously to the FDA through a protocol amendment.

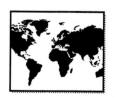

Foreign Marketing Developments. According to the IND regulations, this section should provide a "brief summary of significant foreign marketing developments with the drug during the past year, such as approval of marketing in any country or withdrawal or suspension from marketing in any country."

Request for an FDA Response. If the sponsor requests an FDA meeting, reply, or comment, a log of any relevant outstanding business with respect to the IND should be included.

The FDA revised its IND annual report regulations in February 1998 to require that sponsors tabulate in annual reports the numbers of subjects currently enrolled in their clinical trials according to age group, gender, and race. This new requirement, which became effective in August 1998, is designed to alert sponsors and the FDA to possible demographic deficiencies in trial enrollment that could result in NDA deficiencies.

In a July 1998 report, the Department of Health and Human Services (HHS) Inspector General recommended that FDA consider imposing civil penalties, issuing warning letters, initiating inspections, or issuing clinical holds when companies fail to submit annual reports to active INDs. HHS undertook a study of IND annual reporting compliance after learning that the University of Minnesota sold an unapproved biological product under an IND that was active for more than two decades and under which the university had failed to make annual reports. The center should consider these alternatives, claimed the report, because IND termination, the sole sanction available in such circumstances, may impede important medical research. In responding to the report, the FDA held that the new regulatory sanctions would require new resources and possibly legislative changes.

Information Amendments Often representing the majority of IND amendments, information amendments are used to report to the FDA new information that would not ordinarily be included in a protocol amendment or IND safety report, and information whose importance dictates that it must be reported before the next IND annual report. Information amendments commonly include new data from animal studies, changes or additions to the IND's chemistry, manufacturing, and controls section, and reports on discontinued clinical trials. Such information is more immediately critical than that included in the annual report. The amendments can also be used to provide administrative information, including responses to CDER requests, changes in IND contact persons, and letters of cross reference. Information amendments should be submitted as necessary, but preferably not more frequently than every 30 days.

The principal content requirements for information amendments are: (1) a statement of the nature and purpose of the amendment; (2) an organized submission of the data in a format appropriate for scientific review; and (3) a request for FDA comment on the information amendment (i.e., if the sponsor seeks agency comment).

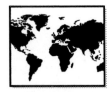

CHAPTER 4

CDER and the IND Review Process

Although most analyses of the U.S. Food and Drug Administration (FDA) focus on the agency's authority to decide which new treatments reach the American market, the FDA plays a regulatory gatekeeper role at another key point in the drug development process. In reviewing investigational new drug applications (IND), the FDA determines which experimental therapies advance from the preclinical to the clinical development phase.

When a drug sponsor submits an IND, the FDA assumes an important role in the development of a new product: From this point forward, the sponsor can do little without at least submitting documents to, and in some cases awaiting the review and approval of, the agency.

In fact, most sponsor activities beyond the preclinical development phase are subject to some form of FDA oversight. This reality is highlighted in the following statement that a sponsor must sign in the IND: "I agree not to begin clinical investigations until 30 days after FDA's receipt of the IND unless I receive earlier notification by FDA that the studies may begin. I also agree not to begin or continue clinical investigations covered by the IND if those studies are placed on clinical hold. I agree that an Institutional Review Board (IRB) that complies with [federal regulations] will be responsible for the initial and continuing review and approval of each of the studies in the proposed clinical investigation. I agree to conduct the investigation in accordance with all other applicable regulatory requirements."

While virtually all other FDA drug review processes have been reformed under the Food and Drug Administration Modernization Act of 1997 (FDAMA) and the reauthorized Prescription Drug User Fee Act (PDUFA), the agency's long-standing IND review process has largely survived the wave of regulatory reform initiatives. In contrast to the NDA review process, which has seen everything from its review timelines to its sponsor communication processes redefined, tightened, or tweaked, it is arguable that only peripheral aspects of the IND review process have been influenced by reform efforts.

Although the IND review process generally is perceived as an efficient and well-designed regulatory process, the FDA's increasing workload in reviewing new IND submissions and in managing active INDs (i.e., INDs under which clinical trials are being conducted) appeared to be an issue as the PDUFA reauthorization discussions began in late 2001. The agency appeared to be using this growing workload as one of several arguments to negotiate increased user fees from the pharmaceutical industry under the next iteration of the user-fee program.

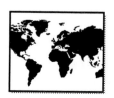

Worldwide Pharmaceutical Regulation Series

CDER and the IND Review Process

Chapter 4

The FDA's Center for Drug Evaluation and Research (CDER) is the regulatory and scientific body that oversees the development and marketing of all new drugs, including the review of IND submissions. Therefore, before outlining the IND review process, it is appropriate to profile CDER, one of several primary program centers within the FDA.

The FDA's Center for Drug Evaluation and Research (CDER)

CDER has functioned in many forms during the past decade. Several restructuring initiatives were undertaken to better distribute workload throughout the center, reflect evolving philosophies and approaches to the drug review process, and respond to emerging issues. At this writing, for example, CDER had just implemented a reorganization designed to streamline the center and to better reflect its focus on risk assessment and management (see discussion below).

The center's current structure is the product of a series of reorganizations in the mid-1990s, the most important of which was a sweeping center-wide restructuring initiative that fundamentally changed the offices and divisions responsible for reviewing INDs and NDAs. Center management stated in 1995 that the initiative was designed to flatten what had become a "pyramidal system" of drug review and approval, to create smaller and more focused and cohesive review teams, and to facilitate intra-center communication.

This October 1995 reorganization created what CDER officials have called two "super offices" within the center:

Office of Review Management. Within its Office of Review Management (ORM), CDER concentrated virtually all the offices and units essential for new drug reviews. In addition, the center reconfigured its 10 previous new drug review divisions into 14 review units, and spread these over 5 Offices of Drug Evaluation, instead of the previous 2 (see organizational chart below). This chapter focuses largely on these 14 new drug review divisions and their activities related to IND reviews. When it was founded, ORM also housed two other offices, including the Office of Post Marketing Drug Risk Assessment (OPDRA), which was ORM's newest office at the time and which was established in 1998 to spearhead CDER's upgraded and higher-profile efforts on post-marketing drug safety surveillance and risk assessment. ORM also housed an Office of Biostatistics, which provides biostatistical expertise for new drug reviews.

Office of Pharmaceutical Science. The Office of Pharmaceutical Science (OPS) was created, in part, to bring all of CDER's generic and new drug review chemists under a single management structure, thereby promoting a greater degree of consistency in chemistry reviews, policies, and approaches. Today, the office oversees four separate offices, including the Office of New Drug Chemistry, the Office of Generic Drugs, the Office of Clinical Pharmacology and Biopharmaceutics, and the Office of Testing and Research.

In May 2001, CDER Director Janet Woodcock, M.D., proposed a series of organizational changes designed to streamline several center units that she felt had become too large to manage, ORM in particular. The most significant element of this restructuring, which was implemented in early 2002, was to shift the Office of Postmarketing Drug Risk Assessment and the Office of Biostatistics from the Office of Review Management (ORM) (as well as CDER's MedWatch Program) under a new Office of

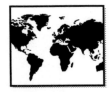

Pharmacoepidemilogy and Statistical Science (OPSS). The shifting of OPDRA and MedWatch (see Chapter 11) under new OPSS Director Paul Seligman, M.D., who joined CDER in July 2001 as a senior advisor for risk management, reflected CDER's intensifying focus on drug safety and risk management. Under the reorganization, OPDRA's name was also changed to the Office of Drug Safety to better reflect its role, and the Office of Biostatistics was renamed the Office of Statistics.

This latest reorganization leaves a streamlined ORM—which was renamed the Office of New Drugs under the restructuring—that could focus more intently on the work of the five new drug review offices and the divisions that function under them. In addition to these five offices, the Office of New Drugs houses CDER's Office of Pediatric Drug Development and Program Initiatives, which was established in October 2001. Although the original proposal did not specify any changes for ORM's 14 new drug review divisions, Woodcock noted that "the senior managers in ORM continue to discuss workload distribution and other operational issues."

Following the reorganization, CDER comprised several principal offices in addition to the Office of Pharmaceutical Science and Office of New Drugs:

The Office of Compliance. CDER's Office of Compliance monitors the quality of marketed drugs through product testing, surveillance inspections, and compliance programs; develops policies and standards for drug labeling, current good manufacturing practice (CGMP), good clinical practices (GCP), and good laboratory practice (GLP); and coordinates actions between CDER's center and field offices (e.g., for regulatory inspections). The Division of Scientific Investigations, which is responsible for CDER's Bioresearch Monitoring Program (see Chapter 14), was recently moved from the Office of Compliance to CDER's Office of Medical Policy for, among other reasons, to more tightly integrate clinical compliance and drug review activities.

The Office of Medical Policy. Led by Robert Temple, M.D., who is also the director of the Office of Drug Evaluation I, CDER's Office of Medical Policy houses the Division of Drug Marketing, Advertising and Communications and the Division of Scientific Investigations.

The Office of Regulatory Policy. This office is responsible for developing and issuing draft and final regulations and policies, handling Freedom of Information Act requests and citizen's petitions, and for coordinating center policies in several areas, including user fees.

The Office of Training and Communications. CDER's Office of Training and Communications was created in 1995 to spearhead the center's various training/personnel development and internal and external communications programs.

The Office of Information Technology. The Office of Information Technology was spun off from CDER's Office of Management, and spearheads the center's IT programs.

Office of Management. The Office of Management leads the center's planning, budgeting, facilities management, and program management efforts.

Office of Executive Programs. The Office of Executive Programs houses CDER's Review Standards Staff (see discussion below), Advisors and Consultants Staff (i.e., advisory committee issues), and executive operations staff.

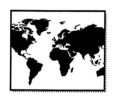

PAGE 66

CDER and the IND Review Process

Chapter 4

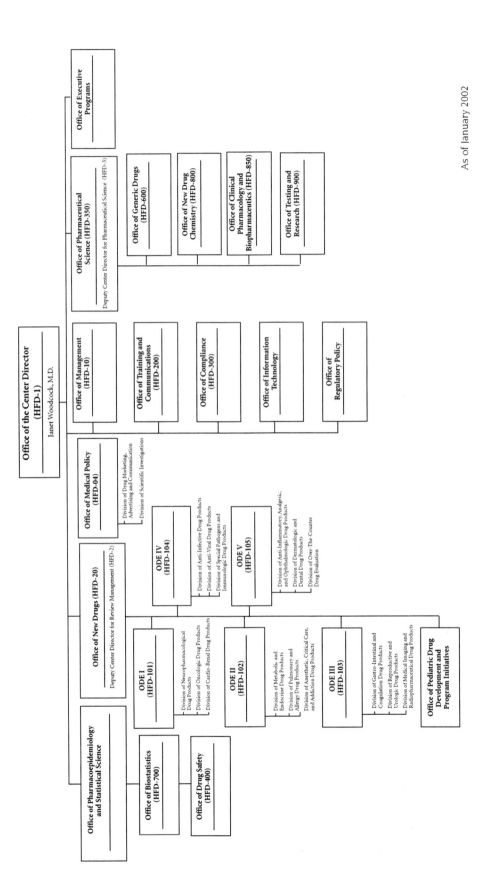

Center for Drug Evaluation and Research

As of January 2002

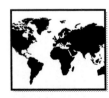

New Drug Approval in the United States

Office of Pharmacoepidemiology and Statistical Science. As noted, this newly created office houses CDER's Office of Drug Safety and Office of Biostatistics.

CDER's organization has also been modified in recent years to respond to emerging public concerns. The most obvious change was CDER's creation of a Quality Assurance Program formed, in part, in response to emerging concerns over drug withdrawals and drug safety and the consistency of the center's drug review processes. The program, whose initial projects included a "lessons learned" review of CDER's withdrawal of Rezulin (troglitazone) and center practices in developing "action packages" (information packages detailing CDER's decisions on NDAs and other submissions), was renamed the Review Standards Staff and was expanded in October 2000. Today, a larger and higher-profile Review Standards Staff includes a quality assurance effort, which evaluates how quality systems can be applied to various CDER process, spearheads the GRP initiative, and has a risk management component, which is designed to spearhead CDER's push in the risk-management area, in part by developing a systems-based approach for risk communication and risk intervention and for communicating risks to important audiences, such as consumers and prescribers.

CDER's Drug Review Divisions

Although each of CDER's offices plays an essential role in drug regulation, this chapter focuses on the Office of New Drugs' five Offices of Drug Evaluation (ODE), which house the 14 new drug review divisions that process and evaluate INDs and NDAs. Since their decisions determine the fates of therapeutically and commercially significant new drugs, these divisions are certainly among the most closely monitored and highly pressured offices within the FDA. With the advent of PDUFA I and PDUFA II, the industry, congressional, and public scrutiny under which the divisions have traditionally operated intensified considerably in the mid- and late 1990s. To meet the review goals established under PDUFA I and II, these divisions absorbed several hundred additional staffers since the early 1990s. Maintaining manageable divisional workloads and creating review groups that evaluate "more focused groups of products" were among CDER's primary motivations in its 1995 restructuring and in several divisional shifts that have taken place since.

As the division titles indicate, the reviewing responsibilities are apportioned to CDER's 14 new drug review divisions by therapeutic area. Each unit has its own areas of expertise, and reviews all new drugs proposed for use in these areas. Not surprisingly, this separation of responsibility creates a disparity in the workloads facing each division and fundamental differences in the scientific and medical issues that each division addresses in reviewing new drugs.

CDER's 14 new drug review divisions differ in other ways. Although the groups function under the same legal and regulatory framework, each division traditionally has had considerable autonomy to establish its own policies and procedures within that general framework. And while the center's drug review groups continue to function independently, at least some of their autonomy has been minimized in recent years by efforts to standardize policies and processes. Since the mid-1990s, for example, the center has maintained a Manual of Policies and Procedures (MaPP), which now comprises dozens of detailed center-wide policies on issues ranging from CDER/sponsor meetings to IND clinical hold procedures. Under its Good Review Practices (GRP) initiative (see Chapter 8), the center is also developing internal guidances and tools designed to add consistency to drug application

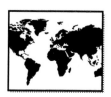

reviews, particularly NDA clinical data reviews. In late 1999, CDER Director Janet Woodcock, M.D., re-emphasized her commitment to standardizing the drug review process, something that she said would be achieved through the GRP initiative, the development of "review templates" for each review discipline, and the implementation of the quality assurance of reviews. Although the movement toward standardization is more focused on NDA reviews, it is likely to affect other reviews as well.

The following sections provide brief profiles of CDER's five ODEs and 14 new drug review divisions, with particular emphasis on the therapeutic categories of drugs that each unit regulates.

CDER's Office of Drug Evaluation I

ODE I comprises the three new drug review divisions profiled below.

Division of Cardio-Renal Drug Products In contrast to most other CDER drug review divisions, the Division of Cardio-Renal Drug Products has maintained its structure, responsibilities, and management team through various center reorganizations during the late 1980s and 1990s. Division Director Raymond Lipicky, M.D., an internist, has headed the division since 1986. Deputy Director Douglas Throckmorton, M.D., Ph.D., is a former medical reviewer within the division.

The primary classes of drugs for which the Division of Cardio-Renal Drug Products is responsible include antihypertensives, agents for the prevention of restinosis, agents for treating renal disease, agents for intermittent claudication, agents used for hypotension and shock, angiographic diagnostic agents, angiotensin converting enzyme inhibitors, antianginal agents, anti-arrhythmics, angiotensin II receptor antagonists, antiplatelet drugs, b-blockers B1 selective, beta blocking agents, botanical products for cardiovascular indications, calcium channel blockers, cardiovascular diagnostics, central alpha-2 agonists, coronary vasodilators, diuretics and renal tubule inhibitors, neutral endopeptidase/angiotensin converting enzyme inhibitors, peripheral vasodilators, potassium channel openers, and potassium salts.

From 1995 through 1999, the division has approved more new molecular entities (NME) than all but one other CDER division, although the division did not approve any new drugs in 2000. Over the same period, the division has markedly improved its average new drug review time—from 21.4 months in 1995 to 13.9 months in 1999.

Division of Oncologic Drug Products In late 1999, the Division of Oncologic Drug Products welcomed a new director, Richard Pazdur, M.D. Pazdur, who is board certified in internal medicine and oncology, joined the division from the M.D. Anderson Cancer Center.

One of CDER's most visible and busiest review units, the Division of Oncologic Drug Products reviews all oncology drugs, including drugs to treat AIDS patients with Kaposi's sarcoma and lymphoma, drugs to treat chronic graft-versus-host disease, antineoplastic hormones, biological response modifiers for cancer treatment, cancer chemotherapeutic agents with or without monoclonal antibodies, cytoxic alkylating agents, cytoxic antimetabolics, cytotoxics, immunomodulators, radiosensitizers, and miscellaneous multi-drug resistance modulators.

In large part due to a 1996 controversy that ultimately brought a greater focus on cancer drug reviews, the division has seen its review staff grow by roughly 20 percent since the mid-1990s. After patient

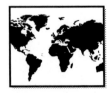

advocacy groups questioned why the agency was expending so many more resources on the review of AIDS treatments than on therapies for cancer or heart disease, CDER unveiled the Oncology Initiative, which the Clinton Administration estimated would reduce cancer drug development times by at least a year and cut oncology NDA review times from an average of 12.4 months to 6 months (see Chapter 15). While the political intensity of cancer drug approvals has faded somewhat in the intervening years, the various elements of the Oncology Initiative either have been incorporated into division practice or were legislated by FDAMA provisions, division staffers point out.

The division has improved its average NME review times substantially in recent years. In fact, the unit is one of only a handful of divisions to approve NMEs in a mean of well under 12 months in 1998, 1999, and 2000. The division approved 5 NMEs in an average of 9.1 months in 1999 and 2 in a mean of 6.3 months in 2000.

Division of Neuropharmacological Drug Products Like the Division of Oncology Drug Products, the Division of Neuropharmacological Drug Products welcomed a new division director in late 1999. Long-time Division Deputy Director Russell Katz, M.D., was named permanent director of the division in November 1999. Katz had served as acting division director since January 1999, when long-time Division Director Paul Leber, M.D., left the agency.

Called CDER's "busiest division" by the center's senior managers, the Division of Neuropharmacological Drug Product's current responsibilities can be divided into two general therapeutic categories:

Neurology Drugs. Anticonvulsants, antiemetics, antinauseants, anti-Parkinson agents, antispasticity agents, cerebral stimulants, vascular agents, drugs to assist memory (Alzheimer's/senility/dementia), and drugs to treat migraine, movement disorders, multiple sclerosis, narcolepsy/sleep apnea, stroke, and tardive dyskinesia.

Psychiatric Drugs. Anorexigenic agents/CNS stimulants, antianxiety agents/anxiolytics, antidepressants, antimanics, antipsychotics, hypnotics, sedatives, and drugs to treat schizophrenia, eating disorders, learning disabilities (dyslexia), minimal brain dysfunction, obsessive compulsive disorder, and panic.

By many measures, the Division of Neuropharmacological Drug Products has CDER's toughest workload. At year-end 2000, for example, the division had the center's second toughest NDA workload, as measured by pending NDAs (17).

Office of Drug Evaluation II

ODE II comprises the three new drug review divisions profiled below.

Division of Metabolic and Endocrine Drug Products CDER's Division of Metabolic and Endocrine Drug Products, which had remained largely intact during sweeping reorganization over the past several years, saw its long-standing senior management team depart in early 2000. Division Director Solomon Sobel, M.D., who headed the unit since 1979, left the division to become the new deputy director of CDER's Office of Review Management. Gloria Troendle, M.D., the division's long-time deputy director and head of one of the division's medical review teams, retired from the agency weeks earlier.

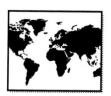

In September 2000, David Orloff, M.D., a medical team leader and the division's acting deputy director, was appointed as the division's permanent director. Board certified in internal medicine and endocrinology and metabolism, Orloff joined the agency in 1994 as a medical officer.

The Division of Metabolic and Endocrine Drug Products classifies its review responsibilities into about a dozen drug and disease areas: adrenal/ACTH, anabolic steroids, bone calcium and phosphorus metabolism developmental disorders, drugs for diabetes (miscellaneous), dopamine agonists, growth hormone and analogs, hyperglycemic agents, oral hypoglycemic agents, oral insulins, large volume parenterals (LVP), lipid-altering agents, metabolic studies and inborn errors of metabolism, nutrients/amino acids, nutritional LVPs, obesity drugs (anorectics), somatostatin, thyroid agents, vasopressin, and vitamins (other than vitamin D).

Despite its considerable NDA workload, which was CDER's third toughest as of January 2001, the Division of Metabolic and Endocrine Drug Products has maintained one of the center's most consistent average new drug review times over the past several years. From 1994 through 2000, for example, its average NME review time has seldom strayed far from the 12-month mark.

Division of Pulmonary and Allergy Drug Products The Division of Pulmonary and Allergy Drug Products was a third CDER unit that obtained a new division director in late 1999. Robert Meyer, M.D., was named to the post in August 1999. Board certified in internal medicine, pulmonary diseases, and critical care medicine, Meyer had been serving as the acting division director since May 1999, when former Division Director John Jenkins, M.D., now the Office of New Drugs director, left the unit to become the director of ODE II.

The Division of Pulmonary and Allergy Drug Products is responsible for reviewing a wide variety of pulmonary and anti-allergic drugs. These include anti-allergy nasal sprays, antiasthmatic dry powder inhalers, antiasthmatic metered dose inhalers, antiasthmatics (nonsteroidal), antihistamines, antitussives, decongestants, beta-2 agonists, bronchodilators, bronchoconstrictors, cough-cold-allergy preparations, inhaled corticosteriods, pulmonary anti-inflammatory agents, antitussives, mucolytic agents, and pulmonary surfactants.

After being founded in May 1995, the division grew to manage one of CDER's larger NDA workloads—as of January 2001, for example, the unit had 16 pending NDAs, the second highest number within the center. Although the division has seen its average NME review time improve during the late 1990s (from 30.7 months in 1996 to 12.0 in 1998), its mean review time jumped to 32.0 in 1999, when the unit approved just 1 NME. From 1997 through 2000, the division has approved just 3 NMEs, one of CDER's lowest rates.

Division of Anesthetic, Critical Care, and Addiction Drug Products Formerly part of ODE III, the Division of Anesthetic, Critical Care, and Addiction Drug Products was moved to ODE II in mid-1999. According to CDER officials, this shift was intended to place the anesthetic and critical care products regulated by the division under the same office (ODE II) responsible for pulmonary drug products (which are regulated by ODE II's Division of Pulmonary and Allergy Drug Products). Because many of these products are inhalation therapies, CDER officials believed that there was value in having all such products regulated under ODE II.

Like a handful of other CDER divisions formed in the mid-1990s, the Division of Anesthetic, Critical Care, and Addiction Drug Products experienced several leadership changes in its early years. The

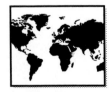

division's current director, Cynthia McCormick, M.D., joined the unit in 1998 from the Division of Neuropharmacological Drug Products, where she was a reviewer on the unit's neurology medical team.

Created in 1995, the Division of Anesthetic, Critical Care, and Addiction Drug Products' current responsibilities can be categorized into two general product groups:

Abusable Drugs. Drugs to treat alcoholism and drug abuse, enkephalin analgesics, hallucinogenic agents, marijuana studies, methadone and other addictives, narcotic antagonist/agonists/analgesics, narcotics in addiction research, and drugs to treat nicotine addiction.

Anesthetic Drugs. Epidural and intrathecal analgesics, neuromuscular blocking agents, preanesthetic sedatives, and general, local, and regional anesthetic agents.

Office of Drug Evaluation III

Like ODE I and II, ODE III oversees three new drug review divisions.

Division of Reproductive and Urologic Drug Products The Division of Reproductive and Urologic Drug Products was moved from ODE II to ODE III in mid-1999. In part, the move was made to create a more even distribution of workload between ODE II and ODE III, CDER officials claim.

Susan Allen, M.D., a reproductive medical team leader within the division, was named division director in June 2000, several months after former Director Lisa Rarick, M.D., now director of CDER's Review Standards Staff, was named deputy director of ODE II. Board certified in preventive medicine and public health, Allen join the division in 1998 as a medical officer.

The Division of Reproductive and Urologic Drug Products is responsible for oral and non-oral contraceptives, dopamine agonists, estrogens, gonadotropins, GnRH agonists and antagonists, oxytocics, androgens/testosterone, progestins, uterine-acting agents, drugs to treat benign prostate disease, drugs for sexual dysfunction, drugs for treatment of preterm labor, IUDs, sclerosing agents, prostaglandins (abortifacients), drugs for premenstrual syndrome, subdermal pellets (testosterone and estrogen), and androgens/anabolic steroids.

The division continues to maintain one of CDER's more challenging NDA workloads. As of January 2001, the division had 13 pending NDAs, the third most within CDER.

Division of Medical Imaging and Radiopharmaceutical Drug Products One of CDER's smaller drug review units, the Division of Medical Imaging and Radiopharmaceutical Drug Products is led by Patricia Love, M.D. A rheumatologist, Love has headed the division since it was founded in October 1995.

The Division of Medical Imaging and Radiopharmaceutical Drug Products oversees a relatively homogeneous group of imaging and therapeutic products, including magnetic resonance image enhancement agents, radioactive diagnostic agents, radioactive therapeutic agents, radiopaque contrast agents, ultrasound imaging agents, positron emission tomography products, and adjuvants used with all of these products (e.g., potassium perchlorate).

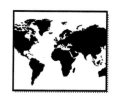

Division of Gastrointestinal and Coagulation Drug Products The Division of Gastrointestinal and Coagulation Drug Products evolved considerably in the late 1990s. The unit transitioned from what its former director characterized in the mid-1990s as "CDER's smallest division with the largest drug review workload," to a somewhat larger unit with a more modest workload. Since 1997, the division has been led by Lilia Talarico, M.D., a hematologist who had served as the division's deputy director since November 1996.

The division's review responsibilities can be broken down into two principal therapeutic areas:

Coagulation Drugs. Anti-anemia drugs, anticoagulants, antifibrinolytics, antiplatelet agents, antithrombin drugs, coagulants, fibrinolytics, hematologics, heparin inhibitors (including protamine sulfate and heparinase), metal chelators, miscellaneous blood drugs (including drugs for hemoglobinopathies, thrombocytopenia, and peripheral vascular disease), prostaglandins, and Vitamin K.

Gastrointestinal Drugs. Antacids, anticholinergics, antidiarrheals, antiemetics, cathartics and laxatives, cholelitholytic agents, GI diagnostics, GI motility modifying agents, H2 receptor antagonists, inflammatory bowel disease agents, irritable bowel syndrome agents, liver agents, metal chelators, miscellaneous gastric secretory agents, miscellaneous GI drugs (including hemorrhoidal preparations), pancreatitis agents, pancreatic enzymes, prostaglandins, proton pump inhibitors, sclerosing agents, sucralfate.

With 6 NME approvals in 2000, the Division of Gastrointestinal Drug Products was easily CDER's most productive in terms of new drug approvals. The unit saw its mean new drug review time spike to roughly the 24-month mark during the year, however.

Office of Drug Evaluation IV

After a May 1997 restructuring, ODE IV comprised three new drug review divisions.

Division of Anti-Infective Drug Products As part of the May 1997 reorganization, the Division of Anti-Infective Drug Products shifted responsibility for several products and product categories to the new Division of Special Pathogens and Immunologic Drug Products, the most significant of which was the quinolones (i.e., other than those for ear/nose/throat indications). Also moved to the new group were antimycobacterials (tuberculosis), vaginal antifungals, tropicals (e.g., anti-malarials), anthelmintics, and H. pylori treatments.

Currently, the Division of Anti-Infective Drug Products regulates aminoglycoides, antibacterial agents, sulfonamides, topical antibiotics, antigonorrheal agents, anti-resistant antimicrobials, antitumor antibiotics, cephalosporins, clindamycins, dermatologics, detergents, erythromycins/systemic macrolides, other topical anti-infectives, other systemic antimicrobial drugs, otic antibiotics in combination, penem antibiotics, penicillins, antibiotic peptides, sulfonamides, gram positive systemic antibiotics, and tetracyclines.

The 1997 reorganization created a somewhat smaller division with more narrow product review responsibilities. After former Division Director Gary Chikami, M.D., left the division on a series of details and then left the agency itself, Janice Soreth, M.D., a former medical team leader, was named

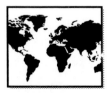

the division's director in December 2001. After joining the division as a medical officer in 1990, Soreth served as a medical team leader and then as acting division director.

Division of Antiviral Drug Products Under ODE IV's 1997 restructuring, the Division of Antiviral Drug Products' responsibilities were narrowed almost exclusively to antiviral products for AIDS and AIDS-related indications. To the new Division of Special Pathogens and Immunology Drug Products, the antivirals unit shifted responsibility for several non-AIDS drugs and drug classes, including solid organ transplantation drugs, drugs for non-viral opportunistic infections in AIDS patients, and wasting agents.

Today, the Division of Antiviral Drug Products is significantly more focused on HIV therapies, although it does review immunomodulators and immunostimulants, and has responsibilities for other indications, such as herpes, hepatitis, CMV, respiratory syncytial virus, and influenza.

Debra Birnkrant, M.D., a former medical officer and the division's deputy director, was named acting director in September 2001 after former director Heidi Jolson, M.D., left the agency. She was named permanent director in December 2001.

Not surprisingly given the nature of the products it regulates, the Division of Antiviral Drug Products maintains CDER's best average new drug review times. For the period 1995 through 2000, for example, the division's average NME approval time has been less than six months.

Division of Special Pathogens and Immunologic Drug Products When it was created in May 1997, the Division of Special Pathogens and Immunologic Drug Products assumed responsibility for several drugs and drug groups previously handled by the two other ODE IV review groups. Today, the division is responsible for aminoglycosides, anthelmintic agents (general), antibacterials (bacterial vaginosis), antibacterial quinolones, antifungal candidiasis, systemic antifungals, systemic anti-infectives, antimycobacterials, antiparasitic agents, antiprotozoal agents, antitrichomonads, antituberculosis, chronic fatigue syndromes, immunomodulators, immunostimulatory agents, macrolides, other drugs for AIDS-related illnesses, other antiparasitic, antimicrobial drugs, drugs to prevent the rejection of transplanted organs, spiramycin, systemic antibiotics (H. pylori indication), and thalidomide.

In October 2001, Mark Goldberger, M.D., M.P.H., who has headed the division since its founding, assumed the latest in a series of recent details, this time as the acting director of ODE IV. Before being named the division director, Goldberger, who is board certified in both internal medicine and infectious diseases, was a medical team leader within the Division of Antiviral Drug Products. Division Deputy Director Renata Albrecht, M.D., is serving as the acting director for the unit.

Office of Drug Evaluation V

ODE V consists of the two new drug review divisions profiled below, in addition to the Division of Over-the-Counter Drug Products, which generally is not considered a new drug review division but which is involved in nonprescription drug issues, including the reviews of NDAs for prescription-to-OTC switches.

Division of Dermatologic and Dental Drug Products After being restructured three times in the mid-1990s, the Division of Dermatologic and Dental Drug Products' organization and responsibilities

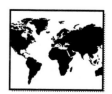

have remained stable over the past several years. Today, the Division of Dermatologic and Dental Drug Products regulates three drug categories:

Dermatological Drugs. Systemic and topical anti-acne drugs, antibacterials for acne, topical antihistamines, topical antimicrobial burn preparations, topical antimicrobials, oral antifungals, antiperspirants, topical antipruritics, anti-seborrheics, topical astringents, topical aural drugs, topical corticosteroids, hair and scalp preparations, miscellaneous topical and systemic immunosuppressants, modulators, pediculicides, pigmenting agents, drugs to treat psoriasis, retinoids, soaps/cleansers, steriods, sunscreens/photoprotectants, thalidomide, and wound cleansing/disinfection agents.

Topical Vaginal Drugs. Topical vaginal drugs.

Dental Drugs. Anticaries preparations (fluorides, etc.), antigingivitis and antiplaque agents, antifibrinolytics, chelating agents, dental tissue adhesives, dental implants, lozenges, mouthwashes, and periodontal treatments, toothpastes, and drugs to treat xerostomia.

The division is headed by Jonathan Wilkin, M.D., a dermatologist.

Division of Anti-Inflammatory, Analgesic, and Ophthalmic Drug Products In terms of its structure and leadership, the Division of Anti-Inflammatory, Analgesic, and Ophthalmic Drug Products has been CDER's least stable since the mid-1990s. After several reorganizations that reshaped the division during the mid-1990s, the unit experienced several leadership changes over the last several years.

In November 2001, Lee Simon, M.D., former head of rheumatology research at Harvard University's Beth Israel Deaconess Medical Center, was named division director. A former associate professor of medicine at Harvard Medical School, Simon will be recused from all deliberations and decision making regarding COX-2 inhibitors for at least 12 months because he was a clinical investigator for Pharmacia/Pfizer's Celebrex.

The Division of Anti-Inflammatory, Analgesic, and Ophthalmic Drug Products is responsible for the three drug categories identified in its title:

Anti-Inflammatory Drugs. Systemic corticosteroids, nonsteroidal cyclooxygenase inhibitors, enzyme blockers, anti-gout drugs, metalloproteinase inhibitors, and immunomodulators for rheumatic diseases.

Neurological Drugs. Non-narcotic analgesics, antipyretics, counterirritants, and muscle relaxants.

Ophthalmics. Alpha adrenergic agonist/blockers, antibiotics, antifungals, antiprotozoals, antivirals, beta adrenergic blockers, carbonic anhydrase inhibitors, corticosteroids, immune system regulators, mast cell inhibitors, nonsteroidal anti-inflammatory agents, prostaglandins, and proteolytic enzymes.

Inside the FDA's Drug Review Divisions

Although CDER's 14 new drug review divisions differ in many ways, they are similar in nature and structure. Each unit is led by a division director who is generally a physician, and has, at its core, a three- or four-discipline review structure. IND and NDA reviews are conducted by individuals from

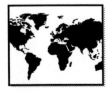

each of the following technical disciplines, who are assisted by consult review disciplines when necessary: medical/clinical; nonclinical pharmacology/toxicology; chemistry; and microbiology (e.g., for anti-infective drugs, sterile products):

Medical/Clinical Discipline Often called medical officers, medical/clinical reviewers are almost exclusively physicians. In some instances, such as in the review of psychiatric and dental products, non-physicians are used as medical officers to evaluate drug efficacy.

Medical reviewers are responsible for evaluating the clinical sections of submissions, such as the safety of the clinical protocols in an IND or the results of clinical testing as submitted in an NDA. Within most divisions, clinical reviewers also take the lead role in IND and NDA reviews, and are responsible for reconciling the results of the chemistry, pharmacology, and clinical reviews to formulate the basis upon which a drug will be approved for marketing or used in early clinical testing.

Generally, medical reviewers are assigned to one or more drug groups, or therapeutically focused teams. In the Division of Gastrointestinal and Coagulation Drug Products, for example, medical officers work on one of two medical teams—the Gastrointestinal Drug Team or the Coagulation/Hematology Drug Team.

Chemistry Discipline Each review division has a group of assigned chemists responsible for reviewing the chemistry, manufacturing, and control sections of drug applications. In general terms, chemistry reviewers address issues related to drug identity, manufacturing and control, and analysis.

Technically, CDER's chemists report into the center's Office of New Drug Chemistry rather than the review divisions in which they work. For practical reasons, however, the chemists are physically located within the respective review divisions.

Pharmacology Discipline The pharmacology review team is staffed by pharmacologists and toxicologists who evaluate the results of animal studies in attempting to relate nonclinical drug effects to potential effects in humans.

Microbiology Discipline Within certain divisions, including the Division of Anti-Infective Drug Products and the Division of Antiviral Drug Products, there is a fourth technical review discipline—microbiology. Since antimicrobial and antiviral drug products are designed to affect microbial or viral—rather than human—physiology, the groups employ microbiologists to evaluate the products' effects on viruses or other microorganisms. In addition, the Office of New Drug Chemistry maintains a team of microbiologists to consult with other divisions on specific drugs (e.g., sterile products).

Project Management Staff/Consumer Safety Officers Within CDER's new drug review divisions, there is at least one other group of individuals critical to the application review process—project management staff. Traditionally called consumer safety officers (CSO), these individuals are now called project managers, or regulatory health project managers, to better reflect their role in the review management process.

CDER's project managers serve as a drug sponsor's primary contact with a division during the product development and application review processes. In addition to a reviewer from each of the primary technical disciplines, a project manager is assigned to each IND and NDA upon its submission.

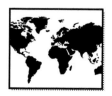

Since most project managers have scientific backgrounds (i.e., primarily in pharmacy), they can provide informed reports on technical issues that arise during the application review process. Their real expertise, however, is their knowledge of the drug review process, and of the policies, procedures, and idiosyncracies of their respective divisions.

The IND Review Process

The IND review is unique among the FDA's application review processes. In many respects, this process and the FDA's treatment of INDs represent a delicate balance between the federal government's responsibility to protect clinical trial subjects from unnecessary risks and its desire to avoid becoming an impediment to the advance of medical research. Given these dual goals, the FDA must perform a safety review of an IND prior to clinical trials, but is given only 30 days in which to reach an initial decision on the application.

The FDA's principal goals during the IND review are: (1) to determine if the preclinical test data show that the drug is reasonably safe for administration to humans; and (2) to determine if the protocol for the proposed clinical studies will expose clinical subjects to unnecessary risks (assuming the protocol proposes only Phase 1 studies).

Although some aspects of the IND review process were addressed by the Food and Drug Administration Modernization Act of 1997, the process has been largely shielded from reform efforts, perhaps due to its efficiency. Because of industry sensitivities regarding the IND clinical hold process, however, FDAMA introduced provisions designed to streamline that process (see discussion below). FDAMA and PDUFA II do attempt to further increase CDER's role as a drug development collaborator with industry, largely by formalizing the process through which early-stage (e.g., pre-IND) meetings are scheduled and held.

In the near term, at least a few initiatives are likely to affect the IND review process to varying degrees:

Submission of eINDs. Although CDER began accepting electronic versions of an IND's pharmacology/toxicology sections in 1994 under its Pharmacology/Toxicology (P/T) Electronic Submission Pilot Project, the center's current plans for eINDs are not based on this effort. Notwithstanding its efforts under this pilot program, CDER has not received or reviewed a completely electronic IND. At this writing, CDER's eIND activities appeared to be advancing on two tracks. First, CDER is party to a CBER effort to develop a formal eIND guidance, which the biologics center hopes to release by early 2002, well before the FDA's October 2002 deadline for implementing a fully electronic, paperless review system for all applications. Once this guidance is published and CDER lists the IND on its e-submissions public docket (92-S-0251), the center will accept eINDs. Meanwhile, however, CDER has proposed an eIND approach and model/prototype that provides a window on how the center wants to approach eNDAs and, ultimately, eCTDs in the future. Specifically, CDER has proposed what it calls an "IND cumulative table of contents" (CTOC), which the center defines as an XML-based "document that would list all the files submitted to an electronic IND, along with information about the type, location, and status of the file and any previously submitted information it references." In part, the CTOC approach addresses one of the considerable document management-related challenges associated with INDs—that is, that INDs comprise many different files and docu-

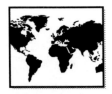

ments submitted over an extended period (i.e., clinical development). An IND reviewer, says the agency, "would use the CTOC files to access, sort, and search the electronic IND submission's content according to multiple criteria (e.g., amended, replaced, or current documents; submission dates; related documents, etc.)...." Following a January 2001 public meeting to discuss the CTOC approach for the eIND, a few companies submitted examples of INDs employing the CTOC.

CDER *Standardization of Review Processes*. As noted above, CDER officials continue to push to standardize the application review process through the ongoing GRP initiative, the development of discipline review templates, and other means. In May 2001, CDER released a reviewer guidance document entitled, P*harmacology/Toxicology Review Format*, to provide the pharmaceutical industry and others "with an understanding of the standard format and content of primary pharmacology/toxicology reviews." The center states that it uses a standardized format for IND and NDA pharmacology/toxicology reviews for several reasons, including that standardization provides for unified communication among multiple audiences, and that it ensures that the most important information is captured in all reviews. Two months earlier, CDER had implemented, on a pilot basis, a standardized NDA review format, or template, for its clinical reviewers centerwide.

Initial Processing of the IND The FDA's early processing of an IND depends on the manner in which the application is shipped to the agency. INDs arriving by regular mail, for example, are forwarded to the general FDA mail room, while applications shipped by courier are sent directly to CDER's Central Document Room.

Once within CDER's Central Document Room, an IND is stamped with the date of receipt, an extremely important event since it starts the 30-day review clock. Staffers within this office assign an identification number to the IND, and then log information about the filing into a computer database—the sponsor's name, the drug's name, and the application's identification number. Finally, staffers package the application (e.g., in review jackets if necessary) before forwarding it to the review division. Generally, sponsors package the IND themselves in appropriately colored jackets that can be purchased from the federal government.

Given the tight IND review time frame, this initial processing occurs extremely quickly. After arriving and being processed by CDER's Central Document Room, most INDs will be forwarded to the relevant review division by the next business day. For treatment INDs, however, the staffers attempt to forward the applications within an hour of receipt.

The IND within the Review Division Once within the relevant review division, the IND is sent to a file or document room, where a staffer creates a history card containing the applicant's name, the IND's date of receipt and identification number, and other information. The division then develops and forwards an "acknowledgement letter," which tells the applicant that the FDA has received the IND. This letter also specifies the IND's identification number and receipt date, and provides the name of the project manager who will act as the sponsor's FDA contact person on matters involving the application.

The assigned project manager will then act as the unofficial coordinator of the review, seeing that the application is forwarded to the relevant individuals. At this stage, the project manager will review the contents of the IND to identify any deficiencies.

Worldwide Pharmaceutical Regulation Series

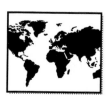

As noted previously, an IND faces reviews by the three or four technical review disciplines within a division—medical/clinical, pharmacology, chemistry, and, in two divisions, microbiology. The first copy of the IND is usually forwarded to a supervisory medical officer, sometimes called a "group leader," who has expertise in the subject drug's therapeutic category. In some review divisions, it is the group leader who analyzes the results of the medical, pharmacology, and chemistry reviews, and recommends whether or not the IND contents are adequate to allow the initiation of clinical trials.

Obviously, each review discipline focuses on the aspect of the IND relevant to its expertise:

Pharmacology Review. The reviewing pharmacologist focuses on the results of animal pharmacology and toxicology testing, and attempts to relate these test results to human pharmacology. As noted above, CDER has provided some insights into the IND pharmacology review in its May 2001 reviewer guidance entitled, *Pharmacology/Toxicology Review Format.*

Chemistry Review. The reviewing chemist evaluates the manufacturing and processing procedures for a drug to ensure that the compound is adequately reproducible and stable in its pure form. If the drug is either unstable or not reproducible, then the validity of any clinical testing would be undermined and, more importantly, the studies may pose significant risks. The chemistry reviewer also evaluates the drug's characterization and chemical structure, and compares the product's structure and impurity profile to those of other drugs (i.e., drugs known to be toxic).

Clinical Review. The medical reviewer evaluates the clinical trial protocol to determine: (1) if the subjects will be protected from unnecessary risks (for all clinical trials proposed in the IND); and (2) if the study design will provide relevant data on the safety and effectiveness of the drug (for Phase 2 and 3 trials). Since the late 1980s, FDA reviewers have been instructed to provide drug sponsors with greater freedom during Phase 1, as long as the investigations do not expose subjects to undue risks. In evaluating Phase 2 and 3 investigations, however, FDA reviewers also must ensure that these studies are of sufficient scientific quality, and that they are capable of yielding data that can support marketing approval.

Microbiology Review. When relevant, a microbiologist evaluates data on the drug's *in vivo* and *in vitro* effects on the physiology of the target virus or other microorganism.

During the drug evaluation process, reviews in the three or four technical areas are supplemented by what are called "consultative reviews" in biostatistics and clinical biopharmaceutics. At the IND review stage, agency biostatisticians may evaluate animal data to determine the statistical significance of drug effects in animals, including tumor rates and dose-response relationships. Further, while FDA biopharmaceutics staffers may not become directly involved in the IND review (except for AIDS drugs and other critical therapies), these staffers can review biopharmaceutics and pharmacokinetic data (i.e., drug concentrations in blood and urine) from initial clinical studies to provide advice on dosing, dosing intervals, and other drug-administration issues for later trials.

During the review process, IND reviewers may contact the applicant via phone, fax, e-mail, or letter to seek clarifications or more information or data (see discussion below). When the reviewers complete their evaluations, each submits a report summarizing his or her findings to the group leader,

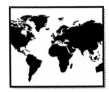

who is left to reconcile these findings and to make a final recommendation to the division director. Recommendations made by group leaders are rarely overturned by division directors.

While a division must complete this safety evaluation within the 30-day period, reviewers may continue to evaluate the IND after the period expires. If new safety concerns arise from this continuing review, the FDA may order that ongoing clinical trials be discontinued until these concerns are addressed and resolved.

The 30-Day Review Clock Except for a narrow class of INDs for emergency research (see discussion below), the FDA has no uniform procedures for informing applicants about the results of routine IND reviews. Most drug review divisions, for instance, do not contact the sponsor if they find no problems with drug safety and the proposed clinical trials. Rather, the divisions just allow the 30-day review period to expire, thereby permitting the sponsor to initiate clinical studies immediately. In this way, INDs are never formally approved, but are passively approved through the center's "administrative silence." Although they are not required to do so, sponsors should contact the agency before beginning clinical trials to confirm that the studies may be initiated.

CDER staffers caution that a firm that has not received an acknowledgement letter should not initiate trials, no matter how long the company believes that an IND has been at the agency. Because INDs can be lost during shipment or misplaced at the agency, applicants should contact the FDA if they have not received an acknowledgement letter within a reasonable period.

When deficiencies are found in an IND, the FDA may place the IND on clinical hold (see discussion below) or permit clinical studies to begin. If the review division decides that an IND deficiency is not sufficiently serious to justify delaying clinical studies, the division may either telephone, or forward an information request letter to, the sponsor. Whichever form the communication takes, the division informs the sponsor that it may proceed with the planned clinical trials, but that additional information is necessary to complete or correct the IND file.

Although there can be considerable variability in the ways that CDER's 14 drug review divisions communicate deficiencies to applicants during the initial IND review process and while clinical studies are being conducted under an IND, center officials have been attempting to standardize these communications recently. Because the initial IND review period is so brief, however, most division/applicant communications regarding IND deficiencies take place via the telephone and less-formal fax communications. If there are problems that reviewers believe need to be addressed before an IND can proceed, the division often will call or fax the applicant to request an amendment (e.g., a protocol amendment) or additional information during the 30-day review period. In many cases, issues can be resolved during this 30-day period, thereby circumventing the need for a formal clinical hold. In certain cases, some divisions also claim that they will permit applicants to begin studies before the submission and agency review of a requested change or information, provided that a company has given its commitment to implement the change or submit the information prior to study initiation.

Once an IND becomes "active," meaning that studies are being conducted under that application (i.e., following the initial 30-day review), there will likely be instances in which a sponsor and CDER will have to communicate to address emerging issues in response to new preclinical and clinical data and

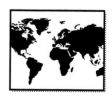

the submission of new clinical protocols. The drug center has attempted to standardize such communications by classifying them into the following types:

Deficiency Letters. Typically, a deficiency letter is sent when a review division identifies problems or deficiencies that might, if not resolved, potentially justify the use of a clinical hold. Rarely is there time during the initial 30-day IND review period to allow for the use of deficiency letters.

Information Request Letters. An information request letter is sent when a review division wants a response from the sponsor (e.g., a clarification or more information on an issue), but when the absence of the information would not typically justify a clinical hold. In virtually all cases, the types of issues that trigger an information request letter can be addressed quickly. For the development and issuance of IND information request letters regarding chemistry/manufacturing/control issues, CDER has developed and released an internal policy manual entitled, *Drafting, Circulating, and Signing Chemistry, Manufacturing, and Controls Letters* (MaPP 5310, October 1998).

Advice Letter. An advice letter is an FDA communication in which a division makes comments to the applicant (e.g., on an ongoing or proposed clinical study or protocol), but when the agency is not seeking any type of response from the clinical sponsor.

Under a mid-1997 regulation, the FDA established that sponsors of INDs for a special class of studies—emergency research conducted under an exemption from informed consent requirements—would require prior FDA authorization before trial initiation (see Chapter 5). For any IND proposing such research, the FDA must provide a written determination before study initiation. In contrast to the submission and review scenario for a traditional IND, therefore, the applicant must await the agency's authorization before it can initiate a study in this special class, even if such authorization is not granted within 30 days.

The Clinical Hold

When CDER discovers serious deficiencies that cannot be addressed before or during the IND review process, the center will contact the sponsor within the 30-day review period to delay the clinical trial. The clinical hold is the mechanism that CDER uses to accomplish this.

Through a clinical hold order, the agency can delay the initiation of an early-phase trial on the basis of information submitted in the IND. Later, clinical hold orders can be used to suspend an ongoing study based on either a re-review of the original IND or a review of newly submitted clinical protocols, safety reports, protocol amendments, or other information. When a clinical hold is issued, a sponsor must address the issue that is the basis of the hold before it can be removed.

The FDA's authority regarding clinical holds is outlined in federal regulations, which specify the clinical hold criteria that the agency applies to the various phases of clinical testing. In addition, CDER has developed a policy guide entitled, IND *Process and Review Procedures* (MaPP 6030.1) to describe the center's policies and procedures for issuing IND clinical holds.

Although Congress addressed clinical holds under the FDA Modernization Act of 1997, the regulation seemed, in most respects, to codify existing FDA practice regarding holds. The law's provisions allow

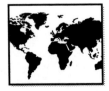

the FDA to issue a clinical hold when it determines that: (1) "the drug involved represents an unreasonable risk to the safety of persons who are the subjects of the clinical investigation, taking into account the qualifications of the clinical investigators, information about the drug, the design of the clinical investigation, the conditions for which the drug is to be investigated, and the health status of the subjects involved;" or (2) for such other reasons as the FDA may by regulation establish.

Clinical Holds and Phase 1 Trials One of the principal goals of the FDA's 1987 IND regulations was to give sponsors "greater freedom" during the initial stages of clinical research. Therefore, the regulations state that the FDA should not place a clinical hold on a Phase 1 study "unless it presents an unreasonable and significant risk to test subjects." In the regulation's preamble, the FDA establishes that it will "defer to sponsors on matters of Phase 1 study design," and will not consider a Phase 1 trial's scientific merit in deciding whether it should be allowed to proceed.

The regulation specified four situations in which the FDA can either delay a Phase 1 study proposed in an IND or discontinue an ongoing Phase 1 trial:

- if human subjects are or would be exposed to an unreasonable and significant risk of illness or injury;
- if the clinical investigators named in the IND are not qualified by reason of their scientific training and experience to conduct the investigation described in the IND;
- if the investigator's brochure (i.e., material supplying drug-related safety and effectiveness information to clinical investigators) is misleading, erroneous, or materially incomplete; or
- if the IND does not contain sufficient information as required under federal regulations to assess the risks that the proposed studies present to subjects.

A June 2000 regulation provided an additional circumstance in which CDER could impose a clinical hold on clinical studies. Under that regulation, CDER can place a clinical hold on a study for a drug intended to treat a life-threatening disease or condition if it finds that the study sponsor has "categorically excluded" otherwise eligible men or women of reproductive potential because of a perceived risk or potential risk of reproductive or developmental toxicity. The regulation is a government response to the previous practice of excluding women of childbearing potential from early clinical trials.

Since the new requirement does not apply to studies that are conducted exclusively in healthy volunteers, it will be irrelevant for many Phase 1 studies. Studies that are pertinent only to one gender (e.g., to evaluate a drug's excretion in semen or its effects on menstrual function) are also exempt from such requirements.

Clinical Holds and Phase 2 and 3 Studies The FDA has greater discretionary powers to delay and discontinue Phase 2 and Phase 3 trials. Current regulations allow the agency to place a clinical hold on a Phase 2 or Phase 3 trial if: (1) any of the Phase 1 clinical hold criteria outlined above are met; or (2) the "plan or protocol for the investigation is clearly deficient in design to meet its stated objectives."

How Clinical Holds Work The FDA acknowledges that the imposition of a clinical hold is a relatively informal and flexible process. Given the nature of product development, the agency has resisted suggestions that it formalize the clinical hold process.

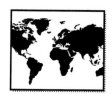

Current regulations state that the hold process will, in many cases, begin with an FDA-sponsor discussion: "Whenever FDA concludes that a deficiency exists in a clinical investigation that may be grounds for the imposition of a clinical hold, FDA will, unless patients are exposed to immediate and serious risk, attempt to discuss and satisfactorily resolve the matter with the sponsor before issuing the clinical hold order." The agency claims that most potential holds, particularly those based on inadequate patient monitoring, can be resolved through such discussions.

In certain situations (e.g., when CDER cannot complete an initial review within 30 days), a division may ask sponsors, on an informal basis, to voluntarily agree to an extension of the 30-day review to avoid a clinical hold order. Called an "informal clinical hold," this mechanism allows the FDA and the sponsor alike to avoid complications associated with formal clinical hold orders (e.g., paperwork). In such cases, the division typically promises to contact the sponsor as soon as a decision is reached. Because increased sponsor/agency communications and development-stage meetings have provided more opportunities for issues to be addressed, FDA officials claim that informal clinical holds are now less common than they once were. Top CDER officials suggested a desire to eliminate informal clinical holds, largely because of uncertainty regarding the regulatory implications of such informal concepts. In addition, industry has proposed that CDER eliminate informal holds because they are not subject to the time and procedural requirements established for formal clinical holds.

CDER's October 2000 *Guidance for Industry: Submitting and Reviewing Complete Responses to Clinical Holds* and its May 1998 MaPP 6030.1 define two types of clinical holds:

Complete clinical hold: "A delay or suspension of all clinical work requested under an IND. If a sponsor submits an initial IND and within the first 30-day period FDA and the sponsor agree on an alternative protocol that is allowed to proceed, this does not constitute a clinical hold provided there are no specific FDA contingencies that require FDA review/approval before further studies are started."

Partial clinical hold: "A delay or suspension of only part of the clinical work requested under the IND (e.g., a specific protocol or part of a protocol is not allowed to proceed; however, other protocols or parts of the protocol are allowed to proceed under the IND). If FDA requires that progress to the next study is contingent (1) on FDA review of additional data and (2) subsequent specific permission for the study to proceed, this represents a partial clinical hold. On the other hand, if the sponsor does not need to wait for FDA review and authorization to proceed before initiating a new protocol, then this is not a partial hold, even if additional data have been requested."

Under CDER policy, the division medical team leader (i.e., the reviewing medical officer's supervisor) is responsible for leading discussions of safety concerns regarding the planned protocol. If these concerns cannot be resolved through the discussions, however, the review division director must be involved in the decision to impose a clinical hold.

According to CDER's MaPP 6030.1, "clinical holds of commercial INDs should be communicated to the appropriate sponsor representative by a telephone call from the division director (or acting division director)." A letter clearly identifying the reasons for the clinical hold must be sent to the sponsor within seven calendar days of this telephone call.

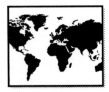

When the hold order is issued, identified studies must be delayed or discontinued immediately. If the study has not yet begun, no subjects may be administered the investigational drug. Ongoing studies placed on clinical hold must be discontinued immediately, and no new subjects may be recruited to the study or placed on the treatment. CDER may, however, permit subjects already on the treatment to continue receiving the experimental drug.

To facilitate CDER's timely review of sponsor responses to clinical holds, applicants should forward their responses by courier to the division document room and fax a copy of the cover letter to the division project manager responsible for the IND. This communication should be clearly identified as a "Clinical Hold Complete Response." When CDER uses a clinical hold letter to communicate issues that are unrelated to the imposition of the clinical hold (i.e., in addition to those issues that are relevant), sponsors should address such issues in a separate amendment to the IND and not in its formal response to the hold, current center guidance states.

CDER policies and regulations call for divisions to respond to complete sponsor responses within 30 calendar days of their receipt. If the division is not able to do so, division staffers must telephone the sponsor and discuss "the review progress to date and what is being done to facilitate completion of the review." Division directors make the final decisions on issuing and lifting all clinical holds. The FDA's PDUFA II commitments also include performance standards affecting this goal: In fiscal years 1999 through 2002, 90 percent of FDA responses must be sent within 30 calendar days.

An applicant must await an FDA response before beginning or resuming a trial placed on clinical hold. According to CDER's October 2000 guidance document, "After an IND has been placed on clinical hold, until the applicant has received a communication (via phone, fax, letter, e-mail) from the Agency allowing the study to proceed, the study may not be initiated."

IND Clinical Hold Rates Within CDER It is well known that CDER's clinical hold rates on commercial INDs declined dramatically in the mid and late 1990s. The agency issued clinical holds on 8 percent of commercial INDs submitted in fiscal year 2000, down from the 11 percent of commercial INDs submitted in fiscal year 1999 and 10 percent in 1998 (*note: these figures can rise over time, since INDs can be placed on clinical hold even after the initial 30-day review period*).

It is important to note, however, that hold rates can vary considerably from division to division. This variability is at least partially influenced by the nature of the drugs that the various divisions review. The Division of Neuropharmacological Drug Products, for example, issued holds on 11 percent (6 of 56) and 31 percent (15/52) of commercial INDs submitted in fiscal years 2000 and 1999, respectively. The Division of Pulmonary Drug Products, on the other hand, has issued clinical hold orders on only 4 of the 96 commercial IND submissions filed over the last four fiscal years (see exhibit below).

There are several potential reasons for the downturn in IND hold rates during the 1990s. Some maintain that all industry submissions have improved in recent years. Others point to CDER's establishment of its Clinical Holds Peer Review Committee, which meets regularly to evaluate all of the center's IND hold decisions. Divisions and reviewers that issue IND holds must be prepared to discuss and defend these actions before the committee, which is composed largely of senior CDER officials. In addition, sponsors are given the opportunity to appear before the committee to discuss the

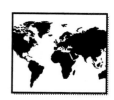

Chapter 4: CDER and the IND Review Process

Clinical Holds* on Commercial IND Submissions by CDER Drug Review Division, 1994–2000

(# INDs placed on hold/# of IND receipts)

	1994	1995**	1996**	1997**	1998**	1999**	2000**
Cardio-Renal Drug Products	0% (0/23)	3% (1/30)	0% (0/26)	8% (2/26)	5% (1/22)	0% (0/23)	19% (5/26)
Neuropharmacological Drug Products	37% (17/46)	45% (19/42)	20% (8/41)	22% (14/65)	35% (19/55)	29% (15/52)	11% (6/56)
Oncologic Drug Products	-	4% (2/55)	3% (2/58)	1% (1/94)	4% (4/105)	5% (3/64)	3% (2/74)
Pulmonary Drug Products	-	9% (2/22)	8% (2/26)	4% (1/25)	4% (1/23)	5% (1/21)	4% (1/25)
Medical Imaging and Radiopharm. Drug Products	-	20% (2/10)	0% (0/5)	0% (0/9)	29% (2/7)	0% (0/11)	0% (0/5)
Gastrointestinal and Coagulation Drug Products	5% (1/19)	8% (2/24)	17% (6/35)	5% (1/22)	12% (3/25)	10% (2/20)	9% (3/32)
Anesthetic, Critical Care and Addiction Drug Products	-	7% (1/15)	0% (0/17)	0% (0/23)	6% (1/18)	12% (3/25)	0% (0/11)
Metabolic and Endocrine Drug Products	18% (8/45)	4% (1/28)	6% (2/34)	9% (3/33)	3% (1/36)	5% (2/37)	18% (9/49)
Anti-Infective Drug Products	5% (1/19)	29% (4/14)	0% (0/7)	15% (2/13)	0% (0/14)	9% (1/11)	0% (0/11)
Anti-Inflammatory, Analgesic and Ophthalmic Drug Products	-	3% (1/30)	9% (3/35)	3% (1/37)	5% (2/39)	21% (7/34)	0% (0/39)
Antiviral Drug Products	7% (2/28)	9% (2/22)	5% (1/20)	9% (2/22)	10% (3/30)	16% (6/37)	4% (1/25)
Reproductive and Urologic Drug Products	-	5% (1/19)	6% (2/29)	9% (3/35)	8% (3/40)	12% (6/52)	11% (4/36)
Special Pathogens and Immunologic Drug Products	-	6% (1/17)	6% (1/18)	0% (0/15)	0% (0/11)	7% (1/14)	0% (0/8)
Dermatological and Dental Drug Products	7% (2/30)	7% (2/30)	12% (3/25)	19% (5/27)	13% (6/46)	3% (1/29)	10% (4/42)
Totals	13% (43/333)	12% (41/358)	8% (30/376)	8% (35/446)	10% (46/471)	11% (48/430)	8% (35/459)

* Holds column in 1995, 1996, 1997, 1998, 1999, and 2000 represents number of INDs received in FY that were placed on hold (full or partial) at any point. Data from previous years represent holds on initial IND submissions.

** 1995, 1996, 1997, 1998, 1999, and 2000 data are for fiscal years.

NA = not available

Source: FDA

holds placed on their INDs. In virtually all cases, the CDER committee has supported the clinical hold orders that it has reviewed.

IND Status

Once the FDA's 30-day review period expires and clinical investigations are initiated, an IND may be classified into any one of five status categories:

Active Status. Generally, an active IND is one under which clinical investigations are being conducted—in other words, the FDA has decided not to delay or suspend the clinical studies proposed under the initial IND or subsequent protocol amendments. However, an IND may remain on active status for extended periods even though no trials are being conducted under the application. In such cases, clinical studies may be re-initiated under the IND without further notification to the FDA.

Inactive Status. An IND on inactive status is one under which clinical investigations are not being conducted. There are two ways through which an IND can be put on inactive status. First, the IND sponsor may ask CDER to place the application on inactive status, thereby eliminating the IND updating and submission requirements applicable to the sponsor. Also, the FDA may place the application on inactive status if the agency finds either: (1) that no subjects are entered into an IND's clinical studies for a period of two years or more; or (2) that all investigations under an application remain on clinical hold for one year or more. CDER may seek to terminate INDs that remain on inactive status for five years or more (see discussion below).

Clinical Hold. As previously discussed, a clinical hold is an FDA order to delay a proposed investigation or to suspend an ongoing investigation. If all investigations covered by an IND remain on clinical hold for one year or more, CDER may place the IND on inactive status.

Withdrawn Status. The sponsor of an IND can withdraw an IND at any time and for any reason. When the sponsor withdraws an IND, all clinical investigations under the IND must be discontinued, the FDA and all investigators must be notified, and all stocks of the drug must be returned to the sponsor or otherwise disposed of at the request of the sponsor.

IND Termination. The FDA will seek to terminate an IND if the agency is unable to resolve deficiencies in an IND or in the conduct of an investigation through a clinical hold order or through a more informal alternative. For example, the agency would pursue IND termination if a sponsor failed to delay a proposed investigation under an IND that had been placed on clinical hold. Except when continuing an investigation will present an immediate danger to clinical subjects, the FDA will issue a proposal to terminate and will offer the sponsor an opportunity to respond before finalizing a termination.

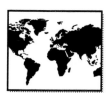

CHAPTER 5

The Clinical Development of New Drugs

By Ronald Keeney, M.D.
PAREXEL International Corporation

Virtually all preclinical work—animal pharmacology/toxicology testing and the development of the IND—is undertaken to obtain the FDA's tacit permission to initiate clinical trials, the ultimate pre-marketing testing ground for unapproved drugs. During these trials, an investigational compound is administered to human subjects and is evaluated for its safety and effectiveness in treating, preventing, or diagnosing a specific disease or condition. The results of this testing will comprise the single most important factor in the FDA's approval or disapproval of a new drug.

As they have in the past, emerging socio-political trends and scientific advances continue to place new demands on, and offer new opportunities to, companies undertaking clinical development programs for experimental drugs. Pharmacoecomics has become a significant new consideration, given the growing concern about health care costs in many countries, including the United States. Increasingly, surrogate clinical markers are being identified and used for expediting the development process ahead of the achievement of definitive clinical endpoints.

The intensifying focus on drug safety by both the U.S. public and U.S. policy makers has put new pressures on clinical development programs and pharmacovigilance activities (e.g., Phase 4 programs and adverse experience reporting efforts) to assure a drug's safety. A series of drug withdrawals in recent years, along with scientific advances in the understanding of specific drug effects, has spotlighted certain adverse drug effects—liver toxicities and QTc prolongation in particular—in the drug development and approval process. This has put growing pressure on drug sponsors to fully characterize drug effects in these and other areas during the development process. In early 2001, for example, CDER Office of Medical Policy Director Robert Temple, M.D., proposed that companies should routinely consider the benefits of "real world" extensions of Phase 3 clinical trials, or Phase 3.5 trials, to study a new drug's risk of causing liver toxicity during the NDA preparation and submission process.

Further, advances in pharmacogenetics have introduced an entirely new paradigm for how diseases are understood and treated and how patients' genotypes might be used to assure both the effective-

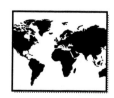

Worldwide Pharmaceutical Regulation Series

ness and safety of drugs. And, at long last, the pediatric population has been granted an entirely new statutory and regulatory base to assure the adequate study of drugs in children (see Chapter 16).

Such major advances have been accompanied by myriad smaller refinements, many of which address FDA review processes and which involve efforts to expedite the availability of new drugs. As these initiatives began to succeed in the mid-1990s, the pharmaceutical industry moved to streamline its drug development processes in response to spiraling product development costs and an increasingly competitive marketplace (i.e., due to managed care, generic competition, etc.). These streamlining efforts seemed to take hold in the late 1990s, reversing a seemingly inexorable rise in clinical development times during the 1980s and 1990s. A 1999 study by the Tufts Center for the Study of Drug Development showed that industry's mean clinical development time for new drugs approved from 1996 through 1998 dipped by 18% compared to drugs approved from 1993 to 1995. In fact, the 5.9-year mean clinical development time for drugs approved during the latter period was the shortest during the 14-year period studied (1984-1998). It is important to note, however, that mean clinical development times varied greatly by therapeutic class—times ranged from 8.0 years for endocrine drugs approved from 1996 through 1998 to 4.4 years for anti-infectives approved during the same three-year span.

Critics of the FDA and the pharmaceutical industry argued, however, that the focus on speed was coming at the expense of drug safety, an argument that they bolstered by pointing to a spate of drug withdrawals in the late 1990s. They also highlighted such practices as industry's use of incentives and finders' fees to speed subject enrollment in clinical trials and the overall commercialization of the clinical research process as evidence that speed and profit were being put before patient safety. This led some to fear a reverse pendulum swing that would produce a series of new government oversight activities. In fact, several recent government initiatives are helping to reshape the clinical development landscape for new pharmaceuticals:

FDA/HHS *"Action Plan" on GCP Compliance.* In response to what then-FDA Commissioner Jane Henney, M.D., called the failure of "some researchers at prestigious [medical and research] institutions...to follow the most basic elements of what it takes to properly conduct clinical studies," the U.S. Department of Health and Human Services (HHS) issued an May 2000 "action plan" comprising a series of initiatives seeking to "heighten government oversight of biomedical research and to reinforce to research institutions their responsibility to oversee their clinical researchers and institutional review boards (IRBs)." The initiatives comprising this action plan included HHS plans to pursue legislation authorizing the FDA to levy civil monetary penalties on clinical investigators and research institutions for violations of informed consent and other important research practices, and new FDA efforts to develop guidances on informed consent and the use of data safety monitoring boards. In November 2001, the FDA released a draft guidance entitled, *Guidance for Clinical Trial Sponsors on the Establishment and Operation of Clinical Trial Data Monitoring Committees* (see discussion below).

FDA *Guidance on Clinical Standards for Drug Approval.* Although the clinical testing process has long been the focus of the plurality of FDA guidelines, the agency added several important guidance documents to this corpus in recent years. Principal among these was a May 1998 guidance entitled, *Providing Clinical Evidence of Effectiveness for Human Drug and Biological Products*, which offers the agency's latest and most detailed views regarding the "quantitative and qualitative standards" for establishing drug effectiveness, including situations in which a single pivotal trial can support drug approval. In an October

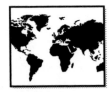

2001 guidance entitled, *Cancer Drug and Biological Products—Clinical Data in Marketing Applications*, CDER clarifies the clinical data necessary for oncology drugs, and notes that those requirements may be less than those for less-serious diseases.

Legislation Regarding Clinical Evidence Necessary for Drug Approval. Several months after the first draft of the guidance cited above was released, Congress passed the FDA Modernization Act of 1997, which revised the Food, Drug and Cosmetic Act to clarify that data from a single adequate and well-controlled study, together with confirmatory evidence, may, at the FDA's discretion, comprise the substantial evidence of effectiveness necessary for approval (see discussion below).

International Guidance on Clinical Trials. Supplementing FDA guidance documents are about a dozen clinically oriented guidelines developed under the International Conference on Harmonization (ICH) initiative, including a final guidance entitled, E8 *General Considerations for Clinical Trials* (December 1997), and a guidance entitled, *Statistical Principles for Clinical Trials* (September 1998). In August 2000, the ICH parties released a draft guideline entitled, *Principles for Clinical Evaluation of New Antihypertensive Drugs*, what is thought to be the first in a series of new ICH guidances that will address clinical testing issues specific to individual therapeutic categories.

FDA Trial-Related Performance Goals. In response to growing clinical development times, many of the FDA performance commitments associated with PDUFA II were designed to expedite processes relevant to clinical trials. These commitments require the FDA to schedule and participate in key sponsor meetings—many critical for clinical development programs—within specific timeframes. Further, PDUFA II brought new and formal procedures under which the FDA will assess and comment on the adequacy of, and enter into agreements regarding, Phase 3 trials.

Initiatives for Testing in Special Populations. Legislative and regulatory initiatives increased pressure on industry to include special populations in clinical trials. As the FDA was pursuing its own regulations to require testing in pediatric populations in specific cases, Congress passed the FDA Modernization Act of 1997, which offers additional marketing exclusivity to sponsors conducting pediatric studies for relevant drugs. Meanwhile, in mid-2000, the FDA implemented a regulation establishing its power to issue clinical holds on any studies that "automatically excluded," because of a possible risk of reproductive or developmental toxicity, women of reproductive potential who suffer from a life-threatening disease. Further, the FDA Modernization Act of 1997 calls on the FDA to consult with the National Institutes of Health (NIH) and the pharmaceutical industry to review and develop guidance on the inclusion of women and minorities in clinical trials. After releasing the results of a 2001 study on the inclusion of gender-related information in new drug applications approved from 1995 to 1999, FDA officials further encouraged clinical trial sponsors to include women in Phase 1 and 2 pharmacodynamic and pharmacokinetic studies on a more routine basis to provide more information on how drugs work differently in men and women and on drug dosing issues. Although the agency issued a February 1998 regulation mandating that IND and NDA sponsors submit efficacy and safety subset analyses based on gender, age, and race, it will use the results of this study, which found that women represent "a relatively small percentage" (just 22%) of subjects enrolled in Phase 1 and 2 studies, to determine the need for further regulations to ensure the inclusion of women and other groups in clinical trials. Overall, however, the study found that women are participating in clinical trials "in approximate proportion to their representation in the population."

Clinical Trial Information Program for Serious and Life-Threatening Diseases. The Food and Drug Administration Modernization Act of 1997 (FDAMA) called on National Institutes of Health (NIH) to establish and maintain a clinical trials data bank designed to provide patients, healthcare providers, and researchers with a central resource for current information on clinical trials for serious and life-threatening diseases. To populate the database, FDAMA required industry sponsors to submit to the Clinical Trials Data Bank a description of the purpose of each qualifying experimental drug, patient eligibility criteria for the trial, the location of clinical trial sites, and a point of contact for trial enrollment. Since FDAMA was somewhat unclear on when trial sponsors had to submit this information for inclusion in the Clinical Trials Data Bank, the FDA clarified submission timeframes in a March 2000 guidance entitled, *Information Program on Clinical Trials for Serious and Life-Threatening Diseases: Establishment of a Data Bank*: "sponsors should submit protocol information to the Clinical Trials Data Bank (1) no later than 21 days after the trial is first opened for enrollment, (2) upon amending the protocol with respect to one of the required data elements, or (3) when recruitment for the study is interrupted, resumed, or completed." In a June 2001 draft guidance entitled, *Information Program on Clinical Trials for Serious or Life-Threatening Diseases; Implementation Program*, the FDA said that companies would not be required to submit trial information until a final guidance is released, although it encouraged firms to submit information as soon as possible through an FDA web-based system. Firms can seek waivers from providing trial information when they can show "specific instances" in which information disclosure would interfere with trial enrollment. While the agency is considering such "specific instances," the agency stated in the June 2001 draft guidance that it had not yet identified such circumstances.

The clinical development program remains, without question, the most complex, time-consuming, and costly element in the pharmaceutical development process. At a minimum, it requires a coordinated effort that involves a sponsor willing to assume the financial, legal, and regulatory responsibilities associated with the program, the commitment and expertise of physicians, nurses, and other health-care professionals, and patients willing to make a contribution to clinical research or to take the chance that an experimental drug will do more for them than either existing therapies or no therapy at all.

The FDA's Role in Clinical Trials

The FDA plays at least three major roles in the clinical testing of a drug. As it does for animal studies, the FDA sets general standards for clinical studies to ensure that data derived from clinical trials are valid and accurate. The agency accomplishes this goal essentially by maintaining and enforcing a set of related guidelines and regulations called Good Clinical Practices, or GCP (see Chapter 6). These documents define the responsibilities of the key figures involved in clinical trials.

The FDA's second role is to protect the rights and, to the degree possible, the safety of subjects participating in clinical trials. Obviously, since such testing involves the administration of pharmacologically active drugs to humans, the agency cannot guarantee the safety of clinical subjects. The FDA's role, then, is to ensure: (1) that clinical subjects are not exposed to any unnecessary risks; (2) that clinical subjects are exposed to the least possible risk given the benefit anticipated from the use of an experimental therapy; and (3) that all clinical subjects give their informed consent before enter-

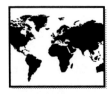

ing a trial. The FDA does this not only through GCP regulations and guidances, but also by reviewing all proposed clinical protocols and all proposed changes to the protocols that may affect the safety of the subjects. The agency also fulfills this role by monitoring the performance of clinical trial monitors, clinical investigators and investigational review boards (see Chapter 14).

Lastly, by deciding the nature and quantity of clinical data necessary to establish a drug's safety and effectiveness, the FDA participates actively in determining what testing is necessary in a clinical development program. Because the scientific and medical issues differ so significantly between various drugs and medical conditions, the agency works with the sponsor to reach such determinations on a case-by-case basis. Ideally, the sponsor initiates this process by providing the FDA with its optimal and comprehensive global development plan for a new drug. At each subsequent meeting, this plan should be reviewed and updated to refine the sponsor's recommended plan of study.

To help drug sponsors design clinical trials that are based upon sound scientific principles and that provide for the protection of clinical subjects, the FDA has developed and published more than two dozen guidelines over the past two decades. More recently, the FDA has released a spate of new draft clinical guidelines necessitated by the evolution of the science and practice of drug development and clinical evaluation (see exhibit below).

In recent years, FDA guidelines have been supplemented by several ICH guidelines that are directly relevant to the design and conduct of clinical trials, including:

- Final E4 *Dose-Response Information to Support Drug Registration* (November 1994);
- Final E1A *The Extent of Population Exposure Required to Assess Clinical Safety for Drugs Intended for Long-Term Treatment of Non-Life-Threatening Conditions* (March 1995);
- Final E6 *Good Clinical Practice: Consolidated Guideline* (May 1997);
- Final E8 *General Considerations for Clinical Trials* (December 1997);
- Final E9 *Statistical Principles for Clinical Trials* (September 1998);
- Final E7 *Studies in Support of Special Populations: Geriatrics* (August 1994);
- Final M3 *Nonclinical Safety Studies for the Conduct of Human Clinical Trials for Pharmaceuticals* (November 1997);
- Final E2B *Guidance on Data Elements for Transmission of Individual Case Safety Reports* (January 1998);
- Final E5 *Ethnic Factors in the Acceptability of Foreign Clinical Data* (June 1998);
- Final E2A *Clinical Safety Data Management: Definitions and Standards for Expedited Reporting* (March 1995);
- Final E2C *Clinical Safety Data Management: Periodic Safety Update Reports for Marketed Drugs* (May 1997);
- Final E11 *Clinical Investigations for Medicinal Products in the Pediatric Population* (July 2000);
- Final E10 *Choice of Control Group in Clinical Trials* (July 2000);

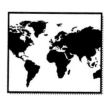

- Draft *Principles for Clinical Evaluation of New Antihypertensive Drugs* (August 2000); and
- Final E3 *Guideline on the Structure and Content of Clinical Study Reports* (July 1996).

The Structure of Clinical Trials

The design of a clinical trial will differ significantly from one drug and disease state to another. The nature of a drug, the product's proposed use, the results of the preclinical testing, principles of medical practice, patient preferences, biostatistical considerations, and the availability and quality of existing standard treatments are among the factors considered in designing a clinical trial or a global drug development program.

Although clinical trials for different drugs can vary greatly in design, they are often similar in structure. Since researchers may know little about a new compound prior to its use in humans, testing the drug through serially conducted investigations permits each phase of clinical development to be carefully designed to use and build upon the information obtained from the research stage preceding it. In its October 1988 *Plan for Accelerated Approval of Drugs to Treat Life-Threatening and Severely Debilitating Illnesses*, the FDA discussed the structure of clinical trials and the basis for this structure:

"[The clinical] drug development process is generally thought of, in simplified terms, as consisting of three phases of human testing to determine if a drug is safe and effective: Phase 1 with 10 to 50 patients to study how the drug is tolerated, metabolized, and excreted; Phase 2 with 50 to 200 patients in which the safety and efficacy of the drug are first evaluated in controlled trials; and Phase 3 with 200 to 1,000 or more patients to confirm and expand upon the safety and efficacy data obtained from the first two phases... The three phases describe the usual process of drug development, but they are not statutory requirements. The basis for marketing approval is the adequacy of the data available; progression through the particular phases is simply the usual means the sponsor uses to collect the data needed for approval. The statute itself focuses on the standard of evidence needed for approval, as derived from adequate and well-controlled clinical investigations, with no mention of phases 1, 2, and 3."

While acknowledging that clinical testing is often classified into these primary "temporal phases," the ICH's final E8 *Guidance on General Considerations for Clinical Trials* (December 1997) also points out that the phases are descriptive rather than prescriptive. For some drugs, this "typical sequence" may be inappropriate or unnecessary, the guidance states (see exhibit below).

When a new drug may offer a significant improvement in the treatment of a serious or life-threatening illness, for example, the traditional phases are, in many cases, supplanted by markedly different approaches, such as those used for new AIDS therapies. During these studies, patient access to the study drug frequently is provided at the same time that the controlled trials are running, something that is done far less often in conventional clinical trial programs (see Chapter 15). In many cases, a new drug that represents a significant therapeutic advance or the first therapy for a serious or life-threatening illness will proceed to the NDA submission stage once the traditional Phase 2 studies have been completed and analyzed. Such an "early" submission would be appropriate only when the data demonstrate a clear and favorable risk/benefit ratio for the therapy. The FDA may require that the applicant conduct a postmarketing Phase 4 study as a condition of such an early approval.

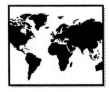

The Clinical Development of New Drugs

Chapter 5

FDA Clinical Guidelines, Points to Consider, and Related Guidelines*

- *General Considerations for the Clinical Evaluation of Drugs* (1977)
- *General Considerations for the Clinical Evaluation of Drugs in Infants and Children* (1977)
- *Guidelines for the Clinical Evaluation of Antidepressant Drugs* (1977)
- *Guidelines for the Clinical Evaluation of Antianxiety Drugs* (1977)
- *Guidelines for the Clinical Evaluation of Anti-Infective Drugs (Systemic)* (1977)
- *Guideline for the Clinical Evaluation of Anti-Inflammatory and Antirheumatic Drugs (Children)* (May 1993)
- *Guideline for the Study and Evaluation of Gender Differences in the Clinical Evaluation of Drugs* (July 1993)
- *Draft Guideline for the Clinical Evaluation of Anti-Anginal Drugs* (January 1989)
- *Draft Guidelines for the Clinical Evaluation of Anti-Arrhythmic Drugs* (July 1985)
- *Guidelines for the Clinical Evaluation of Antidiarrheal Drugs* (1977)
- *Guidelines for the Clinical Evaluation of Gastric Secretory Depressant (GSD) Drugs* (1977)
- *Guidelines for the Clinical Evaluation of Hypnotic Drugs* (1977)
- *Guidelines for the Clinical Evaluation of Antacid Drugs* (1978)
- *Guidelines for the Clinical Evaluation of Motility-Modifying Drugs*
- *Guidelines for the Clinical Evaluation of Laxative Drugs* (1978)
- *Guidelines for the Clinical Evaluation of Psychoactive Drugs in Infants and Children* (1979)
- *Guidelines for the Clinical Evaluation of Bronchodilator Drugs* (1979)
- *Guidelines for the Clinical Evaluation of Drugs to Prevent, Control, and/or Treat Periodontal Disease* (1979)
- *Guidelines for the Clinical Evaluation of Drugs to Prevent Dental Caries* (1979)
- *Guidelines for the Clinical Evaluation of Analgesic Drugs* (Revised 1992)
- *Guidelines for the Clinical Evaluation of Drugs Used in the Treatment of Osteoporosis*
- *Draft Guidelines for the Clinical Evaluation of Lipid-Altering Agents* (1990)
- *Guidelines for the Clinical Evaluation of Antiepileptic Drugs (Adults and Children)* (1981)
- *Guidelines for the Clinical Evaluation of Radiopharmaceutical Drugs* (1981)
- *Guidelines for the Clinical Evaluation of Anti-Inflammatory and Antirheumatic Drugs (Adults and Children)* (Revised April 1988)
- *Guidelines for the Clinical Evaluation of General Anesthetics* (1982)
- *Guidelines for the Clinical Evaluation of Local Anesthetics* (1982)
- *Proposed Guidelines for the Clinical Evaluation of Drugs for the Treatment of Congestive Heart Failure* (December 1987)
- *Proposed Guidelines for the Clinical Evaluation of Antihypertensive Drugs* (May 1988)
- *Guidelines for the Study of Drugs Likely to be Used in the Elderly* (November 1989)
- *Guidelines for the Clinical Evaluation of Drugs for Ulcerative Colitis* (Third Draft)
- *Draft Guidelines for the Development and Evaluation of Drugs for the Treatment of Psychoactive Substance Use Disorders* (February 1992)
- *Draft Guideline for Abuse Liability Assessment* (July 1990)
- *Draft Guidance for the Clinical Evaluation of Weight-Control Drugs* (September 1996)
- *FDA Requirements for Approval of Drugs to Treat Non-Small Cell Lung Cancer* (January 1991)
- *FDA Requirements for Approval of Drugs to Treat Superficial Bladder Cancer* (June 1989)
- *Oncologic Drugs Advisory Committee Discussion on FDA Requirements for Approval of New Drugs for Treatment of Colon and Rectal Cancers*
- *Clinical Development and Labeling of Anti-Infective Drug Products* (October 1992)
- *Points to Consider: Clinical Development Programs for MDI and DPI Drug Products* (September 1994)
- *Draft Points to Consider for OTC Actual Use Studies* (July 1994)
- *Providing Clinical Evidence of Effectiveness for Human Drug and Biological Products* (May 1998)

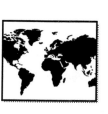

Worldwide Pharmaceutical Regulation Series

FDA Clinical Guidelines, Points to Consider, and Related Guidelines* (continued)

- FDA Approval of New Cancer Treatment Uses for Marketed Drug and Biological Products (December 1998)
- Guidance for Industry on Computerized Systems Used in Clinical Trials (April 1999)
- Guidance on Population Pharmacokinetics (February 1999)
- Draft Guidance on In Vivo Bioequivalence Studies Based on Population and Individual Bioequivalence Studies (December 1997)
- Draft Guidance on Food-Effect Bioavailability and Bioequivalence Studies (October 1997)
- Pharmacokinetics in Patients with Impaired Renal Function—Study Design, Data Analysis, and Impact on Dosing and Labeling (November 1999)
- Clinical Development Programs for Drugs, Devices, and Biological Products for the Treatment of Rheumatoid Arthritis (RA) (January 1999)
- Clinical Evaluation of Combination Estrogen/Progestin-Containing Drug Products Used for Homone Replacement Therapy of Postmenopausal Women
- Content and Format of Pediatric Use Supplements
- Content and Format of Investigational New Drug Applications (IND) for Phase 1 Studies of Drugs, Including Well-Characterized, Therapeutic, Biotechnology-derived Products
- Format and Conent of the Clinical and Statistical Sections of an Application (July 1998)
- Format and Content of the Summary for New Drug and Antibiotic Applications (February 1987)
- Formatting, Assembling and Submitting New Drug and Antibiotic Applications (February 1987)
- Guidance for the Development of Vaginal Contraceptive Drugs (NDA)
- Oncologic Drugs Advisory Committee Discussion on FDA Requirements for Approval of New Drugs for Treatment of Ovarian Cancer (March 1998)
- Postmarketing Reporting of Adverse Drug Experiences (March 1992)
- Preclinical Development of Immunomodulatory Drugs for Treatment of HIV Infection and Associated Disorders
- Preparation of Investigational New Drug Products (Human and Animal) (November 1992)
- Submission of Abbreviated Reports and Synopses in Support of Marketing Applications (August 1998)
- Draft Guidance on Allergic Rhinitis: Clinical Development Programs for Drug Products (July 2000)
- Draft Guidance on Chronic Cutaneous Ulcer and Burn Wounds—Developing Products for Treatment (June 2000)
- Draft Guidance on Clinical Development Programs for Drugs, Devices, and Biological Products Intended for the Treatment of Osteoarthritis (July 1999)
- Draft Guidance on the Clinical Evaluation of Lipid-Altering Agents (October 1990)
- Draft Guidance on Conducting a Clinical Safety Review of a New Product Application and Preparing a Report on the Review (for FDA reviewers) (November 1996)
- Draft Guidance on Developing Medical Imaging Drugs and Biologics (July 2000)
- Draft Guidance on Development of Parathyroid Hormone for the Prevention and Treatment of Osteoporosis (May 2000)
- Draft Guidance on Establishing Pregnancy Registries (June 1999)
- Draft Guidance on Evaluation of Human Pregnancy Outcome Data (June 1999)
- Draft Guidance on Female Sexual Dysfunction: Clinical Development of Drug Products for Treatment (May 2000)
- Draft Guidance for Institutional Review Boards, Clinical Investigators, and Sponsors: Exception from Informed Consent Requirements for Emergency Research (March 2000)
- Draft Guidance on the OTC Treatment of Herpes Labialis with Antiviral Agents (March 2000)
- Draft Guidance on Pediatric Oncology Studies in Response to a Written Request (June 2000)

FDA Clinical Guidelines, Points to Consider, and Related Guidelines* (continued)

- *Draft Guidance on Preclinical and Clinical Evaluation of Agents Used in the Prevention or Treatment of Postmenopausal Osteoporosis* (April 1994)
- *Drug Metabolism/Drug Interaction Studies in the Drug Development Process: Studies In Vitro* (April 1997)
- *Format and Content of the Human Pharmacokinetics and Bioavailability Section of an Application* (February 1997)
- *In Vivo Metabolism/Drug Interaction Studies—Study Design, Data Analysis, and Recommendations for Dosing and Labeling* (November 1999)
- *Average, Population, and Individual Approaches to Establishing Bioequivalence* (August 1999)
- *BA and BE Studies for Orally Administered Drug Products—General Considerations* (August 1999)
- *Statistical Procedures for Bioequivalence Studies Using a Standard Two-Treatment Crossover Design* (July 1992)
- *Bioanalytical Methods Validation for Human Studies* (December 1998)
- *Bioavailability and Bioavailability Studies for Nasal Aerosols and Nasal Sprays for Local Action* (June 1999)
- *General Considerations for Pediatric Pharmacokinetic Studies for Drugs and Biological Products* (November 1998)
- *Acute Bacterial Exacerbation of Chronic Bronchitis—Developing Antimicrobial Drugs for Treatment* (July 1998)
- *Acute Bacterial Meningitis—Developing Antimicrobial Drugs for Treatment* (July 1998)
- *Acute Bacterial Sinusitis—Developing Antimicrobial Drugs for Treatment* (July 1998)
- *Acute or Chronic Bacterial Prostatitis—Developing Antimicrobial Drugs for Treatment* (July 1998)
- *Acute Otitis Media—Developing Antimicrobial Drugs for Treatment* (July 1998)
- *Bacterial Vaginosis—Developing Antimicrobial Drugs for Treatment* (July 1998)
- *Catheter-Related Bloodstream Infections—Developing Antimicrobial Drugs for Treatment* (October 1999)
- *Clinical Considerations for Accelerated and Traditional Approval of Antiretroviral Drugs Using Plasma HIV RNA Measurements* (August 1999)
- *Community Acquired Pneumonia—Developing Antimicrobial Drugs for Treatment* (July 1998)
- *Complicated Urinary Tract Infections and Pyelonephritis—Developing Antimicrobial Drugs for Treatment* (July 1998)
- *Developing Antimicrobial Drugs—General Considerations for Clinical Trials* (July 1998)
- *Empiric Therapy of Febrile Neutropenia—Developing Antimicrobial Drugs for Treatment* (July 1998)
- *Evaluating Clinical Studies of Antimicrobials in the Division of Anti-Infective Drug Products* (July 1997)
- *Lyme Disease—Developing Antimicrobial Drugs for Treatment* (July 1998)
- *Nosocomial Pneumonia—Developing Antimicrobial Drugs for Treatment* (July 1998)
- *Secondary Bacterial Infections of Acute Bronchitis—Developing Antimicrobial Drugs for Treatment* (July 1998)
- *Streptococcal Pharyngitis and Tonsillitis—Developing Antimicrobial Drugs for Treatment* (July 1998)
- *Uncomplicated and Complicated Skin and Skin Structure Infections—Developing Antimicrobial Drugs for Treatment* (July 1998)
- *Uncomplicated Gonorrhea—Developing Antimicrobial Drugs for Treatment* (July 1998)
- *Uncomplicated Urinary Tract Infections—Developing Antimicrobial Drugs for Treatment* (July 1998)
- *Vulvovaginal Candidiasis—Developing Antimicrobial Drugs for Treatment* (July 1998)
- *Acceptance of Foreign Clinical Studies* (March 2001)
- *Cancer Drug and Biological Products—Clinical Data in Marketing Applications* (October 2001)

* list not exhaustive

Phase 1 Clinical Trials

The earliest Phase 1 clinical trials, sometimes called "clinical pharmacology studies," or "first-in-man studies," represent the first introduction of a new drug into human subjects. The focus at this stage is the assessment of clinical safety. Except for extrapolations based on the safety profile obtained from animal studies, investigators may know little about the drug's possible clinical effects prior to these studies.

Phase 1 testing of a new drug is considered highly exploratory because there are often no human safety data available. For this reason, these studies are entered into very cautiously, with the drug being used in an escalating fashion and at fractions of the predicted therapeutic doses in small numbers of subjects, each of whom must submit to close clinical observation for drug effects. Healthy adults whose schedules permit short-term confinement are ideal subjects. In the earliest Phase 1 studies, these subjects are usually males.

Phase 1 clinical trials provide an initial clinical indication of whether a drug is sufficiently safe to be used in further human testing. According to FDA regulations, "Phase 1 includes the initial introduction of an investigational new drug into humans... These studies are designed to determine the metabolism and pharmacologic actions of the drug in humans, the side effects associated with increasing doses, and, if possible, to gain early evidence on effectiveness. During Phase 1, sufficient information about the drug's pharmacokinetics and pharmacological effects should be obtained to permit the design of well-controlled, scientifically valid Phase 2 studies. The total number of subjects and patients included in Phase 1 studies varies with the drug, but is generally in the range of 20 to 80.

"Phase 1 studies also include studies of drug metabolism, structure-activity relationships, and mechanism of action in humans, as well as studies in which investigational drugs are used as research tools to explore biological phenomena or disease processes." These studies can also provide basic pharmacokinetic information, which allows for the comparison of human drug disposition to that of animals so that nonclinical findings can be correlated and verified.

It is worth noting that the term Phase 1 can refer not only to a stage of development (i.e., earliest human exposure), but also to a type of study (i.e., generally any clinical pharmacology study). This type of study may occur at various times throughout a drug's clinical development, and sometimes after the drug has been introduced into the market.

Testing certain drugs in healthy adults is not considered ethical, however. Because of the known toxicity of certain classes of drugs, such as those used in treating AIDS and cancer, some Phase 1 studies are conducted with patients who have, or are at risk of having, the condition for which the drug is being studied. Because healthy volunteers have no opportunity to benefit from the treatment, the administration of highly toxic compounds to such individuals is considered an unacceptable risk. Regardless of the patient population involved, however, these studies are focused on safety issues.

The FDA advises that investigators performing Phase 1 tests involving "normal" volunteers should be skilled in the "initial evaluation of a variety of compounds for safety and pharmacological effect." In those cases in which diseased patients are studied under a Phase 1 protocol, investigators should be,

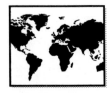

or should work with co-investigators who are, experts in either the particular disease categories to be treated or in the evaluation of drug effects on the disease process. It is also important that such investigators carefully consider the influence of any active disease state on the pharmacokinetic and pharmacodynamic findings. Antiviral drug pharmacodynamics, for example, may be independent of standard blood or plasma concentration-based pharamacokinetic findings. For these drugs, intracellular kinetics, mechanisms of action and trans-membrane, active transport kinetics may be the determinants of successful therapy.

PK/PD and Phase 1 Trials Based on the FDA's reviewing experience in the early 1990s, the selection of the starting dose for clinical trials was recognized as a weakness of many clinical programs. Traditional dose-based comparisons between animals and humans are inadequate largely because of major differences between species in the disposition and metabolism of drugs. Thus, calculations based on animal half-lives and dosing intervals and their relationship to toxicity often led to errors in selecting the starting dose for Phase 1 trials. For these reasons, the "first-in-man" dose is usually a fraction (often as small as one-tenth) of the highest no-effect dose in pertinent animal toxicity studies.

Under former CDER Director Carl Peck, M.D., the FDA advocated the greater use of pharmacokinetic/pharmacodynamic-based methods for the calculation of the starting dose. One such approach, which is supported by National Institutes of Health (NIH) studies of oncologic agents, reduces the number of dose levels required to reach a drug's maximum tolerated dose (MTD), thereby decreasing the number of patients needed for such tests. Termed "pharmacologically guided dose escalation," the technique uses target plasma levels based on preclinical studies to determine the size of doses to be administered during Phase 1 studies. In other cases, the preferred preclinical data are derived from an inter-species model, under which PK data are collected from animals of differing sizes. From a graphic representation, the pharmacokinetisist projects a dose that would theoretically yield predictable plasma concentrations in the target animal—man.

Peck also advocated the incorporation of pharmacokinetic/pharmacodynamic (PK/PD) studies in the first dose-tolerance trials. He maintained that these trials offer a unique, and possibly the only, opportunity to evaluate drug concentration-acute toxic effect relationships of poorly tolerated doses that will be avoided in subsequent trials.

The regulatory focus on early-stage PK/PD studies continued in the years following Peck's departure from CDER. In the ICH's 1994 final guideline entitled, *Dose-Response Information To Support Drug Registration*, the ICH parties stated that dose-response data "are desirable for almost all new chemical entities," and that "assessment of dose-response should be an integral component of drug development with studies designed to assess dose-response as an inherent part of establishing the safety and effectiveness of the drug."

The FDA's efforts to develop additional guidelines provide further evidence of the agency's increasing interest in—and dissatisfaction with—this aspect of clinical research. In a pair of guidances—*In Vivo Drug Metabolism/Drug Interaction Studies-Study Design, Data Analysis, and Recommendations for Dosing and Labeling* (November 1999) and *Drug Metabolism/Drug Interaction Studies in the Drug Development Process: Studies In Vitro* (April 1997)—the agency encourages sponsors to develop information on a drug's metabolic profile early in clinical trials. A May 1998 CDER guidance entitled, *Pharmacokinetics and Pharmacovigilance*

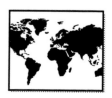

Chapter 5
The Clinical Development of New Drugs

Phases of Clinical Investigation
(from the ICH's December 1997 Final Guideline on General Considerations for Clinical Trials)

Phase 1 (Most typical type of study: Human Pharmacology). Studies in Phase 1 typically involve one or a combination of the following assessments:

- *Estimation of initial safety and tolerability*. The initial and subsequent administration of an investigational new drug into humans is usually intended to determine the tolerability of the dose range expected to be needed for later clinical studies and to determine the nature of adverse reactions that can be expected. These studies typically include both single and multiple-dose administration.

- *Determination of pharmacokinetics* (PK). Preliminary characterization of a drug's absorption, distribution, metabolism, and excretion is almost always an important goal of Phase 1. PK studies are undertaken to assess the clearance of the drug and to anticipate the possible accumulation of parent drug or metabolites and potential drug-drug interactions.

- *Assessment of pharmacodynamics* (PD). Depending on the investigational drug and the endpoint under study, PD studies and studies relating drug blood levels to response (PK/PD studies) may be conducted in healthy volunteer subjects or in patients with the target disease. In some studies involving patients, PD data can provide early estimates of drug activity and potential effectiveness and can guide the dosage and dose regimen in later studies.

- *Early measurement of activity*. Preliminary studies of activity or potential therapeutic benefit may be conducted in Phase 1 as a secondary objective. Such studies may be appropriate when effectiveness is readily measurable with a short duration of drug exposure.

Phase 2 (Most typical kind of study: Therapeutic exploratory). Generally, Phase 2 is considered to comprise studies in which the primary objective is to explore therapeutic effectiveness in patients. Initial therapeutic exploratory studies may use a variety of study designs, such as concurrent controls and comparisons with baseline status. Subsequent trials are usually randomized and concurrently controlled to evaluate the efficacy of the drug and its safety for a particular therapeutic indication. The goals of Phase 2 studies include determining the dose(s) and regimen for Phase 3 studies and the evaluation of potential study endpoints, therapeutic regimens (including concomitant medications), and target populations (e.g., mild versus severe disease) for further study in Phase 2 or Phase 3 trials.

Phase 3 (Most typical kind of study: Therapeutic confirmatory). Usually, Phase 3 is considered to begin with the initiation of studies in which the primary objective is to demonstrate, or confirm, therapeutic benefit. Phase 3 studies are designed to support marketing approval by confirming the preliminary evidence collected in Phase 2 that shows the drug to be safe and effective for use in the intended indication and population. Studies in Phase 3 may also further explore the dose-response relationship, or explore the drug's use in a broader population, in different disease stages, or in combination with another drug.

Phase 4 (Variety of studies: Therapeutic Use). Phase 4 includes all postapproval studies (other than routine surveillance) related to the approved indication. These studies, which are not considered necessary for approval but are often important for optimizing the drug's use, include additional drug-drug interaction, dose-response, or safety studies and studies designed to support use under the approved indication (e.g., mortality/morbidity studies).

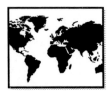

in Patients with Impaired Renal Function: Study Design, Data Analysis, and Impact on Dosing and Labeling specifies when PK studies of patients with impaired renal function should be performed, and discusses the design and conduct of PK/PD studies in such individuals. In a November 1999 draft guidance entitled, *Pharmacokinetics in Patients with Impaired Hepatic Function: Study Design, Data Analysis, and Impact on Dosing and Labeling*, CDER provides recommendations to companies planning to conduct studies to assess the influence of hepatic impairment on the pharmacokinetics and, where appropriate, the pharmacodynamics of experimental drugs. In a February 1999 guidance entitled, *Population Pharmacokinetics*, the agency offers recommendations on the use of population pharmacokinetics to identify differences in safety and effectiveness among population subgroups in drug development programs.

In deciding how the principles of these guidelines should be applied to the design of comprehensive drug development programs, the sponsor and investigator must carefully consider the influence of dynamically different populations on the pharmacokinetics and the pharmacodynamics of the study drug. When evaluating the severely renal compromised patient who needs a drug that is excreted in the urine, for example, one must not only study the new drug's pharmacokinetics at various levels of renal compromise, but also the influence of hemodyalysis and peritoneal dialysis on its pharmocokinetics. A further extension of this logic would include the need to test for unique metabolites that might occur and that might accumulate as a result of prolonged intra-corporeal residence time, and the prolongation of the test drug's duration of exposure to active metabolic systems.

FDA-Sponsor Communication During Clinical Trials Although the clinical program becomes the primary focus of a drug's development once Phase 1 trials begin, other activities continue to support these trials. As clinical trials progress, FDA reviewers continually reassess the safety of these studies. Because the FDA wants these assessments to be based on the latest available data and information, the agency requires that sponsors submit periodic reports on completed and upcoming research. During clinical trials, at least four important types of data and information flow regularly from the sponsor to the FDA:

- New Animal Data. As mentioned previously, animal testing continues during clinical development. Submitted in the form of information amendments to the IND, additional toxicology and pharmacokinetic data may be needed from animal studies to support the safety of new and/or modified clinical studies. For example, longer-term toxicology studies are required as the duration of treatment in humans is extended.

- Protocols and Protocol Amendments. Because protocols for Phase 2 and Phase 3 trials are not normally included in the original IND, protocols for these studies must be forwarded to the FDA subsequently (see Chapter 3). Also, whenever sponsors want to make changes to previously submitted protocols, they must submit protocol amendments.

- Annual Reports. Current regulations require sponsors to submit brief annual reports on the progress of the investigations. These reports must include information on individual studies, provide a summary of the clinical experience with the drug, and provide information on the general investigational plan for the upcoming year, changes in the investigator's brochure, and foreign regulatory and marketing developments (see Chapter 3).

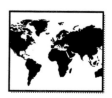

Worldwide Pharmaceutical Regulation Series

- IND Safety Reports. The drug sponsor must notify the FDA and all participating investigators about information that the company receives from any source indicating or suggesting significant hazards, contraindications, side effects, or precautions that are associated with the use of the drug. All significant safety findings must be reported (see Chapter 3).

Ideally, trial sponsors will establish a collegial relationship with the FDA reviewing team, participate in frequent, informal communications to keep the reviewers apprised of developing data, and engage in a progressive exchange of ideas to facilitate the execution of the clinical development program. The FDA has demonstrated that, when such ongoing dialogue drives the process, the data are stronger and cleaner, there are fewer surprises when the NDA is submitted, and NDA time-to-approval is reduced.

Phase 2 Clinical Trials

Phase 2 clinical trials represent a shift away from testing designed almost exclusively for safety to testing designed to provide a preliminary indication of a drug's effectiveness as well. In Phase 2 studies, a drug is used, often for the first time, in patients who suffer from the disease or condition that the drug is intended to prevent, diagnose, or treat.

FDA regulations state that "Phase 2 includes the controlled clinical studies conducted to evaluate the effectiveness of the drug for a particular indication or indications in patients with the disease or condition under study and to determine the common or short-term side effects and risks associated with the drug. Phase 2 studies are typically well-controlled, closely monitored, and conducted in a relatively small number of patients, usually involving no more than several hundred subjects."

In many ways, Phase 2 studies provide the foundation for several key aspects of the study design for the all-important Phase 3 trials. The observed magnitude of the treatment effect in Phase 2 trials is a critical factor in Phase 3 sample size calculations, for example.

As noted above, however, Phase 2 studies may provide the basis on which certain drugs are approved for marketing. When a new drug is the first effective treatment for, or is a significant advance in the treatment of, a serious or life-threatening disease, the sponsor may file an NDA at the completion of Phase 2. In such cases, however, the data must be statistically sound, and a post-marketing surveillance requirement may be a condition of approval. In recent years, this model has been used several times for antiviral treatments directed against herpes viruses and the human immune deficiency virus (HIV) as well as for some of the cancer drugs.

Since Phase 2 trials also involve the first meaningful assessment of a drug's effects on key clinical endpoints (i.e., clinical events or measurements used to assess drug effectiveness), these studies can provide valuable information on the utility of a variety of clinical endpoints and markers. Sponsors and investigators can then use this information to select the most appropriate endpoints—those most reflective of the disease and responsive to therapy, for example—for Phase 3 trials (see discussion of clinical endpoints below).

Generally, Phase 2 study objectives also include the determination of the minimum dose that is maximally effective, or that is sufficiently effective without undue toxicity. Well-conducted Phase 2

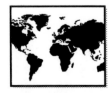

studies of pharmacokinetic and pharmacodynamic parameters may provide useful insights as to whether different subpopulations (e.g., defined by gender, age, or concomitant illness) require different dosing regimens. In diseases whose pathogenesis is dependent upon intracellular disease dynamics, and whose treatment depends upon trans-membrane active transport mechanisms involving potentially toxic drugs, dose-ranging studies may seek the minimal dose that effectively delivers sufficient quantities of the drug to the affected intracellular space.

Because a drug's short-term side effects remain primary concerns during Phase 2 investigations, the compound is administered to a limited number of patients who are closely monitored by the investigators. The use of the drug in larger numbers of subjects (i.e., compared to Phase 1) may reveal less-frequent side effects and provide for better estimates of the dose-toxicity relationships for the more frequently observed adverse effects. Dose-ranging may reveal type 1 target-organ toxicity at the higher doses. Such findings are used to refine the safety surveillance monitoring plans for Phase 3.

When it is both possible and useful, Phase 2 studies should be "controlled" investigations—in other words, the studies should involve the comparison of the experimental drug against a placebo and/or standard therapy. To minimize bias, the studies should employ a randomization and blinding scheme (see discussion below). Generally, the experimental drug is administered to one group of subjects, while the placebo or standard therapy is administered to a similar group. The safety and effectiveness of the two therapies can then be compared. Studies involving special populations, such as children, may require a modified approach, however, since ethical issues in children carry much greater sensitivity and since such issues vary considerably by disease and how "potential benefit" is defined.

Some Phase 2 studies may also employ a parallel design in which study subjects are randomized to one of a limited number of dose levels or regimens. The assessment of response in each treatment group provides the basis for the selection of the optimal doses and regimens to be studied in Phase 3 trials.

Generally speaking, given the comparatively small numbers of patients enrolled in Phase 2 trials, these studies usually are unable to provide the definitive evidence of efficacy and safety necessary to support approval. Under the FDA's expedited development (Subpart E) program, however, Phase 2 trials for products designed to treat life-threatening and severely debilitating diseases may be prospectively designed to support marketing approval (see Chapter 15).

End-of-Phase 2 Meetings and Other Late-Phase FDA-Sponsor Communication Under FDAMA and FDA/industry agreements associated with PDUFA II, the FDA has committed to several goals relevant to both end-of-Phase 2 meetings and other important meetings and communications (e.g., protocol reviews).

End-of Phase 2 Meetings Although the agency had emphasized in the past that end-of Phase 2 meetings are designed primarily for sponsors of NMEs and important new uses of marketed products, the FDA has since made the conferences available to all new drug sponsors, regardless of the classification of their products. Federal regulations state that the purposes of end-of-Phase 2 meetings are to determine the safety of proceeding to Phase 3, to evaluate the Phase 3 plan and protocols and the adequacy of current studies and plans to assess pediatric safety and effectiveness, and to identify any

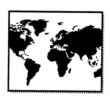

additional information necessary to support a marketing application for the uses under investigation. The ultimate goal of such a meeting is for the sponsor and the FDA to reach agreement on plans for the conduct and design of Phase 3 trials.

Under PDUFA II, the FDA has agreed to respond to meeting requests and hold requested meetings, including end-of-Phase 2 meetings, within specified timeframes. Within 14 calendar days of receiving a formal meeting request (i.e., a scheduled face-to-face meeting, teleconference, or videoconference), CDER should notify the sponsor by letter or fax of the date, time, and place for the meeting, as well as the expected CDER participants. The center will attempt to meet this goal for at least 90% of such requests in FY2001 and FY2002.

The agency's new meetings management system requires CDER to meet with sponsors within specific timeframes based on the type of meeting requested:

Type A Meeting: "A meeting which is necessary for an otherwise stalled drug development program to proceed (a 'critical path' meeting)." These meetings should take place within 30 days of CDER's receipt of a sponsor's request.

Type B Meeting: An end-of-Phase 2, pre-IND, end-of-Phase 1 (i.e., for Subpart E or Subpart H or similar products), or pre-NDA meeting. Type B meetings should occur within 60 calendar days of the agency's receipt of a meeting request.

Type C Meeting: Any other type of meeting. Type C meetings should be held within 75 calendar days of the agency's receipt of a meeting request.

CDER must hold 90% of meetings within these timeframes beginning in FY2000. For a meeting request to qualify under these performance goals, it must be made in writing and meet certain informational standards (e.g., statement of purpose, approximate schedule for submission of supporting documentation). In addition, CDER must agree that the meeting "will serve a useful purpose (i.e., it is not premature or clearly unnecessary)." The agency notes, however, that Type B meetings will be honored "except in the most unusual circumstances."

As its name implies, the end-of-Phase 2 meeting takes place after the completion of Phase 2 clinical trials and before the initiation of Phase 3 studies. Since agency recommendations may bring about significant revisions to a sponsor's Phase 3 trial plans, the agency suggests that these meetings be held before "major commitments of effort and resources to specific Phase 3 tests are made." The FDA adds, however, that such meetings are not intended to delay the transition from Phase 2 to Phase 3 studies.

As they should in all such communications with the FDA, sponsors should attempt to obtain from agency reviewers and officials specific recommendations during the meeting. Agency staffers advise that sponsors develop highly specific questions or well-formulated proposals, and that they focus questions not only on safety issues regarding Phase 3 protocols, but on what studies and data will be necessary for the ultimate approval of the drug as well. Under PDUFA II commitments, the FDA has agreed to prepare the meeting minutes and make them available to the sponsor within 30 days after the meeting. The minutes should "clearly outline the important agreements, disagreements, issues for further discussion, and action items from the meeting in bulleted form and need not be in great detail," the agency states.

Special Protocol Assessment and Agreement Process. As part of a new "special protocol question assessment and agreement" process under PDUFA II, the agency also has agreed to evaluate Phase 3 clinical trial protocols (as well as carcinogenicity and stability protocols) to determine whether a trial's design and size are adequate to meet scientific and regulatory requirements identified by the sponsor. Within 45 days of receiving such a protocol and specific sponsor questions, the agency will provide a written response that includes "a succinct assessment of the protocol and answers to the sponsor's questions." The agency will be called upon to respond to increasing percentages of such requests within this timeframe during PDUFA II's term: 80% in FY2001, and 90% in FY2002.

According to text that accompanied these commitments, "the fundamental agreement here is that having agreed to the design, execution, and analyses proposed in protocols reviewed under this process, the Agency will not later alter its perspective on the issues...unless public health concerns unrecognized at the time of protocol assessment under this process are evident." Related language in the FDA Modernization Act of 1997 seemed to be even stronger: "Any agreement regarding the parameters of the design and size of clinical trials of a new drug...that is reached between the [FDA] and a sponsor or applicant shall be reduced to writing and made part of the administrative record...[and] shall not be changed after the testing begins, except-(i) with the written agreement of the sponsor or applicant; or (ii) pursuant to a decision...by the director of the reviewing division, that a substantial scientific issue essential to determining the safety or effectiveness of the drug has been identified...."

In a December 1999 draft guidance entitled, *Special Protocol Assessment,* the FDA attempts to establish the process through which special protocol assessments will be conducted and agreements will be reached. CDER generally recommends that a sponsor submit a protocol intended for a special protocol assessment to the agency at least 90 days prior to the study's anticipated start date. A separate request in the form of an IND amendment should be forwarded for each protocol that the sponsor wants to have reviewed under this process.

To ensure that the CDER review division "is aware of both the developmental context in which a Phase 3 protocol is being reviewed and the questions that are to be answered," the sponsor should seek an end-of-Phase 2/pre-Phase 3 meeting with the agency. In the request for protocol assessment, the sponsor should pose focused questions concerning specific issues regarding the protocol, protocol design (including proposed size), study conduct, study goal, and/or data analysis for the proposed investigation. The request should also discuss, in reasonable detail, all data, assumptions, and information needed for an adequate evaluation of the protocol.

Within 45 calendar days of receiving an applicant's request for a special protocol assessment, the review team responsible for the drug product should forward its comments to the applicant. If the applicant wants to discuss any remaining issues (e.g., disagreements) or issues regarding the protocol following the special assessment, it can request a meeting (i.e., a Type A meeting). All agency/sponsor agreements and disagreements should be documented clearly in the special protocol assessment letter and/or the minutes of the Type A meeting.

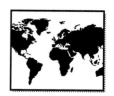

According to the December 1999 draft guidance, "documented special protocol assessments should be considered binding on the review division and should not be changed at any time, except as follows:"

- Failure of a sponsor to follow a protocol that was agreed upon with the agency will be interpreted as the sponsor's understanding that the protocol assessment is no longer binding on the agency.

- If the data, assumptions, or information provided by the sponsor in a request for special protocol assessment change, are found to be false statements or misstatements, or are found to omit relevant facts, the agency will not be bound by any assessment that relied on such data, assumptions, or information.

- A clinical protocol assessment will no longer be considered binding if: (1) the sponsor and FDA agree in writing to change the protocol; or (2) the director of the review division determines that a substantial scientific issue essential to determining the safety or effectiveness of the drug has been identified after the testing has begun. If the director of the review division makes such a determination: (1) the determination should be documented in writing for the administrative record and should be provided to the sponsor; and (2) the sponsor should be given an opportunity for a meeting at which the review division director will discuss the scientific issue involved.

Phase 3 Clinical Trials

In Phase 3 investigations, a drug is tested under conditions more closely resembling those under which the drug would be used if approved for marketing. During this phase, an investigational compound is administered to a significantly larger patient population (i.e., from several hundred to several thousand subjects) to, in the FDA's words, "gather additional information about effectiveness and safety that is needed to evaluate the overall benefit-risk relationship of the drug and to provide an adequate basis for physician labeling."

The larger patient pool and the genetic, lifestyle, environmental, and physiological diversity that it brings allow the investigators to identify potential adverse drug reactions and to determine the appropriate dosage of the drug for the more diverse general population. Patient population criteria for Phase 3 trials may also be expanded to include those with concomitant therapies and conditions.

As defined by a trial's eligibility criteria, the patient population studied in Phase 3 trials will always be a subset of the overall population with a particular disease or condition. The study population in Phase 3 must be sufficiently homogeneous so that variability in response(s) is minimized and so that the study has adequate power to demonstrate an effect. At the same time, the study population must be adequately representative to enable the generalization of the results to the patient population at large.

For certain drugs, principally those for serious and life-threatening illnesses, Phase 3 also marks the point at which clinical trial sponsors must make another important decision: The sponsor often must consider whether to make the study drug available to patients who desperately need therapeutic alternatives and who are unable to enroll in the formal clincial trials. Such availability, sometimes

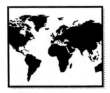

called "expanded access" or "compassionate use," can be provided under several mechanisms that the agency has established, including treatment INDs and emergency use INDs (see Chapter 15). Reached in consultation with the FDA, the decision to make a drug available in this manner is a function, first and foremost, of what is known about a drug's safety and, secondly, what is known about its efficacy. This decision is also based upon the availability of satisfactory therapeutic alternatives in the marketplace and the severity of the disease and its potential for causing disability or death.

Pivotal Clinical Studies Phase 3 testing may produce data from controlled and uncontrolled trials conducted at several hospitals, clinics, or other sites outlined in the protocol. But the clinical data that the FDA will review most closely and upon which the agency will base its approval/disapproval decision are those derived from tests specified in federal regulations as "adequate and well-controlled studies." These are sometimes called "pivotal studies."

The focus on pivotal clinical studies as the primary criterion for approving new drugs is rooted in the Federal Food, Drug and Cosmetic Act, which states that "the term 'substantial evidence' means evidence consisting of adequate and well-controlled investigations...on the basis of which it could fairly and responsibly be concluded by...experts that the drug will have the effect it purports or is represented to have under the conditions of use prescribed, recommended, or suggested in the labeling or proposed labeling thereof."

The concept of substantial evidence has a second important component. With rare exceptions, at least two adequate and well-controlled studies are necessary to obtain FDA approval for a new drug. According to the FDA's *Guideline for the Content and Format of the Clinical and Statistical Sections of an Application*, "the requirement for well-controlled clinical investigations has been interpreted to mean that the effectiveness of a drug should be supported by more than one well-controlled trial and carried out by independent investigators. This interpretation is consistent with the general scientific demand for replicability. Ordinarily, therefore, the clinical trials submitted in an application will not be regarded as adequate support of a claim unless they include studies by more than one independent investigator who maintains adequate case histories of an adequate number of subjects."

It is important to note, however, that the adequate and well-controlled studies submitted in support of a drug need not be identical. In some cases, for example, they might be carried out in patient populations with different expressions of the same target illness to be treated by the investigational drug.

In late 1997 and early 1998, a new FDA guidance and the FDA Modernization Act clarified the concept of the "substantial evidence" of effectiveness necessary for approval. In the November 1997 reform legislation, Congress established that data from a single adequate and well-controlled study, together with confirmatory evidence, may, at the FDA's discretion, comprise substantial evidence of effectiveness.

Then, with its release of a May 1998 *Guidance for Industry - Providing Clinical Evidence of Effectiveness for Human Drug and Biological Products*, the FDA took another important step in clarifying—some might say evolving—this standard. The agency stated that it was appropriate to re-articulate its current thinking concerning the "quantitative and qualitative standards for demonstrating effectiveness of drugs" because "the science and practice of drug development and clinical evaluation have evolved significantly since the effectiveness requirement for drugs was established, and this evolution has implica-

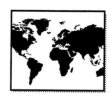

tions for the amount and type of data needed to support effectiveness in certain cases... At the same time, progress in clinical evaluation and clinical pharmacology has resulted in more rigorously designed and conducted clinical efficacy trials, which are ordinarily conducted at more than one clinical site. This added rigor and scope has implications for a study's reliability, generalizability, and capacity to substantiate effectiveness.

"The usual requirement for more than one adequate and well-controlled investigation reflects the need for independent substantiation of experimental results..., [which is] often referred to as the need for 'replication' of the finding. Replication may not be the best term, however, as it may imply that precise repetition of the same experiment in other patients by other investigators is the only means to substantiate a conclusion. Precise replication of a trial is only one of a number of possible means of obtaining independent substantiation of a clinical finding and, at times, can be less than optimal as it could leave the conclusions vulnerable to any systematic biases inherent to the particular study design. Results that are obtained from studies that are of different design and independent in execution, perhaps evaluating different populations, endpoints, or dosage forms, may provide support for a conclusion of effectiveness that is as convincing as, or more convincing than, a repeat of the same study."

This important guidance also identifies situations in which the agency will consider approving new drugs, or new uses of approved medicines, without data from two adequate and well-controlled studies. To the pharmaceutical industry, the guidance's most intriguing aspect was a discussion of the situations in which a single pivotal study could provide the basis for marketing approval. Although the agency had issued a 1995 statement specifying when a single, multicenter study could support approval, the FDA points out that it had not "comprehensively described the situations" in which a single study might be used or the characteristics of a single study that would make it adequate to support approval.

While the FDA contends that none of the characteristics "is necessarily determinative," the presence of one or more of five characteristics can contribute to a conclusion that a single pivotal study would be adequate to support approval: certain large multicenter studies; consistency across study subsets; multiple "studies" in a single study; multiple endpoints involving different events; and statistically very powerful findings.

The guidance also offers several caveats regarding the use of a single pivotal trial for approval. Reliance on a single study, the agency points out, generally will be limited to situations in which a trial has demonstrated a clinically meaningful effect on mortality, irreversible morbidity, or prevention of a disease with a potentially serious outcome, such that confirmation of the result in a second trial would be ethically difficult or impossible.

A 2001 Tufts Center for the Study of Drug Development (CSDD) found that over 80 percent of major pharmaceutical companies surveyed have used or plan to use regulatory provisions allowing the use of a single controlled trial to gain product approval. The study found that 8 of the 15 top worldwide pharmaceutical companies surveyed used the single controlled trial (SCT) approach for product applications submitted in 1998 and 1999. The Tufts CSDD identified 10 approved drug applications employing the SCT approach—6 NDAs, 4 of which were NDAs for new molecular entities, and 4 sup-

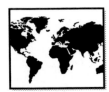

plemental NDAs. Two of the NME-NDAs were submitted to and approved by the Division of Oncologic Drug Products, while the Division of Gastrointestinal and Coagulation Drug Products received four applications using the SCT approach—three supplemental NDAs and 1 original NDA. Many, but not all, of the drugs employing the SCT approach were products for indications for which SCTs "were expected to be acceptable to FDA," including orphan drugs, pediatric indications, and drugs reviewed under the accelerated approval process.

The Tufts CSDD study also notes that 9 of the 12 applications (i.e., 10 NDAs and 2 biologics applications) identified supported data from the SCT with confirmatory evidence from related adequate and well-controlled studies. Five of these 9 applications included data from studies on different doses, regimens, or dosage forms. A third of the applications used just 1 type of related study, 55 percent used 2 or 3 types of related studies, and 11 percent used as many as 5 types of related studies to support the SCT. Interestingly, all 3 of the applications that included data from an SCT alone (i.e., without confirmatory evidence) have been approved. Tufts CSDD notes that the sponsors of these 3 applications all self-rated their SCTs as being very strong in regard to two of the five study characteristics that the FDA claims is of particular importance when an SCT is used: (1) no single site was disproportionately responsible for the positive effect; and (2) there was consistency of important covariates across study subsets.

Standards for Pivotal Trials Because of their central importance to the FDA's approval decision, pivotal studies must meet particularly high scientific standards: "The purpose of conducting clinical investigations of a drug is to distinguish the effect of a drug from other influences, such as spontaneous change in the course of the disease, improvements in supportive care, placebo effect, or biased observation," the agency states. Therefore, adequate and well-controlled trials are designed to isolate the drug's effects from extraneous factors that might otherwise undermine the validity of the trials' results.

Generally, a study must meet four criteria to be considered pivotal:

1. A pivotal study must be a controlled trial. As previously discussed, a controlled trial, in many cases, compares a group of patients treated with a placebo or standard therapy against a group of patients treated with the investigational drug. The FDA specifies in federal regulations, and the ICH parties recognize in a July 2000 guidance (E10 *Choice of Control Group and Related Issues in Clinical Trials*), five types of controls: placebo concurrent controls; dose-comparison concurrent controls; no treatment concurrent controls; active (positive) treatment concurrent controls; and historical (external) controls. The E10 guidance notes that, "the choice of control group is always a critical decision in designing a clinical trial. That choice affects the inferences that can be drawn from the trial, the ethical acceptability of the trial, the degree to which bias in conducting and analyzing the study can be minimized, the types of subjects that can be recruited and the pace of recruitment, the kind of endpoints that can be studied, the public and scientific credibility of the results, the acceptability of the results by regulatory authorities, and many other features of the study, its conduct, and its interpretation" (see exhibit below). The guidance also notes that it is increasingly common for more than one type of control group to be used in a development program. The 2000 guidance has been criticized by industry,

principally because it fails to harmonize the various control group preferences of the ICH regions (e.g., the FDA's preference for placebo controls and European regulators' preference for active comparators). The FDA has acknowledged that the guidance, although it discusses the appropriateness of the various controls in specific situations, does not address the requirements in any of the three regions.

2. A pivotal study must have a blinded design when such a design is practical and ethical. According to the ICH's September 1999 final guideline entitled, *Statistical Principles for Clinical Trials*, "blinding, or masking, is intended to limit the occurrence of conscious and unconscious bias in the conduct and interpretation of a clinical trial arising from the influence that the knowledge of treatment may have on the recruitment and allocation of subjects, their subsequent care, the attitudes of subjects to the treatments, the assessment of end points, the handling of withdrawals, the exclusion of data from analysis, and so on. The essential aim is to prevent identification of the treatments until all such opportunities for bias have passed." Double-blind trials are those in which the subjects and the investigator and sponsor staff involved in treating and evaluating patients are kept from knowing which subjects are receiving the experimental drug and which are receiving the placebo/standard therapy. When double-blind trials are not feasible (e.g., because the pattern of administration differs), studies may employ single blinds, in which only the subjects are kept from knowing which treatment is administered. In some cases, however, only an open-label study is possible because of ethical or practical factors. In certain instances, studies employ a mechanism of blinding often referred to as a "double dummy" design that is intended to eliminate the biases that might otherwise result from the comparison of different formulations or routes of administration. In such a design, each study subject receives two formulations, only one of which would contain the active moiety. This might be used, for example, when an intravenous antibiotic is being compared to an oral antibiotic. Half the subjects might receive the active oral formulation and a placebo intravenous formulation, while the remaining subjects would receive the oral placebo and the active intravenous formulation.

3. A pivotal study must be randomized. This means that clinical subjects are assigned randomly to the treatment and control groups. Therefore, each subject has an equal chance of being assigned to the various treatment and control groups to be studied in a particular trial. In combination with blinding, randomization helps prevent potential bias in the selection and assignment of trial subjects.

4. A pivotal study must be of adequate size. The study must involve enough patients to provide statistically significant evidence that a new drug offers a therapeutic or safety advantage over existing therapies. According to the FDA's *General Considerations for the Clinical Evaluation of Drugs*, the size of a pivotal study is dependent upon factors such as: (1) the degree of response one wishes to detect; (2) the desired assurance against a false positive finding; and (3) the acceptable risk of failure to demonstrate the response when it is present in the population. Sample size calculations require many assumptions about the results to be obtained with the treatment and the population being studied. Because considerable clinical judgement is employed in making these assumptions, FDA officials warn that faulty presumptions frequently result in studies of inadequate statistical power.

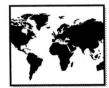

These criteria also are included in FDA regulations, which add that the "characteristics" of adequate and well-controlled studies include the following:

- a clear statement of the objectives of the study;

- a design that permits a valid comparison with a control to provide a quantitative assessment of the drug effect;

- a method of subject selection that provides adequate assurance that subjects have the disease or condition being studied, or that they show evidence of susceptibility and exposure to the condition against which prophylaxis is directed;

- a method of assigning patients to treatment and control groups that minimizes bias and that is intended to assure comparability of the groups with respect to pertinent variables such as age, sex, severity of disease, duration of disease, and the use of drugs or therapy other than test drugs (Author's note: It is important to note that significant improvements in concomitant therapies or mortality rates may drastically alter the conditions of a long-term treatment study involving a chronic disease. The population characteristics of those enrolled near the end of a study may be entirely different from those found in patients enrolled at the beginning of the study);

- adequate measures to minimize bias by the subjects, observers, and analysts of the data;

- well-defined and reliable methods for objectively assessing subjects' responses; and

- an adequate analysis of the study results to assess the effects of the drug (this should not involve so called "data-dredging" to find a positive effect).

The FDA wrote in 1987 that it "has long considered [these] characteristics as the essentials of an adequate and well-controlled study... In general, the regulation on adequate and well-controlled studies has two overall objectives: (1) To allow the agency to assess methods for minimizing bias; and (2) to assure a sufficiently detailed description of the study to allow scientific assessment and interpretation of it."

It is worth noting that federal regulations do not provide a comprehensive discussion of the testing conditions necessary for pivotal trials. Mentions of other standards that the FDA sees as necessary for pivotal studies are scattered throughout a variety of agency guidelines. Although it does not address pivotal trials directly, the ICH's September 1998 guideline entitled, E9 *Statistical Principles for Clinical Trials* offers a useful discussion regarding important aspects of later-phase study design issues, including study configuration (e.g., cross-over and parallel group), trial comparisons (e.g., superiority, equivalence), and sample size.

Completing a Drug's Clinical Study

It is in the best interest of the sponsor, the clinical subjects, and, in many cases, the public that a drug's clinical study be completed as soon as sufficient safety and efficacy data are obtained. If a drug is found during the development process to be unsafe or ineffective, then continuing a trial only

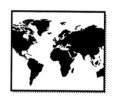

The Choice of Clinical Trial Controls
(from the ICH's July 2000 guidance entitled,
The Choice of Control Group and Related Issues in Clinical Trials)

Placebo Concurrent Control "In a placebo-controlled study, subjects are randomly assigned to a test treatment or to an identical-appearing treatment that does not contain the test drug. The treatments may be titrated to effect or tolerance, or may be given at one or more fixed doses. Such trials are almost always double-blind. The name of the control suggests that its purpose is to control for "placebo" effect (improvement in a subject resulting from thinking that he or she is taking a drug), but that is not its only or major benefit. Rather, the placebo control design, by allowing blinding and randomization and including a group that receives an inert treatment, controls for all potential influences on the actual or apparent course of the disease other than those arising from the pharmacologic action of the test drug. These influences include spontaneous change (natural history of the disease and regression to the mean), subject or investigator expectations, the effect of being in a trial, use of other therapy, and subjective elements of diagnosis and assessment. Placebo-controlled trials seek to show a difference between treatments when they are studying effectiveness, but may also seek to show lack of difference (of specified size) in evaluating a safety measurement."

No-Treatment Concurrent Control "In a no-treatment controlled study, subjects are randomly assigned to test treatment or to no (i.e., absence of) study treatment. The principal difference between this design and a placebo-controlled trial is that subjects and investigators are not blind to treatment assignment. Because of the advantages of double-blind designs, this design is likely to be needed and suitable only when it is difficult or impossible to double-blind (e.g., treatments with easily recognized toxicity) and only when there is reasonable confidence that study endpoints are objective and that the results of the study are unlikely to be influenced by [any of the problems associated with knowledge of treatment assignment (e.g., unblinded subjects on active drug might report more favorable outcomes because they expect a benefit or might be more likely to stay in the trial)]. Note that it is often possible to have a blinded evaluator carry out endpoint assessment, even if the overall trial is not double-blind. This is a valuable approach and should always be considered in studies that cannot be blinded, but it does not solve the other problems associated with knowing the treatment assignment...."

Dose-Response Concurrent Control "In a randomized, fixed-dose, dose-response trial, subjects are randomized to one of several fixed-dose groups. Subjects may either be placed on their fixed dose initially or be raised to that dose gradually, but the intended comparison is between the groups on their final dose. Dose-response studies are usually double-blind. They may include a placebo (zero dose) and/or active control. In a concentration-controlled trial, treatment groups are titrated to several fixed-concentration windows; this type of trial is conceptually similar to a fixed-dose, dose-response trial."

Active (Positive) Concurrent Control "In an active control (or positive control) trial, subjects are randomly assigned to the test treatment or to an active control treatment. Such trials are usually double-blind, but this is not always possible; many oncology trials, for example, are considered

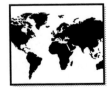

difficult or impossible to blind because of different regimens, different routes of administration, and different toxicities. Active control trials can have two distinct objectives with respect to showing efficacy: (1) To show efficacy of the test treatment by showing it is as good as a known effective treatment or (2) to show efficacy by showing superiority of the test treatment to the active control. They may also be used with the primary objective of comparing the efficacy and/or safety of the two treatments. Whether the purpose of the trial is to show efficacy of the new treatment or to compare two treatments, the question of whether the trial would be capable of distinguishing effective from less effective or ineffective treatments is critical."

External Control (Including Historical Control) "An externally controlled study compares a group of subjects receiving the test treatment with a group of patients external to the study, rather than to an internal control group consisting of patients from the same population assigned to a different treatment... External (historical) control groups, regardless of the comparator treatment, are considered together as the fifth type [of control group] because of serious concerns about the ability of such trials to ensure comparability of test and control groups and their ability to minimize important biases, making this design usable only in exceptional circumstances. The external control can be a group of patients treated at an earlier time (historical control) or a group treated during the same time period but in another setting. The external control may be defined (a specific group of patients) or nondefined (a comparator group based on general medical knowledge of outcome). Use of this latter comparator is particularly trecherous (such trials are usually considered uncontrolled) because general impressions are so often inaccurate. So-called baseline-controlled studies, in which subjects' status on therapy is compared with status before therapy (e.g., blood pressure, tumor size), have no internal control and are thus uncontrolled or externally controlled."

The ICH guidance also notes that it is often possible and "advantageous" to employ more than one type of control in a single study (e.g., using both an active control and a placebo). Some trials might use several doses of a test drug and several doses of an active control with or without placebo. Such a design, says the guidance, may be useful for active drug comparisons when the relative potency of the two drugs is not well established, or when the trial's purpose is to establish relative potency.

exposes more clinical subjects to a dangerous or useless compound, and in some cases, keeps study subjects from using better or safer therapies. On the other hand, if the drug is clearly shown to be safer or more effective than existing therapies, delaying the submission of an NDA to gain additional data needlessly prolongs the development process and denies patients access to a needed drug.

Clinical trials may be discontinued before reaching their subject accrual targets for any one of several reasons, including the following:

- the studies clearly establish a drug's safety and effectiveness;
- an unacceptable adverse effect is discovered; or
- it becomes apparent that the studies are unlikely to establish a drug's safety or effectiveness, or that a drug's apparent safety and effectiveness are less than that of a standard therapy.

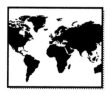

When designing the trial, statisticians will establish what are called "stopping rules." These are rigorous statistical criteria or goals that, if met at some point during the study of a drug, will trigger the end of the clinical trial. To justify discontinuing the trial, the data generally must meet stringent standards to show, for example, that the drug's effects are: (1) statistically significant (i.e., that the drug was tested in a large enough patient population to ensure that observed effects were not due to chance); and (2) clinically significant (i.e., that the test results are sufficient to show that there is a perceptible difference in the clinical effect between the investigational drug and the placebo and/or a standard therapy).

The periodic analysis of accrued data—interim analysis—is undertaken during the clinical trial to determine if any of the pre-established stopping criteria have been met. Because interim analyses can affect the interpretation of the clinical trial, they must be planned and scheduled in advance and disclosed in the clinical protocol. According to the ICH guideline entitled, E9 *Statistical Principles for Clinical Trials*, "most clinical trials intended to support the efficacy and safety of an investigational product should proceed to full completion of planned sample size accrual; trials should be stopped early only for ethical reasons or if the power is no longer acceptable. However, it is recognized that drug development plans involve the need for sponsor access to comparative treatment data for a variety of reasons, such as planning other trials. It is also recognized that only a subset of trials will involve the study of serious life-threatening outcomes or mortality which may need sequential monitoring of accruing comparative treatment effects for ethical reasons. In either of these situations, plans for interim statistical analysis should be in place in the protocol or in protocol amendments prior to the unblinded access to comparative treatment data in order to deal with the potential statistical and operational bias that may be introduced."

For many clinical trials, particularly those involving drugs with major public health significance, the responsibility for monitoring comparisons of efficacy and/or safety outcomes should be assigned to an independent and external group often called a data safety monitoring board (DSMB), the ICH guidance states. The guidance, which calls such boards independent data monitoring committees (IDMC), says that such panels "may be established by the sponsor to assess at intervals the progress of a clinical trial, safety data, and critical efficacy variables and recommend to the sponsor whether to continue, modify or terminate a trial [based on its findings]."

In a November 2001 draft document entitled, *Guidance for Clinical Trial Sponsors on the Establishment and Operation of Clinical Trial Data Monitoring Committees*, the FDA establishes that data monitoring committees (DMC) should be used in all controlled trials employing mortality or major morbidity as a primary or secondary endpoint. DMCs, the agency notes, may also be useful "in settings where trial participants may be at elevated risk of such outcomes even if the study intervention addresses lesser outcomes such as relief of symptoms." The draft guidance defines DMCs, which the FDA requires only when informed consent requirements are waived in studies conducted in emergency settings, as panels of individuals "with pertinent expertise that review on a regular basis accumulating outcome data in certain ongoing clinical trials [and that] advise the sponsor regarding the continuing safety of current participants and those yet to be recruited, as well as the continuing validity and scientific merit of the trial."

In addition to safety considerations (e.g., mortality/major morbidity endpoints, trials in fragile populations, and large/long-duration/multi-center studies), two other factors—practicality and assurance

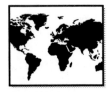

of scientific validity—are relevant in determining whether a sponsor should establish a DMC for a particular trial, says the agency. A DMC may not be practical, for example, for short-term trials in which the trial duration will not give the committee an opportunity to contribute. If a short-term trial presents important safety considerations that justify a DMC, the guidance says that sponsors must develop mechanisms allowing the committee to be informed and convened rapidly when unexpected results are found.

A DMC's likely ability to assure a trial's scientific validity is the third key consideration, the guidance establishes. Trials "of any appreciable duration," the FDA notes, can be affected by changes over time in the understanding of a disease, the affected population, and standard treatments, all of which are changes that may trigger an interest in study modifications as the trial advances. "When a DMC is the only group reviewing unblinded interim data, the trial organizers are free to make changes in the ongoing trial that may be motivated by newly available data outside the trial or by accumulating data from within the trial (e.g., overall event rates)," the guidance states. "In general, recommendations to change the inclusion criteria, the trial endpoints, or the size of the trial are most credibly made by those without knowledge of the accumulating data. When the trial organizers are the ones reviewing the interim data, their awareness of interim comparative results cannot help but affect their determination as to whether these changes should be made. Such changes would inevitably impair the credibility of the study results."

For these reasons and others, the draft guidance touts the advantages of the *independent* DMC, which is defined as "a committee whose members are considered to be independent of those sponsoring, organizing, and conducting the trial" (i.e., have no previous involvement in the trial's design, no current involvement in its conduct other than as the DMC, and have no financial or other important connections to the study sponsor or other trial organizers). A DMC will be considered independent, for example, if the sponsor has no representation on the committee or if the sponsor has a representative only in open meetings, during which enrollment, compliance, and event rates are presented and discussed but during which no study arm-specific data are discussed. The draft guidance acknowledges that DMCs are rarely, if ever, entirely independent of sponsors, given that sponsors typically select and pay the members and establish a committee's goals and responsibilities.

The independence of other individuals interacting with both the sponsor and DMC is equally important, the FDA states. Trial integrity is best maintained when the statistician preparing unblinded data (i.e., interim analyses) for the DMC is external to the sponsor, especially for studies designed to provide the definitive evidence of efficacy, the draft guidance notes. The statistician should have no responsibility for managing the trial and should have "minimal" contact with those who have such involvement.

Although DSMBs have been receiving greater attention in recent years, they have been in use for more than 25 years. One of the earliest uses of DSMBs may have been in conjunction with placebo-controlled herpes encephalitis studies conducted by the NIAID Collaborative Antiviral Substances Study Group in the early 1970s. In these studies, which involved drugs from a historically toxic class of chemicals, it was essential for researchers to know, as early as possible, that the ancient dictum, "First do no harm," was being honored. The ethical dilemma was that the disease itself was highly lethal while the proposed treatment was potentially highly toxic. This clinical study was carefully designed to incorporate monitoring by a DSMB, which would be in a position to detect unacceptable risks in

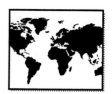

the ongoing trial and to immediately call for the discontinuation of any or all study treatment arms when such risks were identified. So it could be truly independent, none of the DSMB members had any interest in, or connection to, the drug sponsors, investigators or study sites; rather, the board answered only to the FDA. The DSMB's pre-defined, statistical evaluation of the mortality data revealed a 70% mortality in the placebo group (this disease had, prior to these findings, been considered "uniformly fatal"), a suggestion of efficacy with a 50% mortality in one of the investigational drug groups and a whopping 96% mortality in the other investigational drug group. Retrospectively from these findings, it could be concluded that anecdotal use of the "lethal" investigational drug for the preceding 9 years may have inadvertently caused 26% more patient deaths than if the disease had been left to take its natural course. Ever since, the DSMB's role has been valued whenever there is the possibility of serious toxicity in a controlled clinical trial program.

Phase 4 Clinical Studies

In a very real sense, the clinical development process continues long after a product's approval. The further collection and analysis of adverse experience information and other data provide the sponsor and the FDA with a continuing flow of information so that a drug's safety and effectiveness can be reassessed periodically in light of the latest data.

Phase 4 clinical trials, which are studies initiated after a drug's marketing approval, have become an increasingly important and common method through which sponsors obtain new information about their marketed drugs. A drug manufacturer may undertake postmarketing clinical studies for any one of several reasons, including the following:

- To satisfy an FDA request made prior to an NDA's approval that Phase 4 trials be conducted following approval (see Chapter 11). For example, the FDA may want the sponsor to better characterize the drug's safety and/or effectiveness in patient groups that may not have been widely represented in pivotal trials (e.g., children, pregnant women, persons using concomitant medications). Sponsor commitments made at the time of a drug's approval may also become, in effect, postmarketing requirements. Often called "Phase 4 commitments," these commitments—and sponsors' progress in fulfilling them—are actively tracked by the FDA following approval (see Chapter 11).

- To develop pharmacoeconomic, or cost-effectiveness, data that can be used to support marketing claims highlighting the advantages of a drug over competing therapies. Given the emergence of managed care and the increased focus on health care costs, however, growing numbers of companies are incorporating the study of pharmacoeconomic parameters in their premarketing studies.

- Other post-marketing studies are carried out to support the publication of articles in different medical specialty journals and presentations at medical specialty meetings. The goal of these studies, which are often conducted by opinion leaders in various specialties, is to provide information to less-experienced practitioners. These studies are sometimes called "Phase 5" studies.

- Finally, there are Phase 4 studies that characterize new formulations, dose regimens and routes of administration for already proven therapeutic indications.

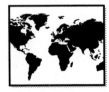

Aside from the fact that they are conducted after approval, Phase 4 studies may differ in a number of important respects from Phase 1, 2, and 3 trials. Phase 4 studies are often of a larger scale than are pre-marketing studies. Also, they may be less rigorously controlled than key, pre-approval studies, although the FDA is monitoring the scientific integrity of these studies, particularly those to be used in support of comparative efficacy and pharmacoeconomic claims (see Chapter 11) and those that become the basis for articles that company sales forces use to promote drug products.

PAGE 115

The Clinical Development of New Drugs

Chapter 5

CHAPTER 6

Good Clinical Practices (GCP)

Because the FDA's approval of a new drug is based largely on clinical data, the agency has a vested interest in these data and the conditions under which they are obtained. Through a set of regulations and guidelines collectively known as "good clinical practices" (GCP), the FDA sets minimum standards for clinical trials.

By identifying and defining the responsibilities of the key personnel involved in clinical trials, the FDA's GCP regulations are designed to accomplish two primary goals: (1) to ensure the quality and integrity of the data obtained from clinical testing so that the FDA's decisions based on these data are informed and responsible; and (2) to protect the rights and, to the degree possible, the welfare of clinical subjects.

Traditionally, GCP has been a term of convenience used by those in government and industry to identify a collection of related regulations and guidelines that, when taken together, define the clinical study-related responsibilities of sponsors, clinical investigators, monitors, and institutional review boards (IRB). For many years, these responsibilities were found primarily in four documents released in the 1980s:

- a 1981 regulation on the informed consent of clinical subjects;
- a 1981 regulation on the responsibilities of IRBs;
- the 1987 IND Rewrite regulations, which define the responsibilities of the investigator and the sponsor; and
- the 1988 *Guideline for the Monitoring of Clinical Investigations*, which outlines the responsibilities of monitors.

While these documents formed the core of GCP, several more recent FDA documents have provided additional information on GCP standards. Among these is a set of so-called *Information Sheets for Institutional Review Boards and Clinical Investigators*, and the FDA compliance program guidance manuals, which specify how FDA investigators ensure that clinical sponsors, monitors, institutional review boards (IRB), and clinical investigators comply with GCP. The information sheets were updated and republished under the title, *Guidance for Institutional Review Boards and Clinical Investigators* in September 1998 (see exhibit below). In late 2001, the FDA was in the process of revising many of these guidances, in part to further emphasize the importance of the informed consent process (see discussion below).

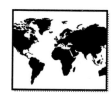

Worldwide Pharmaceutical Regulation Series

Good Clinical Practices (GCP)

Chapter 6

A more recent and significant addition to the FDA's corpus of GCP documents is the International Conference on Harmonization's (ICH) *Good Clinical Practice: Consolidated Guideline*, which was adopted by the ICH parties in 1996 and then as an FDA guidance in May 1997. Designed to provide "a unified standard for designing, conducting, recording, and reporting trials that involve the participation of human subjects," this harmonized guideline provides guidance on IRB, sponsor, investigator, monitoring, and auditing requirements, and offers helpful guidance on the content and format of clinical protocols. Integrated into the consolidated ICH guideline are two guidelines that were issued as separate draft documents in 1994: *Guideline for the Investigator's Brochure*, which specifies the minimum information required in, and recommends a format for, the investigator's brochure; and *Guideline for Essential Documents for the Conduct of a Clinical Study*, which identifies the essential documents that "individually and collectively permit evaluation of the conduct of a clinical study and the quality of the data produced."

FDA officials emphasized at the time of its release that the ICH GCP guideline is entirely consistent with the FDA's established GCP requirements, and that the harmonized documents will supplement, rather than replace, existing regulations and guidelines. Agency officials conceded that, in a few areas, the ICH GCP guideline clarified current U.S. practices and requirements better than the FDA's regulations and earlier guidelines. Other analysts stated that the ICH guideline offers several recommendations that, despite not being mentioned specifically in current FDA documents, reflect typical FDA expectations and industry practices.

Information Sheets: Guidance for Institutional Review Boards and Clinical Investigators

To provide additional guidance on the protection of subjects in clinical trials, CDER makes available what it calls "information sheets" for both clinical investigators and institutional review boards (IRB). The latest versions of these information sheets, which were released in 1998, address various aspects of the investigator and IRB's roles and responsibilities in clinical research, and address various special situations (e.g., emergency drug use) that can arise during clinical trials. The 1998 information sheets are listed in the exhibit below.

- Frequently Asked Questions
    - IRB Organization
    - IRB Membership
    - IRB Procedures
    - IRB Records
    - Informed Consent Process
    - Informed Consent Document Content
    - Clinical Investigations
    - General Questions
- Cooperative Research
- Non-local IRB Review
- Continuing Review After Study Approval
    - Continuing Review Criteria
    - Continuing Review Process
    - Serious Adverse Reactions, Unexpected Events Process
    - Changes During Approval Period Review Process
- Sponsor-Investigator-IRB Interrelationship

–continued–

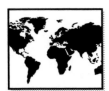

Chapter 6

Good Clinical Practices (GCP)

- Acceptance of Foreign Clinical Studies (Revised March 16, 2001)
- Charging for Investigational Products
- Recruiting Study Subjects
- Payment to Research Subjects
- Screening Tests Prior to Study Enrollment
- A Guide to Informed Consent
  - Consent Document Content
  - IRB Standard Format
  - Sponsor Prepared Model Consent Documents
  - Revision of Consent During the Study
  - General Requirements, 21 CFR 50.20
  - FDA Approval of Studies
  - Non-English Speaking Subjects
  - Illiterate English Speaking Subjects
  - Assent of Children Elements of Informed Consent, 21 CFR 50.25
  - Compensation v. Waiver of Subject's Rights
  - The Consent Process
  - Documentation of Informed Consent, 21 CFR 50.27
- Use of Investigational Products When Subjects Enter a Second Institution
- Personal Importation of Unapproved Products
- Exception from Informed Consent for Studies Conducted in Emergency Settings: Regulatory Language and Excerpts from Preamble
- "Off-Label" and Investigational Use of Marketed Drugs, Biologics and Medical Devices
- Emergency Use of an Investigational Drug or Biologic
  - Obtaining an Emergency IND
  - Emergency Exemption from Prospective IRB Approval
  - Exception From Informed Consent Requirement
  - Planned Emergency Research, Informed Consent Exception
- Treatment Use of Investigational Drugs
- Waiver of IRB Requirements
- Drug Study Designs
- Evaluation of Gender Differences
- FDA Institutional Review Board Inspections
- FDA Clinical Investigator Inspections
- Clinical Investigator Regulatory Sanctions
- Selected Appendices
  - Investigations Which May Be Reviewed Through Expedited Review
  - Significant Differences in FDA and HHS Regulations
  - The Belmont Report
  - Declaration of Helsinki
  - A Self-Evaluation Checklist for IRBs
  - World Wide Web Sites of Interest for Good Clinical Practice and Clinical Trial Information

Source: FDA

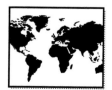

Good Clinical Practices (GCP)

Chapter 6

Recent Developments in GCP Several developments during the late 1990s brought intense scrutiny on all of the key figures involved in the clinical research process, namely whether they were fulfilling their respective roles under GCP and other applicable standards. This scrutiny, particularly the federal government's desire to study and propose action in this area, has not waned in the intervening years, as discussions over possible legislation on human research protections and over revising government guidances on standards for informed consent, clinical trial monitoring, and other GCP areas remain active.

It is important to note, however, that the adequacy of the GCP standards themselves generally was not criticized or questioned because of these developments. More often than not, the discussions have focused not necessarily on developing new standards, but on developing new and clearer guidances to clarify existing standards for those involved in the clinical research process. Still, the developments have had a variety of implications for the FDA's oversight of investigators, sponsors, monitors, and IRBs, particularly as they relate to research subject protection, adverse experience reporting, informed consent, and patient recruitment efforts (see Chapter 14 for a more detailed discussion of these issues):

- In the late 1990s, a series of disclosures shook CDER's confidence in clinical investigators and in the pharmaceutical industry's practices designed to detect investigator noncompliance and even fraud. Chief among these was the case of Southern California Research Institute President and Principal Investigator Robert Fiddes, M.D., who was sentenced in 1998 to 15 months in prison and was fined $800,000 for falsifying and fabricating clinical trial data used in multiple approved NDAs. This case and at least one other like it prompted a series of congressional inquiries into CDER's actions in the Fiddes case, the agency's efforts to detect research fraud and the extent of fraud-related problems in clinical research, the agency's authorities to conduct oversight of, and to discipline, clinical investigators, and the general practices that clinical investigators employ to recruit patients for trials.

- Then, in late 1999, what some FDA officials characterized as "grave and disturbing" clinical investigator noncompliance (e.g., non-reporting of adverse experiences to regulators) in several gene therapy studies, one of which resulted in the well-publicized death of a teenage study participant, galvanized the government to take further action. In May 2000, the FDA and the Department of Health and Human Services (HHS) unveiled a "plan of action" in response to what then-FDA Commissioner Jane Henney, M.D., called the failure of some researchers at prestigious institutions…to follow the most basic elements of what it takes to properly conduct clinical studies." As part of this plan, which seeks to heighten government oversight of clinical research and to reinforce to research institutions their responsibility to oversee their clinical researchers and IRBs, HHS was to pursue legislation authorizing the FDA to levy civil monetary penalties of up to $250,000 per clinical investigator and $1 million per research institution for violations of informed consent and "other important research practices." In addition to this legislative initiative, the FDA/HHS action plan comprised several other moves focusing largely on upgraded training and guidance for clinical investigators: (1) HHS will undertake an "aggressive effort" to improve the education and training of clinical investigators, IRB members, and associated IRB and institutional staff (FDA and NIH will work

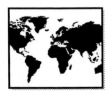

together to ensure that all clinical investigators, research administrators, IRB members and IRB staff receive "appropriate research bioethics training and human subjects research training"); (2) NIH and the FDA will issue specific guidance on informed consent, clarifying that "research institutions and sponsors are expected to audit records for evidence of compliance with informed consent requirements" (for risky or complex trials, IRBs will be expected to take additional measures, which might include requiring third-party observation of the informed consent process); (3) the FDA will issue guidelines for Data and Safety Monitoring Boards (DSMB)—something the agency did in November 2001 (see discussion below)—to define the relationship between DSMBs and IRBs and to establish when DSMBs are appropriate, that they should be independent, and what their responsibilities should be; and (4) the FDA and NIH will develop new conflict of interest policies for the biomedical community, including a requirement "that any researcher's financial interest in a clinical trial be disclosed to potential participants." Although the FDA was in the process of upgrading its informed consent-related and IRB-related guidance documents, by mid-2001 it was facing criticism for not having acted on many of these initiatives, particularly in the informed consent area.

- As the federal government mobilized to respond to the above-mentioned disclosures and perceptions regarding an undermined public confidence in the clinical research process and human subject protections, the NIH and FDA both reorganized to form offices to spearhead initiatives in the human research subject protection area. In March 2001, the FDA formed a GCP-focused office, called the Office of Human Research Trials, within the Office of the FDA Commissioner to coordinate the agency's human subject protection activities and GCP policies, and to direct the agency's international harmonization, outreach and GCP regulation initiatives. Earlier, the NIH's Office for the Protection from Research Risks (OPRR) was renamed the Office for Human Research Protections (OHRP), and was moved to the Department of Heath and Human Services, largely to make the office independent from the NIH-funded studies within its purview. In October 2001, the FDA renamed its Office of Human Research Trials the Office for Good Clinical Practice, in part to differentiate the unit from the NIH's OHRP.

- Beginning in January 1998, CDER's Division of Scientific Investigations (DSI) took steps to examine more closely industry's monitoring practices in a now-completed effort to educate itself about, and establish a baseline of, industry's current monitoring activities. Specifically, all CDER site inspectional assignments contained new instructions for FDA field inspectors to examine specific aspects of sponsor monitoring during inspections of clinical investigators. Further, DSI physicians began to participate in end-of-Phase 2 meetings with sponsors to review and comment on sponsors' planned monitoring and quality assurance programs for Phase 3 trials. Under this pilot program, which was initiated in 1999, DSI hoped to help build quality into the pivotal clinical trial process up front.

- Under a regulation that went into effect in early 1999, CDER now requires NDA sponsors to submit information concerning the financial interests of, and compensation paid to, investigators responsible for key clinical studies. This regulation resulted from concerns regarding the effects of investigators' financial interests on the validity of their research data. When medical reviewers responsible for evaluating NDAs determine that such interests or compensation "raise a serious question about the integrity of the data," CDER can order an audit of the data collected by the clinical investigators in question or take any other action it deems necessary to ensure the data's reliability (see Chapter 7). Reflective of continuing government interest in this area, the Government Accounting Office was developing a report on financial conflict of interest in clinical research after assessing human subject protection issues at several U.S.-based universities.

- In a report entitled, *IRBs: A Time for Reform*, the HHS Inspector General concluded that IRBs are being stretched by the demands and growth of multi-center trials, and that it has become increasingly difficult for IRBs to fulfill their duties. The report, which led to a House subcommittee hearing in mid-1998 and which prompted a follow-up progress report in June 2000 (*Recruiting Human Subjects: Pressures in Industry-Sponsored Clinical Research*), also concluded that the fierce competition for clinical trial participants has promoted the development of recruitment advertising that increasingly presents experimental therapies as proven treatments. In part to implement some of the recommendations in the 1998 HHS report, a House bill entitled the "Human Research Subjects Protection Act" (HR 4605) was introduced in June 2000 but was not passed. This bill would have established standards for IRBs and IRB membership and would have discouraged IRB "shopping" by requiring clinical investigators to disclose prior IRB study protocol rejections. The June 2000 HHS follow-up report focused largely on increasing time-related pressures in the clinical trial process, particularly how such pressures are influencing strategies used to recruit study patients (e.g., enrollment incentives to investigators, referrals, advertising). The HHS encouraged the agency, through its clinicial site inspections, to look into recruitment strategies, particularly the strategies employed by high-enrolling sites.

- In 2000, the HHS and FDA contracted with the Institute of Medicine (IoM) to form an independent panel to examine, and make recommendations for improving, the human subject protection systems in clinical trials. Since beginning its work in December 2000, the panel has issued its first report, which focuses on IRBs and which recommends an accreditation system for such boards. In the second and final phase of its work, the panel is examining other areas, including informed consent, and the work of IRBs and clinical investigators. Its second report, which is expected to include broader recommendations on improving human subject protections in clinical research, is due in September 2002.

Again, while such developments have not changed the core GCP standards, they have certainly helped to sharpen the federal government's focus on human subject protections and CDER's focus on the degree to which sponsors and investigators are fulfilling their responsibilities under GCP requirements.

At this writing, there were multiple pending initiatives and proposals that would affect GCP. For example, the ICH parties were said to be discussing the possibility of harmonizing IRB/ethics committee requirements and standards across the three regions (i.e., U.S., Japan, European Union). In addition, the FDA was considering incorporating into its regulations some of the detailed GCP standards

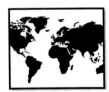

recommended in various guidance documents, including the ICH's Consolidated GCP guidance, as a way to increase industry and investigator awareness of these standards.

International issues stood to affect the GCP area in other ways. A September 2001 HHS report entitled, *The Globalization of Clinical Trials: A Growing Challenge in Protecting Human Subjects* discussed the implications of the ever-increasing number of foreign clinical investigators providing data to be used in NDAs—the number of foreign investigators conducting studies under INDs has grown 16-fold from 1990 to 1999, the report claims. Due to concerns regarding the adequacy of foreign IRBs, and the fact that the FDA's lack of information on foreign IRBs makes it difficult to assure the same level of human subject protections in foreign trials as domestic studies, the HHS report made several recommendations, including that the FDA: (1) work with foreign regulators to obtain more information regarding foreign IRBs; (2) help newly formed foreign IRBs "build capacity" to conduct effective human subject reviews; (3) encourage sponsors to obtain attestations from foreign investigators stating that they will adhere to ethically sound research principles (as is required under IND regulations); (4) encourage more rigorous sponsor monitoring of foreign trials; (5) develop a database to track the growth and location of foreign research; and (6) work with HHS to encourage all IRBs to participate in a voluntary accreditation system.

Responsibilities of the Sponsor

Federal regulations define "sponsor" as "a person who takes responsibility for and initiates a clinical investigation. The sponsor may be an individual or pharmaceutical company, governmental agency, academic institution, private organization, or other organization."

In general, the term "sponsor" refers to a commercial manufacturer that has developed a product in which it holds the principal financial interest. A sponsor may also be a physician, commonly called a "sponsor-investigator," which federal regulations define as "an individual who both initiates and conducts an investigation and under whose immediate direction the investigational drug is administered or dispensed."

The FDA defines sponsor responsibilities in Part 312, Subpart D in the *Code of Federal Regulations* (CFR), which states: "Sponsors are responsible for selecting qualified investigators, providing them with the information they need to conduct an investigation properly, ensuring proper monitoring of the investigation(s), ensuring that the investigation(s) is conducted in accordance with the general investigational plan and protocols contained in the IND, maintaining an effective IND with respect to the investigations, and ensuring that the FDA and all participating investigators are promptly informed of significant new adverse effects or risks with respect to the drug." Sponsor responsibilities can be divided into the following general areas:

- selecting qualified investigators and monitors;
- informing investigators;
- reviewing ongoing studies for compliance with study plans and applicable regulations;
- recordkeeping and record retention; and
- ensuring the return or disposition of unused investigational drug supplies.

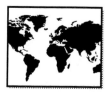

Selecting Investigators and Monitors *Investigator Selection.* The sponsor must select investigators—physicians and other professionals contracted by the sponsor to conduct the clinical study, including supervising the administration of the drug to human subjects—qualified by training and experience as appropriate experts to investigate the drug. Sponsors may ship investigational product only to investigators participating in the investigation (i.e., for studies under an IND, an investigator must have signed a Form FDA-1572 before the sponsor may ship investigational product to the investigator).

To ensure that a clinical investigator is qualified, the sponsor must obtain certain information from the investigator:

- A Completed and Signed Statement of Investigator Form (Form FDA-1572). This form contains information about the investigator, the site of the investigation, and the subinvestigators (e.g., research fellows and residents) who assist the investigator in the conduct of the investigation by directly treating or evaluating study subjects. By signing the form, the investigator also pledges: (1) to conduct the study in accordance with the clinical protocol(s) and to take proper actions should deviations become necessary; (2) to comply with all requirements regarding the obligations of clinical investigators (as described later in this chapter) and other relevant requirements; (3) to personally conduct or supervise the described investigation; (4) to inform patients, or any persons used as controls, that the drug is being used for investigational purposes and to ensure that the requirements related to obtaining informed consent and IRB review and approval (as described elsewhere in this chapter) are met; (5) to report to the sponsor adverse experiences that occur in the course of the investigation in accordance with regulatory requirements; (6) to review and understand the information in the investigator's brochure, including the drug's potential risks and side effects; and (7) to ensure that all associates, colleagues, and employees assisting in the conduct of the studies are informed about their obligations in meeting the above commitments. Through the form, the investigator also pledges that an IRB operating in compliance with regulatory requirements (described later in this chapter) will be responsible for the initial and continuing review and approval of the clinical investigation. In addition, the investigator promises to report to the IRB all changes in the research activity and all unanticipated problems involving risks to human subjects and to not implement any such changes without IRB approval, except when necessary to eliminate apparent immediate hazards to study subjects.

- Curriculum Vitae. The sponsor must obtain a curriculum vitae or other statement of qualifications of the investigator showing the education, training, and experience that qualify the investigator as an expert in the clinical investigation of the drug.

- Clinical Protocol. For Phase 1 investigations, the sponsor must obtain from the investigator a general outline of the planned investigation, including the estimated duration of the study and the maximum number of subjects that will be involved. For Phase 2 or 3 investigations, the sponsor must obtain an outline of the study protocol, including an approximation of the number and characteristics of investigational subjects and controls, the clinical uses to be investigated, the types of clinical observations and laboratory tests to be conducted, the estimated duration of the study, and copies or a description of case report forms to be used.

According to the ICH GCP guideline, the protocol (or other protocol-referenced documents) must identify "any data to be recorded directly on the [subjects' case report forms] (i.e., no prior written or electronic record of data), and to be considered to be source data."

As noted above, a regulation (21 C.F.R. Part 54) that went into effect in early 1999 requires sponsors to collect certain financial information from clinical trial sponsors prior to study initiation. Although this requirement is not considered a factor in determining an investigator's qualifications to participate in a clinical study, the sponsor must collect certain information regarding the investigator's financial interests to permit the company to make a certification or financial disclosure statement in its NDA (see Chapter 7). Specifically, the February 1999 regulations require: (1) that clinical investigators involved in covered clinical studies provide study sponsors with sufficient and accurate financial information to allow a subsequent disclosure or certification by the sponsor; (2) that sponsors maintain complete and accurate records of the financial interests of investigators who are subject to the disclosure regulation; and (3) that applicants submit lists of all clinical investigators who conducted covered clinical studies and that applicants completely and accurately disclose or certify the financial interests of these clinical investigators. Because it addresses potential sources of bias and specifies the above requirements, the FDA's financial disclosure regulation is considered an element of GCP, FDA officials emphasize. To provide further recommendations in this area, the FDA released a March 2001 industry guidance entitled, *Financial Disclosure by Clinical Investigators*.

Selecting Monitors and Monitoring the Clinical Trial. Sponsors are required to monitor clinical investigations to ensure: (1) the quality and integrity of the clinical data derived from clinical trials; and (2) that the rights and welfare of human subjects involved in a clinical study are preserved. The monitoring function may be performed by the sponsor or its employees, or may be delegated to a contract research organization (CRO).

Specific FDA recommendations on proper monitoring duties and procedures are provided in the agency's *Guideline for the Monitoring of Clinical Investigations* (January 1988). In this document, the FDA identifies six different monitoring responsibilities:

- Selection of a Monitor. According to the guideline, a sponsor may designate one or more appropriately trained and qualified individuals to monitor the progress of a clinical investigation. Physicians, clinical research associates, paramedical personnel, nurses, and engineers may be acceptable monitors depending on the type of product involved in the study.

- Written Monitoring Procedures. A sponsor should establish written procedures for monitoring clinical investigations to assure the quality of the study, and to assure that each person involved in the monitoring process carries out his or her duties.

- Preinvestigation Visits. Through personal contact between the monitor and each investigator, a sponsor must assure that the investigator, among other things, clearly understands and accepts the obligations involved in undertaking a clinical study. The sponsor also must determine whether the investigator's facilities are adequate for conducting the investigation, and whether the investigator has sufficient time to honor his or her responsibilities in the trial.

- Periodic Visits. A sponsor must assure, throughout the clinical investigation, that the investigator's obligations are fulfilled and that the facilities used in the clinical investigation are acceptable. The monitor must visit the clinical site frequently enough to provide such assurances. In early 2001, David Lepay, FDA's senior advisor for clinical science and also the director of the FDA's Office for Good Clinical Practice, stated that industry's clinical monitoring efforts should not ignore the trial-related activities of clinical research staff at the various research sites being inspected. Traditionally, sponsor monitoring programs have focused largely on the activities of clinical investigators, he noted.

- Review of Subject Records. A sponsor must assure that safety and effectiveness data submitted to the FDA are accurate and complete. The FDA recommends that the monitor review individual subject records and other supporting documentation and compare these records with the reports prepared by the investigator for submission to the sponsor. The ICH's GCP guideline, which the FDA adopted in 1997, states that the monitor should check "the accuracy and completeness of the [case report form (CRF)] entries, source data/documents and other trial-related records against each other." Specifically, the guideline states that the monitor should verify that: (1) the data required by the protocol are reported accurately on the CRFs and are consistent with the source data/documents; (2) any dose and/or therapy modifications are well documented for each trial subject; (3) adverse events, concomitant medications and intercurrent illnesses are reported in accordance with the protocol on the CRFs; (4) visits that the subjects fail to make, tests that are not conducted, and examinations that are not performed are clearly reported as such on the CRFs; and (5) all withdrawals and dropouts of enrolled subjects from the trial are reported and explained on the CRFs. In many respects, the ICH GCP guideline is considered more comprehensive and detailed than the FDA's *Guideline for the Monitoring of Clinical Investigations*.

- Record of On-Site Visits. The monitor or sponsor should maintain a record of the findings, conclusions, and actions taken to correct deficiencies for each on-site visit.

Informing Investigators The sponsor is responsible for keeping all investigators involved in the clinical testing of its drug fully informed about the investigational product and research findings. Before the investigation begins, a sponsor must supply participating clinical investigators with an investigator's brochure (see Chapter 3), which provides the following: a description of the product; summaries of its known pharmacological, pharmacokinetic, and biological characteristics; potential adverse effects as indicated by animal tests; and, if available, data on clinical use.

Once clinical trials begin, regulations require that sponsors "keep each participating investigator informed of new observations discovered by or reported to the sponsor on the drug, particularly with respect to adverse effects and safe use." This information may be distributed through periodically revised investigator's brochures, reprints or published studies, reports or letters to clinical investigators, or other appropriate means. Safety information must be relayed to all participating investigators and the FDA through written or verbal IND safety reports (see Chapter 3). The sponsor must provide the FDA and all participating investigators a written IND safety report (see Chapter 3) on any adverse experience that is associated with the use of a new drug and that is both serious and unexpected. The sponsor must report any such adverse experience within 15 calendar days of receiving information

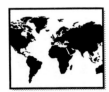

about the experience. If an unexpected adverse drug experience is fatal or life-threatening, the sponsor must also notify the FDA by telephone or facsimile transmission within 7 calendar days.

Review of Ongoing Investigations There are many reasons why the FDA requires sponsors to closely monitor the conduct and progress of their clinical trials. Two of the most important such reasons are to determine whether the investigator is conducting the study in compliance with the protocol, applicable federal regulations, and an acceptable standard of good clinical practice, and whether the new drug study is presenting unreasonable and significant risks to the study subjects.

When a sponsor discovers that an investigator is not in compliance, the company must promptly either secure compliance or discontinue product shipments to the investigator and terminate the investigator's participation in the study. If the latter course is chosen or is necessary, the sponsor must require that the investigator return or dispose of the product in accordance with applicable requirements and must report this action to the FDA. In mid-2001, FDA officials revealed that they were developing a proposed regulation that would require sponsors to report all cases of investigator noncompliance or misconduct, including fraud, data falsification, and human subject protection abuses. Under existing regulations, a sponsor is required to report investigator misconduct only when the investigator is discontinued from a study.

The sponsor must review and evaluate safety and effectiveness data as they are supplied by the investigator. In addition to providing IND safety reports, the sponsor must supply to the FDA annual reports on the progress of the investigation.

Sponsors finding that their drugs or studies present unreasonable and significant risks to subjects must: (1) discontinue the investigations that present the risks; (2) notify the FDA, all IRBs, and all investigators who have at any time participated in the investigations that the studies are being discontinued; (3) assure that the disposition of all outstanding stocks of the drug complies with federal regulations; and (4) furnish the FDA with a full report of its actions.

Recordkeeping and Record Retention A sponsor must maintain adequate records showing the receipt, shipment, or other disposition of the investigational product. The records must include, as appropriate, the name of the investigator to whom the drug is shipped and the date, quantity, and batch or code mark of each shipment. Regulations require that the sponsor retain all specified records and reports for two years after either: (1) the approval of its marketing application; or (2) the discontinuation of drug shipment and delivery and the notification of the FDA.

Disposition of Unused Drug Supplies The sponsor must ensure the return of all unused supplies of the drug from each investigator whose participation is discontinued or eliminated. The sponsor may authorize alternative plans, provided that these do not expose humans to risks from the product. In June 1997, CDER published an updated version of Compliance Policy Guide 7132c.05, entitled, *Recovery of Investigational New Drugs from Clinical Investigators*.

In this and other areas, the ICH GCP guideline provides additional guidance, including the following:

- Recommendations that the sponsor/monitor verify that the disposition of unused investigational product at the trial sites complies with regulatory and sponsor requirements.

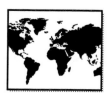

- Recommendations that "electronic trial data handling and/or remote electronic trial data systems" conform to the sponsor's established requirements for completeness, accuracy, reliability, and consistent intended performance (i.e., validation).

- Recommendations that sponsors obtain "all required documentation" (e.g., IRB approval, a signed Form 1572) before providing an investigator with the investigational product. Again, this has been common practice in the United States.

- Recommendations that the sponsor's designated representative document the review and follow-up of the monitoring reports.

Sponsors and Data Safety Monitoring Boards Given the release of new ICH and FDA guidance documents, employing a data safety monitoring board, or what the FDA calls a Data Monitoring Committee, may increasingly be viewed as a GCP-related requirement for certain trials. For many clinical trials, particularly those involving drugs with major public health significance, the responsibility for monitoring comparisons of efficacy and/or safety outcomes should be assigned to an independent and external group often called a data safety monitoring board (DSMB), the ICH's E9 *Statistical Principles for Clinical Trials* guidance states. The guidance, which calls such boards independent data monitoring committees (IDMC), says that such panels "may be established by the sponsor to assess at specific intervals the progress of a clinical trial, safety data, and critical efficacy variables and recommend to the sponsor whether to continue, modify or terminate a trial [based on its findings]."

In a November 2001 draft document entitled, *Guidance for Clinical Trial Sponsors on the Establishment and Operation of Clinical Trial Data Monitoring Committees*, the FDA establishes that data monitoring committees (DMC) should be used in all controlled trials employing mortality or major morbidity as a primary or secondary endpoint. DMCs, the agency notes, may also be useful "in settings where trial participants may be at elevated risk of such outcomes even if the study intervention addresses lesser outcomes such as relief of symptoms." The draft guidance defines DMCs, which the FDA requires only when informed consent requirements are waived in studies conducted in emergency settings, as panels of individuals "with pertinent expertise that review on a regular basis accumulating outcome data in certain ongoing clinical trials [and that] advise the sponsor regarding the continuing safety of current participants and those yet to be recruited, as well as the continuing validity and scientific merit of the trial."

In addition to safety considerations (e.g., mortality/major morbidity endpoints, trials in fragile populations, and large/long-duration/multi-center studies), two other factors—practicality and assurance of scientific validity—are relevant in determining whether a sponsor should establish a DMC for a particular trial, says the agency. A DMC may not be practical, for example, for short-term trials in which the trial duration will not give the committee an opportunity to contribute. If a short-term trial presents important safety considerations that justify a DMC, the guidance says that sponsors must develop mechanisms allowing the committee to be informed and convened rapidly when unexpected results are found.

A DMC's likely ability to assure a trial's scientific validity is the third key consideration, the guidance establishes. Trials "of any appreciable duration," the FDA notes, can be affected by changes over time in the understanding of a disease, the affected population, and standard treatments, all of which are

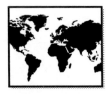

changes that may trigger an interest in study modifications as the trial advances. "When a DMC is the only group reviewing unblinded interim data, the trial organizers are free to make changes in the ongoing trial that may be motivated by newly available data outside the trial or by accumulating data from within the trial (e.g., overall event rates)," the guidance states. "In general, recommendations to change the inclusion criteria, the trial endpoints, or the size of the trial are most credibly made by those without knowledge of the accumulating data. When the trial organizers are the ones reviewing the interim data, their awareness of interim comparative results cannot help but affect their determination as to whether these changes should be made. Such changes would inevitably impair the credibility of the study results."

For these reasons and others, the draft guidance touts the advantages of the *independent* DMC, which is defined as "a committee whose members are considered to be independent of those sponsoring, organizing, and conducting the trial" (i.e., have no previous involvement in the trial's design, no current involvement in its conduct other than as the DMC, and have no financial or other important connections to the study sponsor or other trial organizers). A DMC will be considered independent, for example, if the sponsor has no representation on the committee or if the sponsor has a representative only in open meetings, during which enrollment, compliance, and event rates are presented and discussed but during which no study arm-specific data are discussed. The draft guidance acknowledges that DMCs are rarely, if ever, entirely independent of sponsors, given that sponsors typically select and pay the members and establish a committee's goals and responsibilities.

The independence of other individuals interacting with both the sponsor and DMC is equally important, the FDA states. Trial integrity is best maintained when the statistician preparing unblinded data (i.e., interim analyses) for the DMC is external to the sponsor, especially for studies designed to provide the definitive evidence of efficacy, the draft guidance notes. The statistician should have no responsibility for managing the trial and should have "minimal" contact with those who have such involvement.

Responsibilities of Investigators

A clinical investigator is the individual who actually conducts, or who is the responsible leader of a team that conducts, a clinical investigation. The product is administered or dispensed to a clinical subject under the immediate direction of this individual.

Federal regulations state that an "investigator is responsible for ensuring that an investigation is conducted according to the signed investigator statement, the investigational plan, and applicable regulations; for protecting the rights, safety, and welfare of subjects under the investigator's care; and for the control of drugs under investigation." As part of the investigator's responsibilities in protecting the rights of study subjects, he or she must obtain legally effective informed consents from prospective subjects or their legally authorized representatives prior to involving these subject in a clinical study. Specific investigator responsibilities detailed in GCP provisions include the following:

Control of the Product. The investigator can administer the product only to subjects under his or her personal supervision or under the supervision of a subinvestigator. Regulations do not allow an investigator to supply the drug to persons not authorized to receive it.

Recordkeeping and Record Retention. The investigator must keep adequate drug accountability records, and must prepare and maintain, for each subject, adequate and accurate records of all observations and data pertinent to the investigation. These records must be kept for two years after either a marketing application's approval or a sponsor has discontinued an IND and so notified the FDA. The FDA must be allowed access to these records.

The ICH GCP guideline calls for the investigator to maintain a list of appropriately qualified persons to whom significant trial-related responsibilities have been delegated. In addition, the ICH GCP guideline calls for clinical sites to maintain, and sponsors to document the existence of, a confidential list of the names of all subjects allocated to trial numbers upon trial enrollment.

Investigator Reports. The investigator must provide to the sponsor: (1) reports (e.g., up-to-date CRFs) on the progress of the clinical study; (2) safety reports on all adverse experiences that may reasonably be regarded as caused by, or probably caused by, the drug; and (3) adequate reports shortly after the completion of the investigator's participation in the study—FDA officials indicate that completed case report forms on all subjects usually will suffice. As mentioned above, the FDA has been under some pressure to clarify, and educate clinical investigators on, clinical trial adverse experience reporting requirements following disclosures that certain investigators participating in several gene therapy trials failed to fulfill their responsibilities in this area (see discussion above).

Assurance of IRB Review. The investigator must assure that an IRB complying with regulatory requirements will be responsible for the initial and continuing review and approval of the proposed clinical study. He or she must also promptly report to the IRB all changes in the research activity and all unanticipated problems involving risks to human subjects. The investigator must not make any changes in the research without IRB approval, except when necessary to eliminate apparent and immediate hazards to human subjects.

Handling of Controlled Substances. If the investigational product is subject to the Controlled Substances Act, the investigator must take adequate precautions to prevent theft or diversion of the product.

The Institutional Review Board (IRB)

Except under limited circumstances (e.g., emergency use of a drug or when the FDA exempts a study from IRB review), no clinical study that requires prior agency review (i.e., under an IND) may be initiated unless that study has been reviewed and approved by, and remains subject to continuing review by, an IRB. The IRB's function is to see, through prior and periodic review, that: (1) risks to subjects are minimized and are reasonable in relation to any anticipated benefits to subjects; (2) selection of subjects is equitable; (3) informed consent is sought and documented in accordance with federal regulations; (4) adequate monitoring is provided to ensure subject safety; (5) subjects' confidentiality is adequately protected; and (6) safeguards are provided to protect the rights and welfare of vulnerable subjects. Although the board's main concern is not the adequacy of study design, the board can order that a trial be modified for safety or other reasons.

An IRB must have at least five members, each of whom is chosen by the institution (i.e., assuming that the site has an IRB). FDA regulations allow institutions that do not have IRBs to use "independent" or other institutions' IRBs to review their studies. IRB members must have the professional

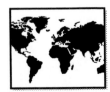

backgrounds necessary to review research activities commonly undertaken by the institution, and have the ability to assess the acceptability of proposed research in terms of institutional commitments and regulations, applicable law, and standards and practices.

IRB members often are physicians, pharmacologists, clergy, and administrative managers from the parent institution. At least one board member must have a primary interest in a nonscientific area. Federal regulations also include several other requirements that are designed to ensure the independence of the IRB and guard against conflicts of interest.

Generally, drug sponsors have limited direct contact with an IRB. The investigator conducting the study at a particular institution usually serves as a liaison between the sponsor and the IRB, and presents the study plans to the IRB for review and approval. Since experienced investigators are often familiar with the particular concerns and priorities of their IRBs, they are often better prepared to deal with them. The FDA does not prohibit direct sponsor-IRB contact, and acknowledges that such contact may help resolve problems in certain cases.

Aside from safety concerns, an IRB may address several issues—including specific standards of the institution, state, and locality—in reviewing a study. To fulfill its responsibilities, an IRB will review research protocols and related materials, including informed consent documents and investigator brochures. Any research program that the board approves must meet several criteria specified in FDA regulations:

- risks to subjects must be minimized;
- risks to subjects must be reasonable in relation to the anticipated benefits and the importance of the knowledge that may be expected to be gained;
- subject selection must be equitable;
- informed consent must be sought from each prospective subject or the subject's legally authorized representative;
- informed consent must be appropriately documented (see discussion below);
- when appropriate, the research plan must make adequate provisions for monitoring the data collected to ensure the safety of subjects; and
- when appropriate, there must be adequate provisions to protect the privacy of subjects and to preserve the confidentiality of data.

As are sponsors, monitors, and investigators, IRBs are subject to operating, reporting, and record-keeping requirements. An IRB must retain adequate minutes of its meetings and copies of all study proposals reviewed, sample approved consent documents, correspondence with investigators, board procedures, and other documents. IRB meeting minutes and records are subject to FDA inspection, and an IRB under FDA jurisdiction may be subject to administrative action for failing to comply with federal regulations.

As noted above, IRBs are finding it increasingly difficult to fulfill all of their responsibilities due to the increasing demands being placed on them. This difficulty caused concern about possible safety and welfare risks to study subjects and prompted government studies, hearings, and proposals in the late

1990s. Although no substantive improvements were made by late 2001, federal officials were continuing to evaluate ways to make IRB workloads more manageable. One of the proposals under evaluation involves reducing the adverse experience-related paperwork that IRBs face.

One proposal that has been implemented is the reorganization of the National Institutes of Health's (NIH) Office for the Protection from Research Risks (OPRR). In June 2000, the office was renamed the Office for Human Research Protections (OHRP), and was moved from the NIH to the office of the HHS assistant secretary for health, largely to make the office independent from the NIH-funded studies within its purview. The OHRP is spearheading the HHS "plan of action" (see discussion above) regarding investigators and IRBs (e.g., new educational programs). With OHRM, the FDA is pursuing the development of a public IRB registry in a consolidated web-based system.

Informed Consent

Informed consent is a concept or process designed to ensure that subjects do not enter a clinical study against their will or without an adequate understanding of the study or the risks involved in the study. Federal regulations require that, except under special circumstances, "...no investigator may involve a human being as a subject in research...unless the investigator has obtained the legally effective informed consent of the subject or the subject's legally authorized representative. An investigator shall seek such consent only under circumstances that provide the prospective subject or the representative sufficient opportunity to consider whether or not to participate and that minimize the possibility of coercion or undue influence. The information that is given to the subject or the representative shall be in language understandable to the subject or the representative."

Clearly, informed consent is a function of an informed subject. Any subject volunteering for a study must be adequately aware of his or her medical condition, alternative treatments, and the purpose of and risks involved in the clinical study.

As noted, upgrading the informed consent process has been a centerpiece of the federal government's efforts to improve the subject protection aspects of clinical research. In late 2001, the FDA was revising its guidance on informed consent to better focus the process on helping subjects understand issues related to the trial and their participation rather than just the mechanical documentation of informed consent itself. Further, as part of its May 2000 "plan of action" on research subject protection, the FDA and NIH announced that they would issue specific guidance on informed consent, clarifying that "research institutions and sponsors are expected to audit records for evidence of compliance with informed consent requirements" (for "risky" or "complex" trials, IRBs will be expected to take additional measures, which might include requiring third-party observation of the informed consent process). In mid-2001, the Government Accounting Office (GAO) criticized the FDA and HHS for not having released new guidance on informed consent, however.

Federal regulations regarding the protection of clinical subjects state that, at a minimum, the following "basic elements of informed consent" must be provided to clinical subjects before involving them in the study:

- a statement that the study involves research, an explanation of the purposes of the research and the expected duration of the subject's participation, a descrip-

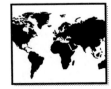

tion of the procedures to be followed, and identification of any procedures that are experimental;

- a description of any reasonably foreseeable risks or discomforts to the subject;
- a description of any benefits that the subject or others may reasonably expect from the research;
- a disclosure of appropriate alternative procedures or courses of treatment, if any, that might be advantageous to the subject;
- a statement that describes the extent, if any, to which confidentiality of records identifying the subject will be maintained and that notes the possibility that the FDA may inspect the records;
- an explanation as to whether any compensation or medical treatments are available if injury occurs during research involving more than minimal risk, and, if so, what the treatments and/or compensation consist of, or where further information may be obtained;
- the identity of the person to contact for answers to pertinent questions about the research and research subject's rights, and the person to contact if the subject suffers a research-related injury; and
- a statement that participation is voluntary, that refusal to participate will involve no penalty or loss of benefits to which the subject is otherwise entitled, and that the subject may discontinue participation at any time without penalty or loss of benefits to which the subject is otherwise entitled.

When appropriate, one or more of the following must also be provided to subjects:

- a statement that a particular treatment or procedure may involve risks to the subject (or to the embryo or fetus, if the subject is or may become pregnant) that are currently unforeseeable;
- anticipated circumstances under which the subject's participation may be terminated by the investigator without regard to the subject's consent;
- any additional costs to the subject that may result from participation in the research;
- the consequences of a subject's decision to withdraw from the research and procedures for ordering termination of participation by the subject;
- a statement that significant new research findings that may affect the subject's willingness to continue his or her participation will be provided to the subject; and
- the approximate number of subjects involved in the study.

While the investigator is directly responsible for obtaining a subject's informed consent and seeing that the subject is truly informed, the IRB and the sponsor/monitor also play roles in ensuring that informed consent requirements are met.

In most cases, informed consent must be obtained by having the subject or the subject's representative sign a written, IRB-approved consent form. Except in the case of FDA-approved "emergency

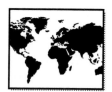

research" (see discussion below), the IRB cannot waive informed consent requirements for FDA-regulated research. Unless the IRB waives the informed consent requirements due to minimal risk, the consent form may take one of two forms: (1) a written consent document that embodies the basic elements of informed consent and that may be read to the subject or the subject's representative, who is then given adequate opportunity to read it before signing; or (2) a "short form" written consent document stating that the basic elements of informed consent have been presented orally to the subject or the subject's representative. If the short form is used, there are several other requirements: there must be a witness to the oral presentation; the IRB must approve a written summary of what will be said to the subject or the representative; the witness must sign both the short form and a copy of the summary; the person obtaining the consent must sign a copy of the summary; and the subject or the representative must sign the short form and must be given a copy of the summary and the consent form.

The FDA notes, however, that the subject's signature, although it provides documentation of his or her agreement to participate in the study, is representative of a larger process. "The entire informed consent process involves giving a subject adequate information concerning the study, providing adequate opportunity for the subject to consider all options, responding to the subject's questions, ensuring that the subject has comprehended this information, obtaining the subject's voluntary agreement to participate, and continuing to provide information as the subject or situation requires," the agency states in its *Guidance for Institutional Review Boards and Clinical Investigators* (1998). "To be effective, the process should provide ample opportunity for the investigator and the subject to exchange information and ask questions."

In late 1996, the FDA issued two final rules that revised its informed consent regulations. The first of these was published in October 1996 and was designed to permit the emergency use of experimental products without prior informed consent. This exception is permitted only for research involving subjects who require emergency medical intervention, who cannot give informed consent due to a life-threatening condition, and who do not have a legally authorized representative available before the drug must be administered. The FDA has established clear and significant regulatory burdens regarding this waiver of informed consent requirements, including special criteria for IRB review and a requirement for the sponsor to submit the study protocol and related materials under a separate IND, even if one is already in place for studies utilizing the conventional consent process. To provide recommendations in this area, CDER released an April 2000 draft guidance entitled, *Guidance for Institutional Review Boards, Clinical Investigators, and Sponsors: Exemption from Informed Consent Requirements for Emergency Research.*

Under changes implemented in December 1996, the FDA revised its informed consent regulations to require that the informed consent form be signed and dated by the subject or the subject's legally authorized representative at the time consent is given. The agency also clarified what adequate case histories must include and that the case histories must document that informed consent was obtained prior to a subject's participation in a study. The agency took this action in response to problems that the FDA has had in verifying that informed consent actually preceded subject participation.

CHAPTER 7

The New Drug Application (NDA)

Since 1938, the new drug application (NDA) has been the vehicle through which drug sponsors formally propose that the FDA approve a new pharmaceutical for marketing and sale in the United States. To obtain this government authorization, a drug manufacturer submits in an NDA thousands of pages of nonclinical and clinical test data and analyses, drug chemistry information, and descriptions of manufacturing procedures in a specific, and fairly well-defined, format that had been revised and refined over the past six decades.

By mid-2001, however, the International Conference on Harmonization (ICH) initiative had produced what many viewed as its most significant achievement: a harmonized core "information package of [clinical, pharmacology/toxicology, and manufacturing] technical data" that could be submitted in the same format and with the same content to obtain marketing authorization in any of the three ICH regions—the United States, the European Union, and Japan. In August 2001, the ICH's "common technical document," or CTD, formally became a regulatory option to the NDA for companies seeking FDA approval of a new drug.

During a "transition period" that will last until July 2003, companies will have the option of submitting original NDAs and even NDA supplements and amendments in either the CTD or conventional NDA format. Beginning in July 2003, the FDA will "highly recommend" that U.S. marketing dossiers be submitted in the CTD format, although the agency will not be able to implement this as a formal requirement until it undertakes a complete revision of its NDA regulations (CFR Part 314).

It is important to note that the CTD and NDA differ primarily in format and not in content. While it is true that the CTD may provide more information in selected areas than a conventional NDA (see discussion below), the FDA's data and information requirements for drug approval will be unaffected by the CTD. In other words, applications in the CTD format must provide the same data and information as those submitted in the conventional NDA format. In many ways, the CTD simply represents, for now, an alternative format or organizational structure into which data and information that otherwise would be provided in the NDA format can be provided to the FDA. For a detailed review of the CTD and the CTD format, see exhibit below.

Even as they were taking their first steps to implement the new CTD model, both the FDA and industry were anxiously looking ahead to, and preparing for, the next evolutionary stage for marketing dossiers internationally. In many ways, industry and the FDA were looking at the paper-based CTD model simply as a bridging mechanism to the electronic CTD, or eCTD, on which the ICH parties were

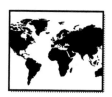

Worldwide Pharmaceutical Regulation Series

busily working and which would dovetail with the FDA's own efforts to move toward electronic NDAs (see discussion below). Although the FDA's August 2001 draft guidance on the CTD emphasizes that the agency will release a guidance when it is prepared to accept electronic submissions in the CTD format, it also noted that industry will, in the interim, be permitted to "adapt the CTD to our current process for electronic submissions...." Meanwhile, following the May 2001 release of a Step 2 eCTD specification, the FDA issued various documents and tools that will, when the eCTD is implemented formally, assist industry in developing Module 1 (the portion specific to the United States) of the eCTD, including a regional DTD for Module 1 and a sample submission in eCTD format.

While fully recognizing the CTD's importance in the future, this chapter focuses largely, but not exclusively, on the conventional NDA. The NDA remains, at this writing and likely for some time into the future, the more frequently used vehicle for obtaining marketing approval in the United States. Since NDA-related requirements are better understood and more defined in current FDA regulations and guidances, and since these requirements must be met by applications regardless of whether they are provided in the CTD or NDA format, such an approach seems wise at this time. For a detailed discussion of the CTD, its format, and its future, see the exhibit below.

Traditionally a paper colossus, the NDA is the largest and most complex premarketing application that the FDA reviews. Given the demands that assembling this regulatory tome put on industry and the demands that reviewing them put on the FDA, there have been some recent efforts attempting to reduce the NDA's size. Under the Food and Drug Administration Modernization Act of 1997, for instance, CDER released a guidance entitled, *Submission of Abbreviated Reports and Synopses in Support of Marketing Applications*, which clarified when NDA sponsors may submit certain clinical trial information in abbreviated reports and synopses rather than full study reports.

Emerging data suggest that NDA size now might be decreasing due to the increasing efficiency of clinical development programs, something that is resulting in fewer and smaller clinical trials for each new drug. A CMR International survey of 14 leading drug companies found that the mean number of trials in 21 marketing dossiers declined from 45 in 1995/1996 to 20 in 1998/1999. At the same time, however, those studying such trends warn that they are accompanied by increasing complexity due to such factors as the need to undertake trials for special patient populations (see discussion below), and that the numbers of subjects enrolled in clinical trials have not declined. A PAREXEL International study of 16 of the 27 NMEs approved by the FDA in 2000 showed that the clinical programs for the approved drugs enrolled a median of 3,840 patients compared to 5,435 for NMEs approved in 1999.

Regardless of its format, size, or complexity, an NDA or CTD must provide sufficient information, data, and analyses to permit FDA reviewers to reach several key decisions, including:

1. Whether the drug is safe and effective in its proposed use(s), and whether the benefits of the drug outweigh its risks.

2. Whether the drug's proposed labeling is appropriate and, if not, what the drug's labeling should contain.

3. Whether the methods used in manufacturing the drug and the controls used to maintain the drug's quality are adequate to preserve the drug's identity, strength, quality, and purity.

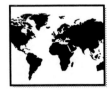

The ICH's Common Technical Document

In mid-1997, the ICH parties agreed to begin work on a project called the common technical document (CTD), what was easily the harmonization program's most ambitious undertaking. The FDA characterized the CTD as "an information package of [clinical, nonclinical, and manufacturing] technical data, in the same format and with the same content, that would be submitted for registering new drugs in all three ICH regions—the United States, the European Union, and Japan." During the CTD's development, the ICH parties noted that the document's common format for an application's technical documentation will "significantly reduce the time and resources needed to compile applications for registration of human pharmaceuticals and will ease the preparation of electronic submissions," while the CTD's "common elements" will facilitate regulatory reviews and applicant/regulator communications and simplify the exchange of regulatory information between regulatory authorities.

Without question, the pharmaceutical industry entered a new and important phase of its history during 2001, when the new CTD format formally became a regulatory option for registering products in the three ICH regions. In the United States, a "transition period" during which the FDA will accept marketing dossiers in either the CTD or conventional NDA format kicked off in August 2001, with the FDA's release of a draft guidance entitled, *Submitting Marketing Applications According to the ICH-CTD Format—General Considerations*. The CTD transition period will last until July 2003, when the use of the CTD format will be "highly recommended" within the United States. Unlike Japan and the European Union, the United States will not mandate the CTD's use in July 2003. To make the CTD a formal requirement, the FDA will have to revamp its NDA regulations, a process that could take years.

The CTD itself provides an optional format in which applicants can submit the data necessary in the marketing dossier, and does not modify the required data and information content for conventional NDAs or the standards traditionally applicable to new drug approval in the United States. The CTD represents a largely harmonized outline or format, although it is designed to accommodate regional differences in submission requirements in several areas.

As the detailed outline below indicates, the CTD format itself comprises five modules: Module 1: Administrative and Prescribing Information, which contains forms and documents specific to each region; Module 2: Common Technical Document Summaries; Module 3: Quality; Module 4: Nonclinical Study Reports; and Module 5: Clinical Study Reports.

To specify the requirements for each section of the CTD, the FDA has released a series of ICH guidances: *Submitting Marketing Applications According to the ICH-CTD Format—General Considerations*, which provides the FDA's recommendations for the U.S.-specific requirements for Module 1; M4: *Organization of the CTD*; M4Q: *The CTD—Quality*; M4S: *The CTD—Safety*; M4E: *The CTD—Efficacy*; and M4S—*The Safety Appendices*.

During the roughly two-year CTD transition period, the FDA will be encouraging CTD submissions in an effort to gain some badly needed experience with the new dossier format. The real-world experience gained during this all-too-brief period will indicate what modifications, if any, might be necessary before the next phase of the CTD's implementation begins in July 2003.

—continued—

The New Drug Application (NDA)

Chapter 7

Worldwide Pharmaceutical Regulation Series

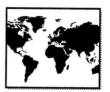

The New Drug Application (NDA)

Chapter 7

Diagrammatic Representation of the CTD

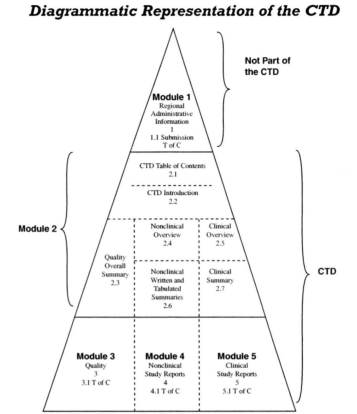

Organization of the CTD: The General Outline*
(Step 4 Guidance)

Module 1: Administrative Information and Prescribing Information

    1.1 Table of Contents of the Submission including Module 1

    1.2 Documents Specific to Each Region (e.g., application forms, prescribing information)

Module 2: Common Technical Document Summaries

    2.1 CTD Table of Contents

    2.2 CTD Introduction

    2.3 Quality Overall Summary

    2.4 Nonclinical Overview

    2.5 Clinical Overview

    2.6 Nonclinical Written and Tabulated Summary
        Pharmacology
        Pharmacokinetics
        Toxicology

    2.7 Clinical Summary
        Biophamaceutics and Associated Analytical Methods

        Clinical Pharmacology Studies
        Clinical Efficacy
        Clinical Safety
        Synopses of Individual Studies

Module 3: Quality

    3.1 Module 3 Table of Contents

    3.2 Body of Data

    3.3 Literature References

Module 4: Nonclinical Study Reports

    4.1 Module 4 Table of Contents

    4.2 Study Reports

    4.3 Literature References

Module 5: Clinical Study Reports

    5.1 Module 5 Table of Contents

    5.2 Tabular Listing of All Clinical Studies

    5.3 Clinical Study Reports

    5.4 Literature References

*a more detailed version of this general outline appears below

—continued—

—continued—

New Drug Approval in the United States

Chapter 7: The New Drug Application (NDA)

Organization of the CTD
(Composite CTD Outline Developed from Various FDA/ICH Guidances)

Module 1: Administrative Information and Prescribing Information* (for U.S. Submissions)

Cover Letter (if applicant wants to submit one, it should be placed here).

FDA Form 356h.

Comprehensive Table of Contents for the Submission Including Module 1. This should include a complete list of all documents provided in the submission, and should specify the location of each document by referring to volume numbers and tab identifiers.

Administrative Documents:

    a. Administrative Documents (e.g., field copy certification, debarment certification)

    b. Prescribing Information (all copies of the labels and all product labeling)

    c. Annotated Labeling Text for NDAs (or labeling comparison for ANDAs).

Module 2: Common Technical Document Summaries

2.1 CTD Table of Contents

2.2 CTD Introduction. This should be "a general introduction to the pharmaceutical, including its pharmacologic class, mode of action, and proposed clinical use. In general, the introduction should not exceed one page."

2.3 Quality Overall Summary. Following the scope and outline of the "Body of Data" in Module 3, the quality overall summary (QOS) should include sufficient information for each section of Module 3 to provide the quality reviewer with an overview of that module. The QOS "should also emphasize critical key parameters of the product and provide, for instance, justification in cases where guidance was not followed... [and] should include a discussion of key issues that integrates information from sections in the Quality module [Module 3] and supporting information from other modules (e.g., qualification of impurities by toxicological studies discussed under the M4S module), including cross-referencing to volume and page numbers in other modules." Generally, the QOS should not exceed 40 pages of text, excluding tables and figures, or 80 pages for biotech products and other products with more complex manufacturing processes.

2.4 Nonclinical Overview. The nonclinical overview, which generally should not exceed 30 pages, should present an integrated and critical assessment of the drug's pharmacologic, pharmacokinetic, and toxicologic evaluation. In contrast to the nonclinical written and tabulated summary, which should be a factual synopsis, the nonclinical overview should provide an interpretation of the nonclinical data, discuss the clinical relevance of the findings, cross-link with the quality aspects of the pharmaceutical, and discuss the implications of the nonclinical findings for the safe use of the drug. It should also discuss and justify the nonclinical testing strategy.

2.5 Clinical Overview. The clinical overview, which should be relatively brief (30 pages, although its length will depend on the application's complexity), should provide a critical analysis of the CTD's clinical data. Although it should refer to data provided in the comprehensive clinical summary, the individual clinical study reports, and other relevant reports, the clinical overview should primarily present the conclusions and implications of those data and should not recapitulate them. In contrast to the clinical summary (see Section 2.7 below), which provides a detailed factual summarization of the CTD's clinical information, the clinical overview should provide "a succinct discussion and interpretation of these findings

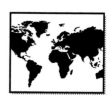

Worldwide Pharmaceutical Regulation Series

together with any other relevant information (e.g., pertinent animal data or product quality issues that may have clinical implications)." In other words, the clinical summary focuses on factual summarization, while the clincial overview focuses on critical analysis and interpretation. Specifically, the clinical overview should: (1) present the strengths and limitations of the development program and study results; (2) analyze the benefits and risks of the medicinal product in its intended use; and (3) describe how the study results support critical parts of the prescribing information.

2.6 Nonclinical Written and Tabulated Summaries.** The primary purpose of the nonclinical written and tabulated summaries is to provide a comprehensive, factual synopsis of the nonclinical data. Because, in some ICH regions, "a review of the Tabulated Summaries (in conjunction with the Written Summaries) represents the primary review of the nonclinical information," the M4S: *The* CTD—*Safety* guidance emphasizes that data presentations in the formats provided as templates and examples "should ensure that a sufficient level of detail is available to the reviewer and should provide concise overviews of related information." In the three written summaries within this section, the applicant should summarize and evaluate the various nonclinical pharmacology, pharmacokinetic, and toxicology studies. The fifth CTD guidance, M4S: *The* CTD—*Safety Appendices*, provides examples of tables and figures for the written summaries, and templates and examples of tables that comprise the three nonclinical tabulated summaries.

    2.6.1 Introduction

    2.6.2 Pharmacology Written Summary

    2.6.3 Pharmacology Tabulated Summary

    2.6.4 Pharmacokinetics Written Summary

    2.6.5 Pharmacokinetics Tabulated Summary

    2.6.6 Toxicology Written Summary

    2.6.7 Toxicology Tabulated Summary

2.7 Clinical Summary.** As noted above, the clinical summary should provide a detailed, factual summarization of all clinical information in the CTD, including clinical study reports, meta-analyses or other cross-study analyses for which full reports have been included in Module 5 (clinical study reports), and postmarketing data for products marketed in other regions. The comparisons and analyses of cross-study results should "focus on factual observations," the CTD guidance documents emphasize. The clinical summary will typically range from 50 to 400 pages (excluding attached tables), although the CTD guidance notes that its size will vary substantially based on the information conveyed.

    Biopharmaceutics and Associated Analytical Methods

    Clinical Pharmacology Studies

    Clinical Efficacy

    Clinical Safety

    Synopses of Individual Studies

Module 3: Quality

As it does for the QOS, the M4Q:*The* CTD—*Quality* establishes the Module 3 format for drug substances and drug products, and for biotech products. The guidance is careful to note that, while

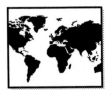

"the content of [Module 3's] sections should include relevant information described in existing ICH guidances,…harmonized content is not available for all sections… Neither the type nor extent of specific supporting data has been addressed…, and both may depend on regional guidance."

    3.1 Module 3 Table of Contents

    3.2 Body of Data. Beyond the fact that this section represents the core of the module, Module 3's Body of Data section is interesting for at least a few reasons. First, it includes the Pharmaceutical Development section (3.2.P.2), which FDA officials have maintained is the CTD's most notable quality- or manufacturing-related departure from traditional NDA submissions. This section, which derives from the development pharmaceutics section in European marketing dossiers, to some degree provides a history of a drug's chemical development and the company's rationale for choosing certain developmental paths (e.g., dosage forms, excipients). In addition, this section includes Section 3.2.R, in which sponsors should provide non-harmonized region-specific information. For U.S. submissions, for example, this would include executed batch records, the methods validation package, and comparability protocols.

    3.3 Literature References

Module 4: Nonclinical Study Reports

    4.1 Module 4 Table of Contents

    4.2 Study Reports

    4.3 Literature References

Module 5: Clinical Study Reports

    5.1 Module 5 Table of Contents

    5.2 Tabular Listing of All Clinical Studies

    5.3 Clinical Study Reports. In addition to the clinical study reports, this section should include the integrated analysis of safety summary (ISS) and integrated efficacy summary (ISE), if they are to be included as separate elements of a CTD to be submitted in the United States. Although neither the ISS or ISE are required elements in the CTD, companies can submit them if that is the applicant's preference, or when the information in these analyses are too voluminous to include within the page-count limitations of the clinical overview and summary.

    5.4 Literature References

*Although the CTD guidances specify a format and document sequence for Module 1, the individual regions dictate what information is to be included in this module and how it is to be presented. Therefore, standards for Module 1 in the United States are provided in the FDA's *Submitting Marketing Applications According to the* ICH-CTD *Format—General Considerations*. Because of this, the sequencing and numbering of Module 1 as presented above reflects the format specified in FDA's *General Considerations* guidance and not the somewhat different outline in the Step 4 CTD guidances.

**Although the CTD guidance says that "applicants should not modify the overall organization of the CTD," it adds that, "however, in the Nonclinical and Clinical Summaries sections of the CTD, applicants can modify individual formats to provide the best possible presentation of the technical information to facilitate the understanding and evaluation of the results."

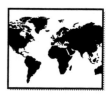

The New Drug Application (NDA)

Chapter 7

The History of the NDA

Given its importance in the drug approval process, the NDA is, as it has always been, a product and a reflection of intersecting medical, political, industry, and public healthcare objectives, priorities, and needs. Because of this, the NDA has evolved considerably during its 62-year history.

For decades, the regulation and control of new drugs in the United States has been based on the NDA. Since 1938, each new drug must have been the subject of an NDA before it could be, for commercial purposes, sold in or imported to the United States.

When the Food, Drug and Cosmetic Act (FD&C Act) was passed in 1938, NDAs were required only to contain information pertaining to the investigational drug's safety. In 1962, the Harris-Kefauver Amendments to the FD&C Act required NDAs to provide evidence that a new drug was effective in its intended use as well. These historic amendments also required, for the first time, that an NDA be approved before a drug could be marketed.

The NDA was again the subject of reform in 1985, when the FDA completed a comprehensive revision of the regulations pertaining to new drug applications. While this revision, commonly called the NDA Rewrite, modified NDA content requirements, it was mainly designed to expedite FDA reviews by restructuring the ways in which information and data were organized and presented in the application.

At this writing, there were several significant regulatory developments that had recently contributed, or were about to contribute, to the continuing evolution of the NDA:

- As noted, CDER continues to lay the regulatory groundwork for computer-assisted new drug applications, or electronic NDAs (eNDA), to replace the paper-based NDA—that is, in those cases in which sponsors want to use an electronic submission in lieu of the hardcopy alternative. This process began with the release of a March 1997 final regulation, which established the agency's criteria for accepting electronic records, including eNDAs, and electronic signatures as equivalent to paper records and handwritten signatures (previously, electronic records and submissions could only supplement paper-based records and filings, which were required by regulation). The migration to electronic submissions is expected to accelerate going forward: Under PDUFA II commitments, the FDA agreed to develop a paperless, electronic application submission system for all applications, including INDs and NDAs, by fiscal year 2002. With the March 1997 final regulation in place, CDER is making various types of applications (e.g., INDs and NDAs) formally eligible for electronic submission by publishing guidances that address each type of submission. At this writing, CDER had released a handful of formal guidances and related documents applicable to electronic NDAs: *Regulatory Submissions in Electronic Format: General Considerations* (January 1999), which discusses general issues associated with electronic submissions, including the formats in which certain data should be provided and the types of media that should be used; *Regulatory Submissions in Electronic Format: New Drug Applications* (January 1999), which provides recommendations for providing the complete archival copy of the NDA in electronic format (see discussion below); and *Example of an Electronic New Drug Application Submission* (February 1999). These guidances established CDER's willingess to accept certain elements of the NDA in electronic-only form: the complete archival copy of

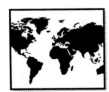

the NDA, Section 11 (case report tabulations), and Section 12 (case report forms). While these documents address the archival NDA copy, they do not fully address the review copies of the NDA submission (the technical sections actually evaluated by CDER reviewers). CDER officials point out that, since drug reviewers can waive the requirement for paper-based review copies of the NDA (the above-mentioned guidances already establish that some review-copy elements can be submitted electronically), fully electronic NDAs are possible today. The only elements of the NDA that cannot be submitted electronically are those forms requiring original signatures, they note. Since the publication of the NDA-related guidances, the numbers of eNDAs submitted and the numbers of companies developing them have increased markedly. Of the first 61 original NDAs submitted in FY2001, for example, 35 percent (21 applications) were fully electronic (i.e., the complete archival copy in electronic format) and another 36 percent were mixed paper/electronic submissions. In eNDAs, text-based documents are submitted as PDF files, while datasets are provided in SAS transport file format. CDER officials claim to be considering new regulations to require electronic submissions in the future due to the high costs of maintaining dual electronic and paper-based review systems.

- In 2000, industry experts were beginning to speak of a consensus that NDAs may be becoming smaller due to more efficient and focused drug development programs, and the fewer clinical trials that were being conducted as part of such programs. A CMR International study of 21 submissions developed by 14 leading drug firms revealed that the mean number of trials decreased from 45 in 1995-1996 to 20 in 1998-1999. Experts point out, however, that regulatory dossiers also may be more complex today, given such factors as the need to address pharmacoeconomic issues and to test in special populations (e.g., elderly, children). Further, an increasing focus on drug safety in the United States—which is, in part, a product of a spate of drug withdrawals in the late 1990s—has the potential to reverse the trends that may be leading to smaller NDAs. In 2001, in fact, there were several reports of major drug companies delaying their NDA submissions to conduct additional safety studies following the completion of their pivotal efficacy studies. Typically, these studies were designed to further characterize drug effects and safety issues that had been spotlighted by regulators due to recent withdrawals and advances in medical knowledge (e.g., liver toxicity, QTc prolongation).

- In August 1997, the FDA made a controversial proposal that companies submitting NDAs for new drugs that are considered "therapeutically important and/or likely to be used in children" provide pediatric clinical study data to support pediatric use at the time of, or soon after, approval. Subsequently, the agency published a December 1998 final rule "that created a presumption" that all new drugs would be studied in pediatric patients, but that allowed manufacturers to obtain a waiver of the requirement if the product does not represent a meaningful therapeutic benefit over existing treatments for pediatric patients and is not likely to be used in a substantial number of pediatric patients. Unless an applicant obtains a deferral or waiver relative to such requirements (or has an automatic exemption because it is an orphan drug), an NDA or supplemental NDA submitted on or after December 2, 2000, for a new active ingredient, new indication, new dosage form, new dosing regimen, or new route of administration must "contain data that are adequate to assess the safety and effectiveness of the drug product for the claimed indications in all relevant pediatric subpopulations, and to support dosing and administration for each pediatric subpopulation for which the drug is safe and effective." A new "pediatric use section" within the NDA should provide a summary of the required pediatric assessment reports (submitted in full with the NDA), in addition to information "describing the investigation of the drug for use in pediatric populations, including an integrated summary of the information (the clinical pharmacology studies, controlled clinical studies, or uncontrolled clinical studies, or other data or information) that is relevant to the safety and effectiveness and benefits and risks of the drug in pediatric populations for the claimed indications, [and] a reference to the full descriptions of such studies provided in the [NDA's Human Pharmacokinetic and Bioavailability Section and Clinical Data Section]." (Note: Although the pediatric use section is specified in FDA regulations, it had not been incorporated into the NDA Form (356h) as of this writing). A November 2000 FDA draft guidance entitled, *Recommendations for Complying with the Pediatric Rule (21 CFR 314.55 (a) and 601.27 (a))* discusses the FDA's interpretation of the rule, describes how companies can obtain waivers (e.g., because a drug does not offer meaningful benefits over existing treatments for pediatric patients) or deferrals (e.g., if the drug is ready for approval before pediatric studies are completed), and specifies what applicants must do to comply with the pediatric rule. Although the agency emphasizes that it can take regulatory and legal actions when firms refuse to comply with the pediatric rule, the guidance states that the "FDA does not intend to deny or withdraw approval of a product for failure to conduct pediatric studies except in rare cases, because removal of a product from the marketplace could deprive other patients of the benefits of a useful medical product." For a detailed analysis of the December 1998 pediatric final rule, see Chapter 16.

NDA Content and Format Requirements

Although submission requirements are, to some degree, a function of a drug's nature, the NDA must, in each case, provide all relevant data and information that a sponsor has collected during the product's research and development. FDA regulations provide the most fundamental description of NDA content and format requirements: "Applications…are required to be submitted in the form and contain the information, as appropriate for the particular submission… An application for a new chemical entity will generally contain an application form, an index, a summary, five or six technical sections, case report tabulations of patient data, case report forms, drug samples, and labeling. Other applications will generally contain only some of those items and information will be limited to that needed to support the particular submission… The application is required to contain reports of all investigations of the drug product sponsored by the applicant, and all other information about the drug pertinent to an evaluation of the application that is received or otherwise obtained by the applicant from any source. The Food and Drug Administration will maintain guidelines on the format and content of applications to assist applicants in their preparation."

In addition to FDA regulations, a large and growing number of agency and ICH guidance documents drive NDA submission requirements. In many cases, particularly in areas in which the FDA's guidelines are several years old, the ICH guidances provide a better account of the agency's current views

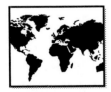

on submission requirements. In fact, some of the agency's more recent guidance documents refer directly to ICH guidance documents rather than the relevant FDA guidances that predated them. Some of the newer FDA guidances simply incorporate large sections of text from relevant ICH guidances addressing the same subject. The FDA and ICH guidances relevant to NDA submissions are discussed below.

The Fundamentals of NDA Submissions

Although the quantity of information and data submitted in NDAs can vary considerably, the component parts of drug applications are somewhat more uniform. According to *Form FDA-356h, Application To Market A New Drug, Biologic, or an Antibiotic for Human Use* (see sample form below), NDAs can comprise as many as 20 different sections in addition to the form itself:

1. Index
2. Labeling
3. Summary
4. Chemistry Section
    A. Chemistry, manufacturing and controls information
    B. Samples
    C. Methods validation package
5. Nonclinical Pharmacology and Toxicology Section
6. Human Pharmacokinetics and Bioavailability Section
7. Clinical Microbiology Section
8. Clinical Data Section
9. Safety Update Report
10. Statistical Section
11. Case Report Tabulations
12. Case Report Forms
13. Patent Information on any patent that claims the drug
14. A Patent Certification with respect to any patent that claims the drug
15. Establishment Description
16. Debarment Certification
17. Field Copy Certification
18. User Fee Cover Sheet (Form FDA 3397)

19. Financial Information

20. Other Information

Editor's Note: Although the listing above identifies 20 sections, Section 15-Establishment Description is relevant only for biological products.

The components of any NDA are, in part, a function of the nature of the subject drug and the information available to the applicant at the time of submission. For example, the safety update report section is not submitted in the original NDA, but is forwarded 120 days after the NDA submission (see discussion below).

An instruction sheet that accompanies Form 356h made clear that the form's numbered listing of contents is not designed to dictate the NDA's format. "It should be noted that the numbering of the items on [Form 356h's] checklist is not intended to specify a particular order of the inclusion of those sections into the submission," the FDA states. "The applicant may include sections in any order, but the location of those sections within the submission should be clearly indicated in the index." Each NDA section is discussed further below.

Although the user-fee program put a renewed focus on the need for an NDA to include all necessary sections, data, and information at the time of its submission, it is worth noting that, under some circumstances, the agency will accept incomplete, or "rolling," NDAs. While certain CDER divisions have accepted incomplete, or "partial," applications in an effort to expedite the review of selected high-priority products, FDAMA formally called on the agency to do so in some cases. Under the legislation's "fast track" review procedure, the FDA can agree to accept and begin the review of an incomplete NDA for a designated fast track product. In such cases, however, the partial NDA must provide the "letter date" of the FDA's agreement to accept the incomplete submission as well as the applicant's schedule for submitting all remaining sections of the NDA. The "fast track" process applies only to drugs that have the potential to address unmet medical needs for serious and life-threatening conditions (see Chapters 8 and 15).

The Archival, Review, and Field Copies of the NDA

Since October 1993, drug sponsors have been required to submit three different copies of an NDA to the agency. The NDA's review and archival copies have been regulatory requirements for years, while the field copy of the application is a more recent NDA requirement.

The FDA provides specific guidance on content requirements for the archival and review copies in its *Guideline on Formatting, Assembling, and Submitting New Drug and Antibiotic Applications* (February 1987). This guidance provides a detailed table outlining the content requirements for archival and review copies. It is important to note, however, that the NDA has evolved considerably since this guidance was published, and that several new sections (e.g., debarment certification, financial information, field copy certification) are now required in the NDA. Although no subsequent agency guidance addresses content requirements as directly as the February 1987 guideline, a January 1999 guidance entitled, *Regulatory Submissions in Electronic Format: New Drug Applications* (see discussion below) does provide a more up-to-date discussion on the archival and review copies of the NDA.

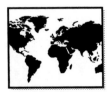

The roles and content of the archival, review, and field copies of the NDA differ considerably. The archival copy, which is stored by the FDA as a reference document, must contain all the relevant sections identified above. It must also include cover letters confirming FDA-applicant agreements, identifying company contact persons, and providing other information relevant to the NDA review. The purpose of the archival copy is to permit individual reviewers to refer to information not included in their review copies, to give other agency personnel access to the complete application for official business, and to maintain in a single file a complete copy of the entire NDA.

The review copy is a less comprehensive version of the application. It comprises the NDA's five or six technical sections—clinical, nonclinical pharmacology/toxicology, chemistry, statistics, biopharmaceutics, and, for anti-infective drugs, microbiology as well. Each of these technical sections is packaged for distribution to, and evaluation by, reviewers in the corresponding technical disciplines. Therefore, these sections must be bound separately, and be accompanied by a table of contents and a copy of the NDA's application form, index, and summary.

NDA sponsors must also submit what is called a "field" copy of the NDA. To be used by FDA inspectors during preapproval manufacturing inspections, the field copy consists of an NDA's chemistry, manufacturing, and controls section, the NDA application form (Form FDA 356h), and the NDA summary. In addition, the field copy must include a certification indicating that it includes an exact copy of the chemistry, manufacturing, and control section "contained in the archival and review copies of the application." U.S.-based applicants must submit the field copy directly to their respective "home" FDA district offices. Foreign-based applicants should submit field copies to FDA headquarters along with their archival and review copies.

In a November 1996 draft guideline, CDER indicated that the NDA's archival copy would be among the first application components that the agency would seek to accept in electronic-only format (i.e., without a paper-based version). In September 1997, the FDA released a final guideline entitled, *Archiving Submissions in Electronic Format—NDAs* to provide recommendations on the submission of certain records (i.e., specifically, case report forms and case report tabulations) in electronic form. This final guidance has been superseded by a January 1999 guidance entitled, *Regulatory Submissions in Electronic Format: New Drug Applications*.

Although the January 1999 electronic submissions guidance applies only to the NDA's archival copy, a sponsor's decision to submit an electronic version of the archival copy can have implications for the accompanying review copy of the submission. If a company provides the NDA's archival copy in electronic format, for example, the agency will exempt the sponsor from having to submit certain elements of the NDA's review copy in paper format. According to the guidance document, these would include the methods validation reports from the chemistry, manufacturing and controls section, the individual animal line listings from the nonclinical section, and certain study report appendices from the clinical sections. Certain review divisions may permit NDA applicants to avoid submitting other sections of the NDA's review copy, the guidance points out.

Application Form All three versions of the NDA must contain an NDA application form, called Form FDA 356h (see exhibit below). This form, which serves as the NDA's cover sheet, provides a comprehensive checklist of the elements that each application should include. The latest version of the form was implemented in April 2000.

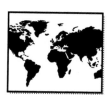

The application form must be completed and signed by the applicant or the applicant's authorized U.S. agent. If the sponsor does not have a residence or place of business within the United States, the application form must provide the name and address of, and be countersigned by, an authorized agent who resides or maintains a place of business in the United States. By signing this form, the sponsor agrees to comply with a variety of legal and regulatory requirements, including current good manufacturing practice (CGMP) standards, advertising and labeling regulations, safety update reporting requirements, and local, state, and federal environmental impact laws.

The Index Perhaps the most critical factor in an NDA's user-friendliness is the speed and ease with which a reviewer can locate specific information during the review process. Since it is the reviewer's "roadmap" to an application that can be hundreds of volumes long and because it can influence the speed and efficiency of the review as well, the NDA's index is an important element of the application.

While the FDA states that the various NDA components may be submitted in any order, the agency emphasizes that the index should clearly indicate the location of each section within the application. Therefore, the agency recommends that, particularly for large submissions, the index "be the first item following the Form FDA 356h."

The archival copy of the NDA must provide a comprehensive index by volume number and page number to the NDA summary, each of the five or six technical sections, and the case report forms and tabulations section. FDA guidelines state that the index should serve as a detailed table of contents for the entire archival NDA.

Each of the separately bound technical sections comprising the review copies must include a copy of the NDA index as well. In addition, each section should include its own individual table of contents based upon the portions of the larger NDA index relevant to that technical section.

Labeling The NDA's archival copy must contain copies of the label and all labeling proposed for the drug product. In the NDA, applicants must submit either 4 copies of a product's draft labeling or 12 copies of the final printed labeling (FPL).

If a sponsor submits draft labeling, one copy should be bound in the archival copy, with single copies placed in the review copies of the clinical, chemistry, and pharmacology sections (labeling in the review sections may be bound separately in the appropriate colored jacket for the respective review sections).

When a sponsor provides FPL and carton labeling, one copy should be mounted, bound, and inserted in the archival copy. The remaining 11 copies should be mounted, bound, and submitted in a separate jacket clearly marked "Final Printed Labeling" (see Chapter 8 for a more detailed discussion of drug labeling requirements).

The NDA Summary In many respects, the NDA summary is an abridged version of the entire application. The summary is designed to provide an overview of the NDA, explaining its intent—to establish the drug's safety and effectiveness for a specific use—and highlighting the studies and analyses that support the product's use.

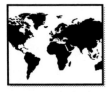

PAGE 149

The New Drug Application (NDA)

Chapter 7

DEPARTMENT OF HEALTH AND HUMAN SERVICES
FOOD AND DRUG ADMINISTRATION
APPLICATION TO MARKET A NEW DRUG, BIOLOGIC, OR AN ANTIBIOTIC DRUG FOR HUMAN USE
(Title 21, Code of Federal Regulations, 314 & 601)

Form Approved: OMB No. 0910-0338
Expiration Date: March 2003
See OMB Statement on page 2.

FOR FDA USE ONLY
APPLICATION NUMBER

APPLICANT INFORMATION

NAME OF APPLICANT

DATE OF SUBMISSION

TELEPHONE NO. *(Include Area Code)*

FACSIMILE (FAX) Number *(Include Area Code)*

APPLICANT ADDRESS *(Number, Street, City, State, Country, Zip Code or Mail Code, and U.S. License number if previously issued):*

AUTHORIZED U.S AGENT NAME & ADDRESS *(Number, Street, City, State, ZIP Code, telephone & FAX number)* IF APPLICABLE

PRODUCT DESCRIPTION

NEW DRUG OR ANTIBIOTIC APPLICATION NUMBER, OR BIOLOGICS LICENSE APPLICATION NUMBER (if previously issued)

ESTABLISHED NAME *(e.g., Proper Name, USP/USAN name)*

PROPRIETARY NAME *(trade name)* IF ANY

CHEMICAL/BIOCHEMICAL/BLOOD PRODUCT NAME *(if any)*

CODE NAME *(If any)*

DOSAGE FORM: STRENGTHS: ROUTE OF ADMINISTRATION:

(PROPOSED) INDICATION(S) FOR USE:

APPLICATION INFORMATION

APPLICATION TYPE
(check one)   ☐ NEW DRUG APPLICATION (21 CFR 314.5)   ☐ ABBREVIATED NEW DRUG APPLICATION (ANDA, 21 CFR 314.94)
☐ BIOLOGICS LICENSE APPLICATION (21 CFR part 601)

IF AN NDA, IDENTIFY THE APPROPRIATE TYPE   ☐ 505 (b) (1)   ☐ 505 (b) (2)

IF AN ANDA, OR 505(b)(2), IDENTIFY THE REFERENCE LISTED DRUG PRODUCT THAT IS THE BASIS FOR THE SUBMISSION
Name of Drug   Holder of Approved Application

TYPE OF SUBMISSION
(check one)   ☐ ORIGINAL APPLICATION   ☐ AMENDMENT TO A PENDING APPLICATION   ☐ RESUBMISSION
☐ PRESUBMISSION   ☐ ANNUAL REPORT   ☐ ESTABLISHMENT DESCRIPTION SUPPLEMENT   ☐ EFFICACY SUPPLEMENT
☐ LABELING SUPPLEMENT   ☐ CHEMISTRY MANUFACTURING AND CONTROLS SUPPLEMENT   ☐ OTHER

IF SUBMISSION IS A PARTIAL APPLICATION, PROVIDE LETTER OF AGREEMENT TO PARTIAL SUBMISSION: _____

IF A SUPPLEMENT, IDENTIFY THE APPROPRIATE CATEGORY: ☐ CBE   ☐ CBE-30   ☐ PRIOR APPROVAL (PA)

REASON FOR SUBMISSION

PROPOSED MARKETING STATUS (check one)   ☐ PRESCRIPTION (Rx)   ☐ OVER THE COUNTER PRODUCT (OTC)

NUMBER OF VOLUMES SUBMITTED   THIS APPLICATION IS   ☐ PAPER   ☐ PAPER AND ELECTRONIC   ☐ ELECTRONIC

ESTABLISHMENT INFORMATION (Full establishment information should be provided in the body of the Application.)
Provide locations of all manufacturing, packing and control sites for drug substance and drug product (continuation sheets may be used if necessary). Include name, address, contact, telephone number, registration number (CFN), DMF number, and manufacturing steps and/or type of testing (e.g., Final dosage form, Stability testing) conducted at the site. Please indicate whether the site is ready for inspection or, if not, when it will be ready.

Cross References (list related License Applications, INDs, NDAs, PMAs, 510(k)s, IDEs, BMFs, and DMFs referenced in the current application)

FORM 356h (4/00)

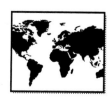

Worldwide Pharmaceutical Regulation Series

The New Drug Application (NDA)

Chapter 7

This application contains the following items: *(Check all that apply)*		
1. Index		
2. Labeling (check one) ☐ Draft Labeling ☐ Final Printing Labeling		
3. Summary (21 CFR 314.50 (c))		
4. Chemistry section		
A. Chemistry, manufacturing, and controls information (e.g., 21 CFR 314.50 (d) (1); 21 CFR 601.2)		
B. Samples (21 CFR 314.50 (e) (1); 21 CFR 601.2 (a)) (Submit only upon FDA's request)		
C. Methods validation package (e.g., 21 CFR 314.50 (e) (2) (i); 21 CFR 601.2)		
5. Nonclinical pharmacology and toxicology section (e.g., 21 CFR 314.50 (d) (2); 21 CFR 601.2)		
6. Human pharmacokinetics and bioavailability section (e.g., 21 CFR 314.50 (d) (3); 21 CFR 601.2)		
7. Clinical Microbiology (e.g., 21 CFR 314.50 (d) (4))		
8. Clinical data section (e.g., 21 CFR 314.50 (d) (5); 21 CFR 601.2)		
9. Safety update report (e.g., 21 CFR 314.50 (d) (5) (vi) (b); 21 CFR 601.2)		
10. Statistical section (e.g., 21 CFR 314.50 (d) (6); 21 CFR 601.2)		
11. Case report tabulations (e.g., 21 CFR 314.50 (f) (1); 21 CFR 601.2)		
12. Case report forms (e.g., 21 CFR 314.50 (f) (2); 21 CFR 601.2)		
13. Patent information on any patent which claims the drug (21 U.S.C. 355 (b) or (c))		
14. A patent certification with respect to any patent which claims the drug (21 U.S.C. 355 (b) (2) or (j) (2) (A))		
15. Establishment description (21 CFR Part 600, if applicable)		
16. Debarment certification (FD&C Act 306 (k)(1))		
17. Field copy certification (21 CFR 314.5 (k) (3))		
18. User Fee Cover Sheet (Form FDA 3397)		
19. Financial Information		
20. OTHER (Specify)		

CERTIFICATION

I agree to update this application with new safety information about the drug that may reasonably affect the statement of contraindications, warnings, precautions, or adverse reactions in the draft labeling. I agree to submit safety update reports as provided for by regulation or as requested by FDA. If this application is approved, I agree to comply with all laws and regulations that apply to approved applications, including, but not limited to the following:

1. Good manufacturing practice regulations in 21 CFR Parts 210 and 211, or applicable regulations, Parts 606, and/or 820.
2. Biological establishment standards in 21 CFR Part 600.
3. Labeling regulations in 21 CFR 201, Parts 606, 610, 660 and/or 809.
4. In the case of a prescription drug product or biological product, prescription drug advertising regulations in 21 CFR 202.
5. Regulations on making changes in application in FD&C Act Section 506A, 21 CFR 314.71, 314.72, 314.97, 314.99, and 601.12.
6. Regulations on reports in 21 CFR 314.80, 314.81, 600.80 and 600.81.
7. Local, state, and Federal environmental impact.

If this application applies to a drug product that FDA has proposed for scheduling under the Controlled Substances Act, I agree not to market the product until the Drug Enforcement Administration makes a final scheduling decision.

The data and information in this submission have been reviewed and, to the best of my knowledge are certified to be true and accurate.

Warning: a willfully false statement is a criminal offense, U.S. Code, title 18, section 1001.

SIGNATURE OF RESPONSIBLE OFFICIAL OR AGENT	TYPED NAME AND TITLE	DATE
ADDRESS (Street, City, State, and ZIP Code)	Telephone Number ( )	

Public reporting burden for this collection of information is estimated to average 24 hours per response, including the time for reviewing instructions, searching existing data sources, gathering and maintaining the data needed, and completing and reviewing the collection of information. Send comments regarding this burden estimate or any other aspect of this collection of information, including suggestions for reducing this burden to:

Department of Health and Human Services
Food and Drug Administration
CBER, HFM-99
1401 Rockvillle Pike
Rockville, MD 20852-1448

Food and Drug Administration
CDER, HFD-94
12420 Parklawn Drive, Rm 3046
Rockville, MD 20852

An agency may not conduct or sponsor, and a person is not required to respond to, a collection of information unless it displays a currently valid OMB control number.

FORM FDA 356h (4/2000)

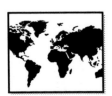

New Drug Approval in the United States

The New Drug Application (NDA)

Chapter 7

Given that the summary is one of the few elements of the application that all reviewers receive, its importance cannot be overstated. A well-prepared summary, which should include a balanced, unbiased presentation and analysis of a drug's beneficial and adverse effects, can build a reviewer's confidence in the applicant, the drug, and the validity and completeness of the information in the NDA.

As evidence of the importance that is placed on the NDA summary, the FDA dedicated an entire guideline to the topic—*Guideline for the Format and Content of the Summary for New Drug and Antibiotic Applications* (February 1987). According to this document, "each full application is required...to contain a summary, ordinarily 50 to 200 pages in length, that integrates all of the information in the application and provides reviewers in each review area, and other agency officials, with a good general understanding of the drug product and of the application. The summary should discuss all aspects of the application and should be written in approximately the same level of detail required for publication in, and meet the editorial standards generally applied by, refereed scientific and medical journals... To the extent possible, data in the summary should be presented in tabular and graphic forms... The summary should comprehensively present the most important information about the drug product and the conclusions to be drawn from this information. The summary should avoid any editorial promotion of the drug product, i.e., it should be a factual summary of safety and effectiveness data and a neutral analysis of these data. The summary should include an annotated copy of the proposed labeling, a discussion of the product's benefits and risks, a description of the foreign marketing history of the drug (if any), and a summary of each technical section."

Specifically, federal regulations require the NDA summary to provide the following:

- the proposed text of the labeling for the drug, with annotations to the information in the summary and technical sections of the application that support the inclusion of each statement in the labeling, and, if the application is for a prescription drug, statements describing the reasons for omitting a section or subsection of the labeling format;

- a statement identifying the pharmacologic class of the drug and a discussion of the scientific rationale for the drug, its intended use, and the potential clinical benefits of the drug product;

- a brief description of the marketing history, if any, of the drug outside the United States, including a list of the countries in which the drug has been marketed, a list of any countries in which the drug has been withdrawn from marketing for any reason related to safety or effectiveness, and a list of countries in which applications for marketing are pending (the section must describe marketing by the applicant and, if known, the marketing history of other persons);

- a summary of the chemistry, manufacturing, and controls section of the application;

- a summary of the nonclinical pharmacology and toxicology section of the application;

- a summary of the human pharmacokinetics and bioavailability section of the application;

- a summary of the microbiology section of the application (for anti-infectives only);

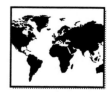

- a summary of the clinical data section of the application, including the results of statistical analyses of the clinical trials; and

- a concluding discussion that presents the benefit and risk considerations related to the drug, including a discussion of any proposed additional studies or surveillance the applicant intends to conduct following approval.

Chemistry Section In the NDA's first technical component, the chemistry section, the sponsor describes, and provides data regarding, the composition, manufacture, and specifications of both the drug substance (i.e., the active ingredient) and the final drug product, including their physical and chemical characteristics and stability.

The 1997 revision to the new Form 356h restructured this NDA section to some degree. Essentially, the outline provided in Form 356h folds the NDA's samples and methods validation package sections into the new chemistry section. Under the previous iteration of the form, these components were independent of the chemistry section.

Historically, deficiencies have been more common in the NDA's chemistry, manufacturing, and controls (CMC) section than in other aspects of the application. This is probably due to several factors, including the fact that sponsors cannot develop final product formulations and commercial-scale manufacturing processes until late in the drug development process.

Recognizing this, the FDA released, in the mid-1980s, a spate of guidelines that provide agency advice on preparing chemistry, manufacturing, and controls sections for NDAs and other applications: *Guideline for the Format and Content of the Chemistry, Manufacturing, and Controls Section of an Application* (February 1987); *Guideline for Submitting Documentation for the Manufacture of and Controls for Drug Products* (February 1987); *Guideline for Submitting Documentation for Packaging for Human Drugs and Biologics* (February 1987); *Guideline for Submitting Documentation for the Stability of Human Drugs and Biologics* (February 1987); and *Guideline for Submitting Supporting Documentation in Drug Applications for the Manufacture of Drug Substances* (February 1987). A few years later, these were supplemented by the agency's *Draft Guideline for Submitting Supporting Chemistry Documentation in Radiopharmaceutical Drug Applications* (November 1991), *Guidance for the Submission of Chemistry, Manufacturing, and Controls for Synthetic Peptide Drug Substances* (November 1994), and *Guideline for Drug Master Files* (September 1989).

Although the FDA has invested much of its most recent CMC guidance development effort into the ICH harmonization process (see discussion below), the agency did publish a handful of formal and draft guidances in the late 1990s, including: *Guidance for Industry: Container Closure Systems for Packaging Human Drugs and Biologics* (May 1999); *Environmental Assessment of Human Drug and Biologics Applications* (July 1998), which superseded the *Guidance for Industry for the Submission of an Environmental Assessment in Human Drug Applications and Supplements* (1995); *Draft Guidance for Industry on Stability Testing of Drug Substances and Drug Products* (June 1998), which will, when it is published as a new guidance, supersede CDER's *Guideline for Submitting Documentation for the Stability of Human Drugs and Biologics* (February 1997); *Draft Guidance for Industry: NDAs: Impurities in Drug Substances* (December 1998); *Draft Guidance for the Submission of CMC Information for Nasal Spray and Inhalation Solution, Suspension, and Spray Drug Products* (June 1999); and *Draft Guidance for the Submission of CMC Information for Metered Dose Inhaler (MDI) and Dry Powder Inhaler (DPI) Drug Products* (September 1999).

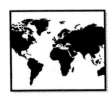

As noted above, the ICH initiative has produced numerous guidelines relevant to the NDA's chemistry section. These documents are cited in the more detailed discussions below.

Form 356h's listing of the NDA contents indicates that the chemistry section should comprise three elements:

A. Chemistry, manufacturing and control information;

B. Samples; and

C. Methods validation package.

A. Chemistry, Manufacturing, and Control Information. According to FDA regulations, an NDA's chemistry, manufacturing, and control section should comprise four principal elements: (1) a description of the drug substance; (2) a description of the drug product; (3) an environmental impact analysis report (or request for a waiver); and (4) a field copy certification.

A *Description of the Drug Substance*. The sponsor's description of the drug substance should include the following:

The Substance's Stability and Physical and Chemical Characteristics. Provide the substance's chemical name and related names (if available and appropriate), structural formula, physicochemical characteristics, the physical and chemical data necessary to elucidate and confirm the substance's chemical structure, and a description of the studies (including results) on the substance's stability. Regarding drug substance stability requirements for NDAs, applicants should refer to the ICH's final revised 2001 guideline entitled, Q1A(R) *Stability Testing of New Drug Substances and Products* and, if applicable, to a pair of annexes to this guideline, Q1B *Guideline for the Photostability Testing of New Drug Substances and Products* (November 1996) and Q1C *Stability Testing for New Dosage Forms* (May 1997). In October 2001, the ICH released a draft guidance entitled, Q1D *Reduced Bracketing and Matrixing Designs for Stability Testing in Drug Substances and Drug Products*. Applicants should also refer to the FDA's draft guidance entitled, *Stability Testing of Drug Substances and Drug Products* (June 1998), which is consistent with the ICH's Q1A guidance and which will, when published as a final guidance, supersede the FDA's *Guideline for Submitting Documentation for the Stability of Human Drugs and Biologics* (1987).

The Name and Address of the Manufacturer. Provide the name and address of each facility (i.e., besides those of the applicant) that participates in manufacturing the drug substance (e.g., performs the synthesis, isolation, purification, testing, packaging, or labeling), and describe the operation(s) that each facility performs.

Method(s) of Manufacture and Packaging. Provide a full description of the materials and method(s) used in the synthesis, isolation, and purification of the drug substance, including a list of starting materials, reagents, solvents, and auxiliary materials. Also, describe the process controls used at various stages of the manufacturing, processing, and packaging of the drug substance, and provide information on the characteristics of, and the test methods used for, the container-closure system. In addition, the original application should provide a full description of the preparation of any reference standard substance used, including a description of the purification steps.

Specifications and Analytical Methods for the Drug Substance. Provide a full description of the acceptance specifications and test methods used to assure the identity, strength, quality, and purity of the drug substance and the bioavailability of drug products made from the drug substance, including specifications relating to stability, sterility, particle size, and crystalline form. It is also typical to include data from the validation of these studies in this section as well. For additional guidance, applicants can refer to the following ICH final guidelines: Q3A *Impurities in New Drug Substances* (a draft revised guidance, Q3A(R), was issued in July 2000); Q2A *Text on Validation of Analytical Procedures: Definitions and Terminology* (1995); Q2B *Validation of Analytical Procedures: Methodology* (1997); and Q3C *Impurities: Residual Solvents* (1997). In January 2001, the ICH parties also released final guidance entitled, Q6A *Specifications: Test Procedures and Acceptance Criteria for New Drug Substances and New Drug Products: Chemical Substances*, which provides recommendations on the selection and justification of acceptance criteria for new drug substances and the new drug products produced from these substances.

In December 1998, CDER issued a draft guidance for industry entitled, NDAs: *Impurities in Drug Substances*. CDER uses this brief draft guidance to recommend that applicants refer to the ICH's Q3A *Impurities in New Drug Substances* (1996) when seeking guidance on the identification, qualification, and reporting of impurities in drug substances that are not considered new drug substances. While CDER acknowledges that the Q3A document was developed to provide guidance on providing information on impurities in NDAs for new drug substances, the center emphasizes that applicants submitting NDAs for products that are not considered new drug substances should refer to it as well. The applicants to which this recommendation applies would include firms submitting NDAs for new dosage forms for already approved drug products, for changes in drug substance synthesis or process, and for products containing two or more active moieties that are individually used in already approved drug products but that have not previously been approved or marketed together in a drug product. In July 2000, the ICH parties issued a draft revision to Q3A, entitled Q3B(R) *Impurities in New Drug Products*, to provide modified and new text on threshold limits, degradation products, and rounding.

Solid State Drug Substance Forms and Their Relationship to Bioavailability. Provide appropriate specifications characterizing the drug substance (e.g., particle size) to assure the bioavailability of the drug product.

The sponsor may provide for the use of alternatives in meeting any of the applicable requirements, including alternative sources, process controls, methods, and specifications. In some cases, reference to the current editions of the U.S. *Pharmacopeia* and the *National Formulary* may satisfy the content requirements outlined above.

Often, applicants utilize components (e.g., drug substances, nonstandard excipients, containers) manufactured by other firms. In such cases, the contract manufacturer may want to preserve the confidentiality of its manufacturing processes. Since an NDA must provide information on these processes, contract manufacturers will often submit this information directly to the FDA in a drug master file (DMF). This allows drug sponsors using the company's products to meet submission requirements by incorporating by reference information provided in the DMF. Because the drug sponsor never sees the information in the DMF, the confidentiality of the contract facility's manufacturing processes is maintained.

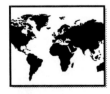

An incorporation by reference should be made in the section of the NDA in which the referenced information would normally appear. The reference must identify specifically where the agency can find the information in the DMF (or other referenced document), and must identify the file by name, reference number, volume, and page number (i.e., the FDA stores DMFs and reviews the information in the file only when referenced in a pending drug application). When the applicant cross-references a DMF submitted by another firm (e.g., a bulk drug manufacturer), the NDA must include a letter of authorization from the DMF's owner in addition to the information specified above. For more information on DMFs, sponsors should refer to CDER's *Guideline for Drug Master Files* (September 1989).

In a January 2000 final rule, CDER eliminated Type I DMFs, which traditionally had been used to incorporate by reference information on manufacturing sites, facilities, operating procedures, and personnel in INDs, NDAs, and other applications. Under the final rule, which took effect in July 2000, information formerly provided in Type I DMFs are to be provided in Type II, Type III, and Type V DMFs. CDER first proposed eliminating Type I DMFs in July 1995 in response to the recommendations of an internal task force, which concluded that information in Type I DMFs was often outdated, that such DMFs were not always easily accessible to FDA investigators, and that facility-related information in Type I DMFs was typically available to agency investigators at manufacturing facilities.

A *Description of the Drug Product*. In many ways similar to the drug substance section, this part of the NDA should include the following:

A List of Components. Provide a list of all components used in the manufacture of the drug product (regardless of whether they appear in the final product).

A Statement of Drug Product Composition. Provide a statement of the product's quantitative composition, indicating the weight or measure for each substance used in the manufacture of the dosage form. Also, provide the batch formula to be used in the product's manufacture.

Specifications and Analytical Methods for Inactive Components. Provide a full description of the acceptance specifications and test methods used to assure the identity, quality, and purity of each inactive ingredient.

Name and Address of Manufacturer(s). Provide the name and address of each facility involved in manufacturing the drug product (e.g., the drug processing, packaging, labeling, or control applications), and describe the operations that each will perform.

Method(s) of Manufacture and Packaging. Provide a copy of the master/batch production and control records or a comparably detailed description of the production process (a schematic diagram of the production process is often helpful). Also, provide complete information on the characteristics of, and test methods used for, the container-closure system or other component parts of the drug product package to assure their suitability for packaging the drug product. To provide recommendations on meeting NDA submission requirements for information on drug product packaging materials, CDER released a final *Guidance for Industry: Container Closure Systems Used for the Packaging of Human Drugs and Biologics: Chemistry, Manufacturing, and Controls Documentation* (May 1999). For further guidance on specific issues relevant to this subsection, applicants can refer to an ICH guideline entitled, *Q3C Impurities: Residual Solvents* (December 1997) and CDER's *Guidance for Industry for the Submission of*

Documentation for Sterilization Process Validation in Applications for Human and Veterinary Drug Products (November 1994).

Specifications and Analytical Methods for the Drug Product. Provide a full description of the specifications and analytical methods necessary to assure the product's identity, strength, quality, purity, homogeneity, and bioavailability throughout its shelf life. The methods and standards of acceptance should be sufficiently detailed to permit FDA laboratories to duplicate them. Typically, applicants include data on the validation of the analytical methods in this section as well. For recommendations on impurities-related submission requirements, applicants can refer to final ICH guidances entitled, Q3B *Impurities in New Drug Products* (a proposed revision to this 1997 guidance was released in July 2000) and Q3C *Impurities: Residual Solvents* (December 1997). In January 2001, the ICH parties also released a final guidance entitled, Q6A *Specifications: Test Procedures and Acceptance Criteria for New Drug Substances and New Drug Products: Chemical Substances*, which provides recommendations on the selection and justification of acceptance criteria for new drug substances and new drug products produced from these substances.

Stability. Provide a complete description of, and data derived from, studies of product stability, including information establishing the suitability of the analytical method(s) used.

In this section as well, the sponsor may provide alternatives for meeting relevant requirements, including alternative components, manufacturing and packaging procedures, in-process controls, methods, and specifications. Reference to the current editions of the U.S. *Pharmacopeia* and the *National Formulary* may satisfy relevant requirements. Regarding drug product stability requirements for NDAs, applicants can refer to the ICH's final revised 2001 guideline entitled, Q1A(R) *Stability Testing of New Drug Substances and Products* and, if applicable, to a pair of annexes to this guideline, Q1B *Guideline for the Photostability Testing of New Drug Substances and Products* (November 1996) and Q1C *Stability Testing for New Dosage Forms* (May 1997). In October 2001, the ICH released a draft guidance entitled, Q1D *Reduced Bracketing and Matrixing Designs for Stability Testing of Drug Substances and Drug Products*. Applicants should also refer to the FDA's draft guidance entitled, *Stability Testing of Drug Substances and Drug Products* (June 1998), which is consistent with the ICH's Q1A guidance and which will, when published as a final guidance, supersede the FDA's *Guideline for Submitting Documentation for the Stability of Human Drugs and Biologics* (1987).

A September 1993 final regulation modified content requirements for this portion of the chemistry, manufacturing, and controls section. The regulation mandates that applicants provide certain information about the batches of the drug product used to conduct the "pivotal" bioavailability and bioequivalence studies and the "primary" stability studies: (1) the batch production record; (2) the specifications and test procedures for each component and for the drug product itself; (3) the names and addresses of the sources of the active and noncompendial inactive components and of the container and closure system for the drug product; (4) the name and address of each contract facility involved in the manufacture, processing, packaging, or testing of the drug product, and identification of the operation performed by each contract facility; and (5) the results of tests performed on the drug product and on the components used in the product's manufacture.

In addition, the 1993 regulation requires that this section provide the "proposed or actual master production record, including a description of the equipment, to be used for the manufacture of a

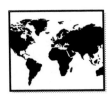

commercial lot of the drug product or a comparably detailed description of the production process for a representative batch of the drug product."

It is worth noting that CDER chemists often find it helpful when applicants submit developmental pharmaceutics information beyond that called for in current FDA regulations and guidelines. Reviewers claim that the information can give CDER chemists a greater "comfort level" with the application because it describes the product's formulation development history and the company's rationale on formulation-related issues (e.g., methods, ranges, inactive ingredients). FDA officials strongly recommend, however, that sponsors ask CDER chemists about the utility of such information on a case-by-case basis, and about where the information should be located in the NDA if it is to be provided. It is interesting to note, however, that developmental pharmaceutics information is called for in the harmonized CTD document (see discussion above).

Environmental Impact Analysis Report. Like all applications and petitions requesting formal FDA action, an NDA must include either an environmental assessment (EA) or a claim for a categorical exclusion from the EA submission requirement. Fulfilling a promise made under a 1995 Clinton Administration regulatory reform initiative, the agency released a July 1997 final regulation to establish that EAs would be required only under "extraordinary circumstances" (e.g., when available data indicate that the expected level of exposure could seriously harm the environment).

Through this change, the FDA grants categorical exclusions, or exemptions, from EA requirements to all but a "fairly narrow category" of drugs and biologics. According to the July 1997 final regulation, an NDA will not "ordinarily" require the preparation of an EA in the following circumstances: (1) the application's approval will not increase the use of the active moiety; (2) the NDA's approval will increase the use of the active moiety, but the estimated concentration of the substance at the point of entry into the aquatic environment will be below 1 part per billion; or (3) the NDA is for a substance that occurs naturally in the environment and the application's approval does not alter significantly the concentration or distribution of the substance, its metabolites, or degradation products in the environment. A claim for categorical exclusion must include a statement of compliance with the categorical exclusion criteria, and must state that, to the applicant's knowledge, no "extraordinary circumstances" exist.

To provide further guidance regarding the changes brought by the July 1997 regulation, CDER released a formal guidance entitled, *Environmental Assessment of Human Drug and Biologics Applications* (July 1998), which superseded CDER's *Guidance for Industry for the Submission of an Environmental Assessment in Human Drug Applications and Supplements* (November 1995).

Field Copy Certification. U.S.-based applicants must include in this section a statement "certifying that the field copy of the application has been provided to the applicant's home district office." Since foreign applicants must provide the field copy with the archival and review copies, no such certification is needed in their applications.

Given the nature and detail of the chemistry, manufacturing, and control section, the FDA allows sponsors to submit the completed section 90 to 120 days before the anticipated filing of the entire NDA. In some cases, the agency claims, this may speed the NDA review process.

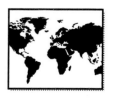

For such early submissions, both the archival and review copies of the section are required, while the field copy may be forwarded when the full NDA is submitted. The early submission should provide a cover letter, the application form, an index to facilitate the location of the information within the section, and the identification of a sponsor contact person with whom the FDA may discuss the data. If any information required for the section is unavailable at the time of the advance submission, this should be noted in the cover letter.

B. *Samples*. Drug samples should not accompany the NDA submission, but should be submitted only in response to an FDA request. The FDA may request these samples to validate the adequacy of the analytical methods that the sponsor uses to identify the drug product and drug substance. Typically, the FDA requests that applicants submit samples directly to "two or more" agency laboratories that will perform the validation work.

Upon such a request, the applicant must submit "four representative samples of the following, with each sample in sufficient quantity to permit FDA to perform three times each test described in the application to determine whether the drug substance and the drug product meet the specifications given in the application:" the drug product proposed for marketing; the drug substance used in the drug product from which the samples of the drug product were taken; and reference standards and blanks (except that reference standards recognized in an official compendium need not be submitted).

Upon an FDA request, sponsors must also provide samples of the product's "finished market package." The FDA may ask for two copies of the package, although one generally suffices.

For FDA recommendations regarding samples, applicants should refer to an agency guidance entitled, *Submitting Samples and Analytical Data for Methods Validation*. When issued as a final guidance, an August 2000 FDA draft guidance entitled, *Analytical Procedures and Methods Validation Chemistry, Manufacturing, and Controls Documentation*, will supercede that guidance.

C. *Methods Validation Package*. The archival copy of the NDA must include a methods validation package, which provides information that allows FDA laboratories to validate all of the analytical methods for both the drug substance and drug product. It should provide a listing of all samples to be submitted, including lot number, identity, package type and size, and quantity. In addition, the package usually includes descriptive information copied from pertinent sections of the NDA. FDA regulations state that "related descriptive information includes a description of each sample; the proposed regulatory specifications for the drug; a detailed description of the methods of analysis; supporting data for accuracy, specificity, precision and ruggedness; and complete results of the applicant's tests on each sample." To aid the reviewing chemist, these copies should retain the original pagination of the NDA sections from which they were copied.

The FDA provides specific advice on the development of this section in its *Guideline for Submitting Samples and Analytical Data for Methods Validation* (February 1987). In March 1995, the ICH published a final guideline entitled, Q2A *Text on Validation of Analytical Procedures*, which discusses "the characteristics that should be considered during the validation of the analytical procedures included as part of registration applications." More recently, the ICH parties published a final guideline entitled, Q2B

Validation of Analytical Procedures: Methodology (May 1997), which provides recommendations on how manufacturers should consider the various validation characteristics for each analytical procedure, as well as guidance on the data that should be presented in a marketing application.

Four copies of the methods validation package should be included with the initial submission. Although FDA regulations state that three of the copies should be submitted in the archival copy, agency guidelines recommend submitting one copy with the archival copy and three additional copies with the chemistry, manufacturing, and controls section of the review copy. If the applicant does the latter, the submission should include a statement indicating that this option was selected.

Nonclinical Pharmacology and Toxicology Section Federal regulations state that this section should "describe, with the aid of graphs and tables, animal and in vitro studies with [the] drug." The section should provide all nonclinical animal and laboratory studies involving the drug, including data from preclinical studies originally submitted in the IND; data compiled and submitted during clinical investigations (e.g., long-term testing such as carcinogenicity and reproductive testing); and, in some cases, nonclinical studies not submitted previously.

The FDA reviews these studies to evaluate their adequacy and comprehensiveness, and to ensure that there are no inconsistent or inadequately characterized toxic effects. According to federal regulations, the principal content requirements for this section are:

1. Studies of the pharmacological actions of the drug in relation to its proposed therapeutic indication, and studies that otherwise define the pharmacologic properties of the drug or that are pertinent to possible adverse side effects.

2. Studies of the toxicological effects of the drug as they relate to the drug's intended clinical use(s), including, as appropriate, studies assessing the drug's acute, subacute, and chronic toxicity, carcinogenicity, and studies of toxicities related to the drug's particular mode of administration or conditions of use.

3. Studies, as appropriate, of the drug's effects on reproduction and on the developing fetus.

4. Any studies of the absorption, distribution, metabolism, and excretion of the drug in animals.

5. For each nonclinical laboratory study, a statement that it was conducted in compliance with good laboratory practice (GLP) regulations, or if the study was not conducted in compliance with those regulations, a brief statement of the reason for the noncompliance.

As part of its continuing effort to standardize the NDA review process, CDER has released a May 2001 reviewer guidance entitled, *Pharmacology/Toxicology Review Format*. By providing NDA applicants with what the FDA calls an "understanding of the standard format and content of primary pharmacology/toxicology [NDA] reviews," the guidance can provide some insights into this section of the application and how it will be evaluated and used. CDER is implementing such a standardized format for pharmacology/toxicology and other discipline reviews for several reasons, including that standardization provides for unified communication among multiple audiences and that it ensures that the most important information is captured in all IND and NDA reviews.

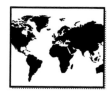

The FDA is sensitive to organizational problems regarding the presentation of toxicological, pharmacological, and other data from nonclinical studies. Therefore, drug sponsors should refer to specific recommendations in the FDA's *Guideline for the Format and Content of the Nonclinical Pharmacology/Toxicology Section of an Application* (February 1987). Although it concedes that nonclinical data are collected over several years and are submitted in varying formats, the guideline recommends that the data be reorganized for the NDA submission. NDA applicants should also refer to a May 2001 FDA guidance entitled *Bioanalytical Method Validation*, which provides recommendations on developing validation information on bioanalytical methods for nonclinical pharmacology/toxicology studies as well as clinical studies.

Human Pharmacokinetics and Bioavailability Section The NDA must include a section providing data and analyses from all human pharmacokinetic and bioavailability studies (or information supporting a waiver of *in vivo* bioavailability data). The section should include data from and descriptions of any of the five general types of biopharmaceutic studies that were relevant for the investigational drug:

1. Pilot and background studies, which are conducted to provide a preliminary assessment of absorption, distribution, metabolism and/or elimination (ADME) of a drug as a guide in the design of early clinical trials and definitive kinetic studies.

2. Bioavailability/bioequivalence studies, including bioavailability, bioequivalence, and dosage form proportionality studies (this discussion should include a description of the analytical and statistical methods used in each study).

3. Pharmacokinetic studies, descriptions of which must include a discussion of the analytical and statistical methods used in each study.

4. Other *in vivo* studies using pharmacological or clinical endpoints.

5. *In vitro* studies designed to define the release rate of a drug substance from the dosage form (obviously, such dissolution tests are not relevant for drug forms such as injectables and some others).

According to FDA regulations, this section should consist of as many as three elements:

- "A description of each of the bioavailability and pharmacokinetic studies of the drug in humans performed by or on behalf of the applicant that includes a description of the analytical and statistical methods used in each study and a statement [that it was conducted according to relevant federal regulations]."

- "If the application describes in the chemistry, manufacturing, and controls section specifications or analytical methods needed to assure the bioavailability of the drug product or drug substance, or both, a statement in this section of the rationale for establishing the specification or analytical methods, including data and information supporting this rationale."

- "A summarizing discussion and analysis of the pharmacokinetics and metabolism of the active ingredients and the bioavailability or bioequivalence, or both, of the drug product."

The FDA provides its most detailed recommendations on the development and presentation of this section in its *Guideline for the Format and Content of the Human Pharmacokinetics and Bioavailability Section of*

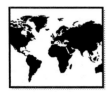

an Application (February 1987). In November 1994, the ICH published a final guideline entitled, E4 *Dose-Response Information to Support Drug Registration*, which describes the importance of dose-response information and the types of studies that sponsors can use to obtain such information (i.e., parallel-dose response, cross-over dose response, forced titration, and optional titration). More recently, the FDA published *Guidance for Industry-Drug Metabolism/Drug Interaction Studies in the Drug Development Process: Studies In Vitro* (April 1997), which provides recommendations on current approaches to *in vitro* studies of drug metabolism and interactions, and a variety of other final guidances, including *Population Pharmacokinetics* (February 1999) and *Pharmacokinetics in Patients with Impaired Renal Function* (May 1998). In the late 1990s, the center has released a spate of draft guidances relevant to this section of the NDA, including *In Vivo Drug Metabolism/Drug Interaction Studies-Study Design, Data Analysis, and Recommendations for Dosing and Labeling* (November 1998), *General Considerations for Pediatric Pharmacokinetic Studies for Drugs and Biological Products* (November 1998), *BA and BE Studies for Orally Administered Drug Products—General Considerations* (August 1998), *Draft Guidance on Food-Effect Bioavailability and Bioequivalence Studies* (October 1997), *Bioanalytical Methods Validation for Human Studies* (December 1998), *Bioavailability and Bioequivalence Studies for Nasal Aerosols and Nasal Sprays for Local Action* (June 1999), *Topical Dermatological Drug Product NDAs and ANDAs—In Vivo Bioavailability* (June 1998), and *Waiver of In Vivo Bioavailability and Bioequivalence Studies for Immediate Release Solid Oral Dosage Forms Containing Certain Active Moieties/Active Ingredients Based on a Biopharmaceutics Classification System* (January 1999). The most recent in this area include *Bioanalytical Method Validation* (May 2001), which provides recommendations on developing validation information on bioanlytical methods for pharmacokinetic evaluation of human clinical pharmacology, bioavailability, and bioequivalence studies, and a February 2001 draft guidance entitled, *Statistical Approaches to Establishing Bioequivalence*, which discusses the use of average, population, and individual bioequivalence approaches and which replaces several earlier guidance documents in this area.

Microbiology Section This section is required only in NDAs for anti-infective/antibiotic, antiviral, special pathogen, sterile and certain nonsterile drug products. Since anti-infective, antiviral, and special pathogen drugs affect microbial—rather than clinical—physiology, reports on the drug's *in vivo* and *in vitro* effects on the target microorganisms are critical for establishing product effectiveness.

For sterile and certain nonsterile drugs (e.g., aqueous dosage forms that can support microbiological growth), applicants must also provide information to permit CDER microbiologists to conduct a product quality assessment. However, such information should be provided in the chemistry, manufacturing and controls section of the NDA.

Current regulations require that an NDA's microbiology drug section include microbiology data describing: (1) the biochemical basis of the drug's action on microbial physiology; (2) the drug's antimicrobial spectra, including results of *in vitro* preclinical studies demonstrating concentrations of the drug required for effective use; (3) any known mechanisms of resistance to the drug, including results of any known epidemiologic studies demonstrating prevalence of resistance factors; and (4) clinical microbiology laboratory methods needed to evaluate the effective use of the drug. Full reports of the studies, summary tables, and a summary narrative should be included for each portion of this section.

Specific guidance on developing the microbiology component of the NDA is available from the FDA's *Guideline for the Format and Content of the Microbiology Section of an Application* (February 1987). While they

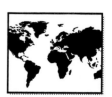

Worldwide Pharmaceutical Regulation Series

are not directly applicable to the NDA's microbiology section, it is worth noting here that CDER has released a spate of guidances as part of a series of documents to assist industry in conducting clinical trials on antimicrobial drugs for various infections. In 1998 alone, for example, the center released 20 such draft guidances for specific categories of antimicrobial drugs, including those for acute bacterial meningitis and sinusitis, acute otitis media, bacterial vaginosis, community-acquired pneumonia, Lyme disease, nosocomial pneumonia, uncomplicated gonorrhea, and uncomplicated urinary tract infections. The series also includes a general guidance entitled, *Developing Antimicrobial Drugs—General Considerations for Clinical Trials* (July 1998).

Clinical Data Section Since the FDA's conclusions regarding a new drug's safety and effectiveness are based largely on the data and analyses provided in the clinical data section, it is clearly the single most important element of the NDA. When taken together with the NDA's statistical component (see discussion below), the clinical section is also the application's most complex and voluminous.

Throughout the mid- and late 1990s, CDER's requirements for the NDA's clinical data section have been revised and clarified by several agency and ICH initiatives:

- Continuing CDER interest in standardizing the NDA review process has had implications for a few sections of the NDA, including the clinical data section. In October 1999, CDER Director Janet Woodcock, M.D., emphasized her desire to further standardize the review process, in part through the development and use of review "templates," which might ultimately reshape the presentation of clinical data. Woodcock also mentioned that she had a plan for the completion of CDER's Good Review Practices (GRP) initiative, which in part seeks to provide "some level of standardization in clinical reviews of NDAs" and which could also influence clinical safety and efficacy data presentations in new drug applications. In March 2001, CDER implemented, on a pilot basis centerwide, a standardized NDA review format, or template, for its clinical reviewers. Although the clinical review format, or template, was introduced on a pilot basis, it is mandatory within the center and is expected to be formally implemented by early 2002. CDER officials have also noted that the center is developing new GRP-related guidances to standardize the collection and analysis of clinical safety data in such areas as QTc prolongation and liver toxicity.

- In an August 1999 guidance entitled, *Submission of Abbreviated Reports and Synopses in Support of Marketing Applications*, CDER clarifies that NDA sponsors may submit specific trial information in different "formats"—full study reports, abbreviated reports, and synopses—depending on the information's importance. According to the agency, the guidance is intended to address industry uncertainty that has prevented many companies from submitting "less-than-full" studies, an option that FDA officials claim has been available to firms under the agency's *Guidelines for the Format and Content of the Clinical and Statistical Sections of New Drug Applications* (1988) and the ICH's E3 *Guidelines for the Structure and Content of Clinical Study Reports* (1996). The August 1999 guidance emphasizes that abbreviated study reports and synopses are more applicable to the submission of efficacy data, and that full reports on safety will be required in most cases.

- In releasing two guidances under its New Use Initiative - Primary and Supplemental Approvals, the FDA has provided perhaps its most detailed discussion of the clinical

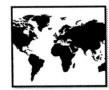

efficacy data necessary to support drug approval (see Chapter 5). A May 1998 guidance entitled, *Providing Clinical Evidence of Effectiveness for Human Drug and Biological Products* offers the agency's latest and most detailed views regarding the "quantitative and qualitative standards" for establishing drug effectiveness, including situations in which a single pivotal trial can support drug approval. In an October 2001 guidance entitled, *Cancer Drug and Biological Products—Clinical Data in Marketing Appliations*, CDER clarifies the clinical data necessary for oncology drugs, and notes that those requirements may be less demanding than those for less-serious diseases.

Given the complexity and importance of the clinical and statistical sections, it is not surprising that the FDA's most detailed NDA-related guideline addresses these two sections of the NDA. The agency's 125-page *Guideline for the Format and Content of the Clinical and Statistical Sections of an Application* (July 1988) provides recommendations on formatting and organizing these sections and on presenting the clinical and statistical information and accompanying documentation. The guideline also describes a fully integrated clinical and statistical report for documenting the results of individual studies. An ICH final guideline entitled, E3 *Structure and Content of Clinical Study Reports* (July 1996) supersedes Section III of the FDA guideline, and provides format and content standards for "an integrated full report of an individual study."

As specified in the FDA's 1988 guideline, the first two elements in the clinical data section are: (1) a list of investigators supplied with the drug or known to have studied the drug, INDs under which the drug has been studied, and NDAs submitted for the same drug substance; and (2) a background/overview of the clinical investigations (i.e., the general approach and rationale used in developing clinical data). According to FDA regulations and the guideline referenced above, the NDA's clinical data section should consist of as many as 11 additional elements:

1. A description and analysis of each clinical pharmacology study of the drug, including a brief comparison of the results of the human studies with the animal pharmacology and toxicology data.

2. A description and analysis of each controlled clinical study pertinent to a proposed use of the drug, including the protocol and a description of the statistical analyses used to evaluate the study. If the study report is an interim analysis, this must be noted and a projected completion date provided. Controlled clinical studies that have not been analyzed in detail should be provided, along with a copy of the protocol and a brief description of the results and status of the study.

3. A description of each uncontrolled study, a summary of the results, and a brief statement explaining why the study is classified as uncontrolled.

4. A description and analysis of any other data or information relevant to an evaluation of the safety and effectiveness of the drug product obtained or otherwise received by the applicant from any foreign or domestic source. This might include information derived from commercial marketing experience, reports in scientific literature, unpublished scientific papers, and controlled and uncontrolled studies of uses of the drug other than those proposed in the application.

5. An integrated summary of the data demonstrating substantial evidence of effectiveness for the claimed indications. Evidence is also required to support the

dosage and administration section of the labeling, including support for the dosage and dose interval recommended, and modifications for specific subgroups of patients (e.g., pediatrics, geriatrics, patients with renal failure).

6. An integrated summary of all available information about the safety of the drug product, including pertinent animal data, demonstrated or potential adverse effects of the drug, clinically significant drug/drug interactions, and other safety considerations, such as data from epidemiological studies of related drugs. Unless provided under section 2 above, the integrated safety summary should also describe any statistical analyses used in analyzing the safety data.

7. For drugs that might be abused, a description and analysis of studies or information related to abuse of the drug, including a proposal for scheduling and a description of any studies related to overdosage.

8. An integrated summary of the benefits and risks of the drug, including a discussion of why the benefits exceed the risks under the conditions stated in the labeling.

9. A statement noting that each human clinical study was conducted in compliance with the IRB regulations and with the informed consent regulations. If the study was not subject to IRB regulations, the applicant must state this fact.

10. If the sponsor transferred any of its regulatory obligations regarding the conduct of a clinical study (e.g., monitoring) to a contract research organization (CRO), a statement providing the name and address of the CRO, the identity of the clinical study, and a listing of the responsibilities transferred. When a sponsor transfers all of its obligations, the NDA may provide a "general statement of this transfer" in lieu of an itemized listing.

11. If the sponsor reviewed or audited original subject records during the course of monitoring any clinical study to verify the accuracy of the case report forms submitted by the investigator, the NDA must provide a list identifying each clinical study audited or reviewed.

Because it is designed, in part, to assist companies in assessing clinical data and preparing clinical summaries for marketing applications, the ICH's September 1998 E9 *Statistical Principles for Clinical Trials* should also be consulted by applicants. Applicants might also review the ICH's E9 *General Considerations for Clinical Trials* (December 1997).

During the early 1990s, the FDA became increasingly concerned with gender-, age-, and race-related drug response differences, particularly following a study showing that many NDAs lacked this information. Such information was already requested in the agency's 1988 *Guideline for the Format and Content of the Clinical and Statistical Sections of New Drug Applications*. In 1993, then-CDER Director Carl Peck, M.D., wrote to industry to emphasize the importance of this information and to announce that NDAs would no longer be accepted for review without it.

The pressure on sponsors to test their drugs in, and provide clinical data on, special populations has increased considerably during the mid- and late-1990s. The ICH, for example, has published *Guideline on Studies in Support of Special Populations: Geriatrics* (August 1994). In February 1998, the FDA released a final regulation to explicitly require gender, age, and racial subgroup data in NDAs. Under the regu-

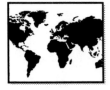

lation, which became effective in August 1998, an NDA's integrated summaries of safety and effectiveness must each include demographic subset analyses by gender, age, and racial subgroups and, when appropriate, other relevant subgroups.

In June 1998, the ICH parties released E5 *Ethnic Factors in the Acceptability of Foreign Clinical Data*, which provides guidance on regulatory and development strategies to allow clinical data collected in one region to be used to satisfy data requirements in other regions while permitting sponsors and regulatory bodies to adequately assess the impact of ethnic factors on a drug's safety, efficacy, dosage, and dose regimen. The ICH parties emphasize, however, that the E5 guidance is not designed to modify data requirements in the three participating regions, but rather to recommend when such requirements can be satisfied with foreign clinical data.

Safety Update Report Section As implied by its title, the safety update report is not filed with the original NDA, but is submitted in the form of updates at specific points in the application review process. Applicants must submit safety update reports four months after the NDA's submission, following the receipt of an approvable letter, and at other times requested by CDER.

In these reports, the applicant must update its pending NDA "with new safety information learned about the drug that may reasonably affect the statement of contraindications, warnings, precautions, and adverse reactions in the draft labeling." The updates must include the same types of information (from clinical studies, animal studies, and other sources), and must be submitted in the same format, as the NDA's integrated safety summary. They must also include case report forms for each patient who died during a clinical study or who did not complete the study because of an adverse event (unless this requirement is waived). Federal regulations encourage applicants to consult with the FDA on the form and content of these reports prior to the submission of the first report.

Statistical Section As evidenced by the fact that the FDA addressed the NDA's clinical and statistical sections in a single guideline, the two components are closely related. In fact, the core of the statistical section comprises data and analyses taken directly from the application's clinical data section.

According to the agency's *Guideline for the Format and Content of the Clinical and Statistical Sections of New Drug Applications* (July 1988), the core of the statistical section should include the following sections taken verbatim from the NDA's clinical section: (1) a list of investigators supplied with the drug or known to have investigated the drug, INDs under which the drug has been studied, and NDAs submitted for the same drug substance; (2) a background/overview of clinical investigations; (3) the controlled clinical studies section; (4) the integrated summary of effectiveness data; (5) the integrated summary of safety data; and (6) the integrated summary of benefits and risks.

The ICH guidance entitled, E9 *Statistical Principles for Clinical Trials* (September 1998) is the latest guidance addressing issues related to the statistical component of marketing applications. The guideline provides recommendations to sponsors regarding the design, conduct, analysis, and evaluation of clinical trials of an investigational product in the context of its overall clinical development. More germane to this discussion, the guidance also provides recommendations on preparing application summaries and assessing efficacy and safety evidence, principally from late Phase II and Phase III clinical

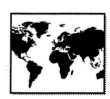

trials. For additional guidance, applicants should also consult the ICH guideline entitled, E3 *Structure and Content of Clinical Study Reports* (July 1996).

The FDA encourages applicants to meet with CDER—specifically, with the assigned biostatistical reviewer(s) within CDER's Office of Biostatistics—before an NDA's submission to discuss the section's format, tabulations, statistical analyses, and other important issues. In some cases, the agency permits applicants to submit, for review and comment, the preliminary tabulation of patient data and the materials on the statistical analyses of controlled clinical studies and/or safety data (see discussion of pre-NDA meetings below).

Case Report Tabulations Section During the FDA's most recent overhaul of its NDA regulations, the agency declared that "an efficient agency review of individual patient data should be based primarily on well-organized, concise, data tabulations...." Reviews of the "more lengthy patient case report forms" should be reserved for those instances in which a more detailed review is necessary, the agency stated (see discussion below).

In its *Guideline on Formatting, Assembling, and Submitting New Drug and Antibiotic Applications* (February 1987), however, the agency advises sponsors to "meet with FDA to discuss the extent to which tabulations of patient data in clinical studies, data elements within tables, and case report forms are needed. Such discussions can also cover alternative modes of data presentation and the need for special supporting information (for example, electrocardiograms, x-rays, or pathology slides)."

According to agency regulations and guidelines, the NDA must provide data tabulations on individual patients from each of the following: (1) the initial clinical pharmacology studies (Phase 1 studies); (2) effectiveness data from each adequate and well-controlled study (Phase 2 and Phase 3 studies); and (3) safety data from all studies.

Current regulations state that these tabulations should include "the data on each patient in each study, except that the applicant may delete those tabulations that the agency agrees, in advance, are not pertinent to a review of the drug's safety or effectiveness." The FDA is willing to discuss appropriate deletions from these tabulations at a "pre-NDA" conference.

Given that case report tabulation (CRT) and case report form submissions (see discussion below) can be voluminous, it is not surprising that CRTs and CRFs were the first elements of the NDA to be accepted in electronic form without their paper-based counterparts. In May 1996, CDER published a policy formally establishing a waiver process through which applicants could obtain permission to do so. In reality, however, this waiver process was a stopgap measure to be used until the FDA could finalize its proposed rule on electronic records and signatures, something that the agency did in March 1997. Under this regulation, all sections of an NDA can be submitted electronically without accompanying paper-based submissions.

In its related actions, however, the agency indicated that it planned to ease into the era of electronic-only filings, and that some of its early steps would be taken with electronic CRT and CRF filings. In September 1997, the agency released a guidance document entitled, *Archiving Submissions in Electronic Format—NDAs*, which provided guidance to applicants that wanted to make electronic submissions of CRFs and CRTs as part of the NDA's archival copy. A January 1999 guidance document entitled,

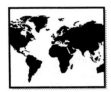

Providing Regulatory Submissions in Electronic Format—NDAs then superseded the September 1997 guidance, and provided information on how applicants could submit the entire archival copy of the NDA in electronic format. This document was accompanied by another guidance, *Providing Regulatory Submissions in Electronic Format—General Considerations* (January 1999), which addresses some of the more technical aspects of electronic submissions for CRTs and other NDA elements.

In more recent guidances, the FDA has stated its preference that CRTs be submitted in electronic data sets. In an October 2001 guidance entitled, *Cancer Drug and Biological Products—Clinical Data in Marketing Applications*, for example, the agency notes that the electronic CRT "is the preferred form of data submission for most oncology submissions, because data submitted electronically can generally be reviewed more rapidly and thoroughly."

Case Report Forms Section As stated above, the FDA does not require the routine submission of patient case report forms. Rather, an NDA must include CRFs for: (1) patients who died during a clinical study; and (2) patients who did not complete a study because of any adverse event, regardless of whether the adverse event is considered drug-related by the investigator or sponsor.

The FDA may request that the sponsor submit additional case report forms (and tabulations) that the agency views as important to the drug's review. Typically, the agency requests all case report forms for the pivotal studies. In doing so, the review division attempts to designate the critical studies for which case report forms are required approximately 30 days after the NDA's receipt. If a sponsor fails to submit the CRFs within 30 days of the FDA's request, the agency may view the eventual submission as a major amendment and extend the review period as appropriate.

Patent Information Applicants must provide information on any patent(s) on the drug for which approval is sought, or on a method of using the drug.

Patent Certification Applicants must provide a patent certification or statement regarding "any relevant patents that claim the listed drug or that claim any other drugs on which investigations relied on by the applicant for approval of the application were conducted, or that claim a use for the listed or other drug." According to the FDA's *Guideline on Formatting, Assembling, and Submitting New Drug and Antibiotic Applications* (February 1987), the patent certification and patent information sections should be attached to the application form (Form 356h) in the NDA submission.

Establishment Description The establishment description section is relevant for certain biological products only. Its incorporation in Form 356h is a function of the FDA's effort to develop a harmonized application form for both drugs and biologics.

Debarment Certification Since mid-1992, the FDA has required that all NDAs include a certification that the applicant did not and will not use the services of individuals or firms that have been debarred by the FDA. Under the Generic Drug Enforcement Act of 1992, the FDA is authorized to debar individuals convicted of crimes relating to the development, approval, or regulation of drugs or biologics from providing any services to applicants. The statute requires that applications for drug products include "a certification that the applicant did not and will not use in any capacity the services of any person debarred…in connection with such application." To address some of industry's most frequently asked questions about debarment certification and information requirements,

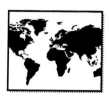

CDER released a September 1998 guidance for industry entitled, *Submitting Debarment Certification Statements*.

Field Copy Certification As stated earlier, U.S.-based NDA sponsors must submit a "field" copy of the NDA's chemistry, manufacturing, and controls section, application form, and summary directly to the relevant FDA district office for use during the pre-approval manufacturing inspection (see discussion above). The applicant is also required to certify in its NDA that an exact copy of the application's chemistry, manufacturing, and controls section has been forwarded to the district office.

User Fee Cover Sheet (Form FDA 3397) Since January 1994, the FDA has required every new drug application to include a copy of the User Fee Cover Sheet. This form provides information that allows the FDA to determine whether the application is subject to user fees and, if so, whether the appropriate fee for the application has been submitted (a check in the appropriate amount must be mailed to a specified FDA account at the same time that the NDA is forwarded to the agency). The agency issued a new version of the form in mid-1998. The User Fee Cover Sheet should be included with the NDA application form in the first volume of the application.

Financial Information Section In April 2000, the FDA revised its Form 356h to accommodate the new information required under its February 2, 1998, and December 31, 1998, final rules on investigator financial disclosure and certification. The agency issued these regulations for drug, biologics, and medical device applicants to ensure that investigator financial interests and sponsor/investigator financial arrangements that could affect the reliability of data submitted in premarketing applications are disclosed to the agency. Under these regulations, an applicant must submit, in the NDA, a list of clinical investigators who conducted covered clinical studies and, for each clinical investigator, must provide one of the following:

1. A certification on Form 3454 that: (1) no financial arrangements with the investigator have been made under which study outcome could affect compensation; (2) the investigator has no proprietary interest in the tested product; (3) the investigator does not have a significant equity interest in the sponsor of the covered study; and (4) the investigator has not received "significant payments of other sorts" (see discussion below).

2. A disclosure on Form 3455 of specific financial arrangements between the investigator and sponsor and any steps that the sponsor has taken to minimize bias. Under the agency's regulations, disclosable financial arrangements include the following:

    A. Compensation made to the investigator in which the value of compensation could be affected by study outcome. This requirement applies to all covered studies that are ongoing or completed as of February 2, 1999, or later.

    B. A proprietary interest in the tested product, including, but not limited to, a patent, trademark, copyright, or licensing agreement. This requirement applies to all covered studies that are ongoing or completed as of February 2, 1999, or later.

    C. Any equity interest in the sponsor of a covered study (i.e., any ownership interest, stock options, or other financial interest whose value cannot be

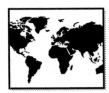

readily determined through reference to public prices). This requirement applies to all covered studies that are ongoing or completed as of February 2, 1999, or later.

D. Any equity interest in a publicly held company that exceeds $50,000 in value must be disclosed only for covered clinical studies that are ongoing on or after February 2, 1999. The requirement applies to interests held during the time the clinical investigator is carrying out the study and for 1 year following the completion of the study.

E. Significant payments of other sorts, which are payments that have a cumulative monetary value of $25,000 or more made by the sponsor of a covered study to the investigator or the investigator's institution to support activities of the investigator exclusive of the costs of conducting the clinical study or other clinical studies (e.g., a grant to fund ongoing research, compensation in the form of equipment or retainers for ongoing consultation or honoraria) during the time the clinical investigator is carrying out the study and for 1 year following completion of the study. This requirement applies to payments made on or after February 2, 1999.

If, upon reviewing such information in the NDA, agency reviewers determine that the financial interests raise a serious question about the integrity of the data, the FDA may initiate an audit of the data provided by the clinical investigator in question, request that the applicant conduct further data analyses or that additional studies be conducted to confirm the results of the questioned study, refuse to use the investigator's data as a basis for agency action, or take other appropriate action. According to CDER officials, when reviewers find that an investigator has a financial interest in a sponsor or the product under review, they will consider such information by more carefully scrutinizing the number of subjects the investigator enrolled and whether there were any outliers in terms of the adverse reactions reported by the investigator.

A disclosure or certification must be provided for each investigator of a "covered" clinical trial, FDA regulations state. Covered trials are defined as "any study of a drug, biological product, or device in humans submitted in a marketing application or reclassification petition that the applicant or FDA relies on to establish that the product is effective (including studies that show equivalence to an effective product) or any study in which a single investigator makes a significant contribution to the demonstration of safety. This would, in general, not include phase 1 tolerance studies or pharmacokinetic studies, most clinical pharmacology studies (unless they are critical to an efficacy determination), large open safety studies conducted at multiple sites, treatment protocols and parallel track protocols." In a March 2001 guidance document entitled, *Financial Disclosure by Clinical Investigators*, the FDA states that the sponsor must consider the potential role of a particular study based on study size, design, and other considerations, and that studies other than controlled effectiveness studies could also be considered critical, such as a pharmacodynamic study in a population subset or a bioequivalence study supporting a new dosage form."

With regard to the lengths to which companies should go in collecting this information from investigators, the guidance states that, "sponsors and applicants should use reasonable judgement in deciding how much effort needs to be expended to collect this information. If sponsors/applicants

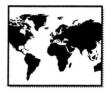

find it impossible to obtain the financial information in question, applicants should explain why this information was not obtainable and document attempts made in an effort to collect the information."

In mid-2000, CDER released data characterizing its experiences in the first year under the financial disclosure regulation. Perhaps most importantly, the center had not declined to review a study as a pivotal study because of any investigator's financial ties to a sponsor or product in the regulation's first 14 months. Of the applications that the agency received from February 1999 through April 2000, 33 included financial disclosures for one or more investigators, according to the data. Most of the remaining submissions dealt with the disclosure requirements in other ways, such as claiming that the studies included in the applications were not "covered" studies to which such requirements were relevant. Agency officials noted that they have been flexible with firms that have experienced problems in collecting financial information from investigators, provided that such firms have been able to show "due diligence" in attempting to obtain the information. Although a handful of the applications failed to make any reference to the financial disclosure requirements, agency officials noted that they have attempted to work with companies and had not refused to file any of the initial 129 applications submitted under the new regulation.

Other Information If necessary, the sponsor may use this portion of the application to incorporate by reference any information submitted prior to the NDA filing. The sponsor must also provide an accurate and complete English translation of a foreign language document for any information originally written in a foreign language.

Pre-NDA Meetings

Because of the NDA's complexity and because the FDA wants to avoid investing scarce resources reviewing deficient NDAs, the agency offers pre-submission conferences, called pre-NDA meetings, to all drug sponsors. Federal regulations state that the primary purpose of pre-NDA meetings "…is to uncover any major unresolved problems, to identify those studies that the sponsor is relying on as adequate and well-controlled to establish the drug's effectiveness, to acquaint FDA reviewers with the general information to be submitted in the marketing application (including technical information), to discuss appropriate methods for statistical analysis of the data, and to discuss the best approach to the presentation and formatting of data in the marketing application."

As is true for end-of-Phase 2 conferences, a sponsor must request a pre-NDA meeting with the division responsible for a drug's review. Although federal regulations establish that all drug sponsors have access to such conferences, the importance of the drug, the time constraints facing the relevant drug review division, and the significance of the scientific and regulatory issues at hand will do much to determine whether the FDA grants a pre-NDA meeting. CDER officials note that pre-NDA meeting requests are generally granted. In its PDUFA II commitments, the agency states that pre-NDA meetings and other Type B meetings (see Chapter 5 for a detailed discussion of the various types of meetings) "will be honored except in the most unusual circumstances." The pre-NDA meeting can take place any time before an NDA submission, but should not be held before Phase 3 studies near completion. According to CDER officials, such meetings generally are held six months prior to the planned NDA submission date.

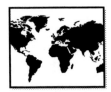

FDA commitments associated with PDUFA II have, in many cases, re-affirmed, and in other cases changed, CDER's standards for meetings as expressed in a 1996 policy entitled, *Formal Meetings Between CDER and CDER's External Constituents* (MaPP 4512.1). According to this MaPP, written requests for meetings should include at least six elements: a brief statement of the purpose of the meeting; a listing of the specific objectives/outcomes the requestor expects from the meeting; a proposed agenda, including the estimated time needed for each agenda item; a listing of planned external attendees; a listing of requested participants from CDER; and the approximate time at which supporting documentation (i.e., the "backgrounder") for the meeting will be sent to CDER (i.e., "x" weeks prior to the meeting, but should be received by CDER at least 2 weeks in advance of the scheduled meeting).

In a February 2000 guidance entitled, *Formal Meetings with Sponsors and Applicants for PDUFA Products*, the agency recommends a similar, but slightly more detailed, list of contents for meeting requests: (1) product name and application number; (2) chemical name and structure; (3) proposed indication(s); (4) the type of meeting being requested (in this case, a Type B meeting); (5) a brief statement of the purpose of the meeting, possibly including a discussion of the types of completed or planned studies or data that the sponsor or applicant intends to discuss at the meeting, the general nature of the critical questions to be asked, and where the meeting fits in the overall development plans; (6) a list of the specific objectives/outcomes expected from the meeting; (7) a preliminary proposed agenda, including estimated amounts of time needed for each agenda item and designated speaker(s); (8) a draft list of specific questions grouped by review discipline (e.g., clinical, chemistry); (9) a list of individuals (including titles) who will attend the proposed meeting from the sponsor's or applicant's organization and consultants; (10) a list of agency staff that the sponsor requests participate in the proposed meeting (if the applicant is uncertain as to what agency officials should attend, it does not need to include specific individuals in the request, but should include requested disciplines if known); (11) the approximate date on which the sponsor will forward supporting documentation (i.e., the information package) to the review division; and (12) suggested dates and times (i.e., morning or afternoon) for the meeting.

Within 14 days of receiving the request, the reviewing division must notify the requestor in writing (either by letter or fax) of the date, time, and location at which the meeting will be held, as well as the likely CDER participants. Under CDER's PDUFA II commitments, the pre-NDA meeting should occur within 60 calendar days of the agency's receipt of the meeting request. If such a meeting is immediately necessary for an otherwise "stalled" drug development program to proceed, a sponsor can request an earlier, "critical path meeting." Such meetings, FDA notes, generally will be reserved for dispute resolution, to discuss clinical holds, and to address special protocol assessments following the agency's initial evaluation. CDER must fulfill its meetings management system goals for at least 80% of meeting requests received in FY2000 and 90% in subsequent fiscal years (see Chapter 5 for a more detailed discussion of CDER's meetings management system).

The success of a pre-NDA meeting depends largely on sponsor preparation. To help FDA staffers prepare and to ensure that there will be a "meaningful discussion" at the meeting, sponsors should submit to the reviewing division an "information package" at least four weeks in advance of the formal pre-NDA meeting. This information package, which the agency recommends in its guidance should be a fully paginated document with a table of contents, indices, appendices, cross references, and

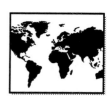

tabs, should generally include the following elements: (1) product name and application number; (2) chemical name and structure; (3) proposed indication(s); (4) dosage form, route of administration, and dosing regimen (frequency and duration); (5) a brief statement of the purpose of the meeting, possibly including a discussion of the types of completed or planned studies or data that the sponsor or applicant intends to discuss at the meeting, the general nature of the critical questions to be asked, and where the meeting fits in the overall development plans; (6) a list of the specific objectives/outcomes expected from the meeting; (7) a proposed agenda, including estimated amounts of time needed for each agenda item and designated speaker(s); (8) a list of specific questions grouped by review discipline (e.g., clinical, chemistry); (9) a clinical data summary (as appropriate); (10) a preclinical data summary (as appropriate); and (11) chemistry, manufacturing, and controls information (as appropriate). Although the applicant will have provided much of this information in the meetings request, it should be updated for the information package, the agency notes.

Recently, CDER has begun to develop industry guidances for discipline-specific aspects of sponsor/applicant meetings. In a February 2000 draft guidance entitled, IND *Meetings for Human Drugs and Biologics: Chemistry, Manufacturing, and Controls Information*, for example, CDER outlines considerations relevant to the elements of pre-NDA meetings focused on CMC issues.

FDA staffers stress that a particularly important element of pre-NDA meetings is the portion devoted to the statistical review. To make optimal use of the meeting, the sponsor should send, or have present at the meeting, sample mock-ups or computer printouts of data to provide FDA statisticians the opportunity to offer advice on data organization and presentation.

Under CDER's PDUFA II commitments, final minutes of the formal meeting should be distributed to FDA and sponsor attendees within 30 days of the meeting. Applicants can submit their own draft minutes to the agency for consideration in developing the formal meeting minutes, provided that they are forwarded promptly. After reviewing the agency's formal minutes, the applicant can seek clarification or amendment of the minutes.

Assembling and Submitting the NDA

The FDA has extremely specific requirements for the NDA's assembly, many of which are provided in the agency's *Guideline on Formatting, Assembling, and Submitting New Drug and Antibiotic Applications* (February 1987). This 32-page document offers general guidance on such issues as content requirements, and more detailed specifications on such issues as paper size, maximum volume size, volume identification, and pagination.

In mid-1997, CDER stopped supplying application binders to industry, and firms had to provide for the printing of their own binders. In November 1997, CDER issued a guidance entitled, *Required Specifications for FDA's IND, NDA, ANDA, and Drug Master File Binders* to provide companies with detailed specifications on application binders.

Due to difficulties that industry experienced in having commercial printers develop binders that met agency specifications as well as resources that CDER had to invest in rejacketing NDAs that included out-of-specification binders, the agency announced in April 1998 that industry could purchase official

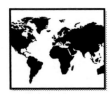

binders from the Government Printing Office. Applicants can obtain specific details on binder specifications and information on ordering binders through the FDA's website at www.fda.gov/cder/ddms/binders.html.

Amending the NDA

Either at its own initiative or in response to an FDA request, an applicant may seek to clarify or augment the information provided in the original NDA during the review process. For example, the applicant may submit a new analysis of previously submitted data, new data not available at the time of the NDA submission, or information necessary to address a deficiency in the drug application. As noted above, the FDA is now permitting NDA applicants to develop and submit NDA amendments in the common technical document (CTD) format (see discussion above). NDA applicants can provide amendments in the CTD format even when the conventional NDA format was used for the original application.

Regardless of the format in which it is submitted, any such information provided for an unapproved application is considered an NDA amendment. Depending on its timing, the submission of a significant amendment—a major reanalysis of clinical data, for example—may trigger an extension in the FDA's timeline for the application's review (see Chapter 8).

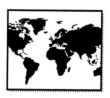

CHAPTER 8

The NDA Review Process

During the 1990s, no other aspect of the U.S. drug development and approval system evolved as significantly as the FDA's new drug application (NDA) review and approval process. So fundamental were these changes—and the improvements in drug review times that resulted from them—that CDER's NDA review performance was transformed from one of the most harshly criticized of FDA activities into what was perhaps the agency's best defense against various regulatory reform proposals advanced in the mid-1990s.

The driving force behind this evolution, of course, was the Prescription Drug User Fee Act (PDUFA I and II), and the changes that CDER has implemented to meet the evolving review timelines associated with the legislation. In the early and mid-1990s, CDER management instituted tight controls for managing and tracking drug reviews, and reorganized the center's drug review divisions into smaller, more therapeutically focused units (see Chapter 4).

But CDER's success in approving record numbers of new drugs in record time drew considerable criticism in light of other developments during the late 1990s. After three approved drugs (Redux, Posicor, and Duract) were withdrawn within a nine-month span from late 1997 through mid-1998, agency critics quickly and openly charged that the focus on the speed of drug approvals had come at the expense of drug safety, which they claimed was contributing to the estimated 100,000 U.S. deaths each year related to adverse drug reactions. More recent drug withdrawals, including Rezulin, Lotronex, Raplon, and Baycol, continued to feed such perceptions as the FDA and industry headed into all-important discussions for PDUFA reauthorization in late 2001.

True or not, these perceptions seemed to be supported, at the time, by public comments from CDER reviewers. In what was likely the most public criticism of the FDA's user fee program by a CDER reviewer, Division of Metabolism and Endocrine Drug Products Medical Officer Robert Misbin, M.D., wrote in a letter to the *Washington Post*, "Considering such cases [of the questionable use of washout periods in clinical studies for diabetes and other indications] along with recent examples of unsafe drugs that had to be pulled from the market soon after approval, an observer might conclude that the pharmaceutical industry is conspiring with university-based medical researchers to bring new drugs to market as quickly as possible, and that the FDA is failing in its duty to protect the public." In offering possible explanations for "this state of affairs," Misbin noted that "the program by which drug companies pay fees for review of their new drug applications has enabled FDA to hire new physician reviewers (including myself) and to reduce the time needed for review. But an unfortunate consequence is a linking of the productivity of FDA reviewers with the approval of new products. The more new drugs approved, the more productive the FDA appears, even if the new drugs are not as good as what is available today."

In December 1998, the Public Citizen's Health Research Group (HRG) released the results of a survey of 52 CDER medical officers in which some claimed that, under the prescription drug user fee program, certain drugs had been approved too quickly, some approved drugs should never have been approved, "inappropriate pressure" in the form of phone calls from Congress and senior FDA employees was being applied to encourage drug approvals, and reviewers were being pressured to alter their review opinions in some cases.

CDER officials responded to the resultant press, congressional, and public pressure by emphasizing that, during the PDUFA years, its record of drug withdrawals "compared favorably" with its record in earlier years. Emerging data that include the latest round of drug withdrawals suggest that the agency's drug withdrawal rates may be at least as high in more recent years. After withdrawing 3.2 percent and 4.4 percent of new molecular entities approved in 1979-1983 and 1984-1988 respectively, the agency withdrew just 2.4 percent of those NMEs approved from 1989-1993. The agency's withdrawal rates appear to be rising at least somewhat during the years in which the prescription drug user fee program really took hold: To date, the agency has withdrawn 2.9% of the NMEs approved from 1994-1998 and 3.3 percent of the new drugs approved from 1999-2000.

While insisting that drug withdrawal rates had not increased, FDA officials openly acknowledged the growing need for a particularly efficient and well-conceived post-marketing drug risk surveillance, assessment, and management program in the face of the speedier and rising numbers of new drug approvals. Therefore, CDER officials announced a reinvigorated postmarketing drug surveillance program under a newly named Office of Post-Marketing Drug Risk Assessment (OPDRA). In addition, the agency spoke about the need to apply "a new systems framework" to medical product risk management, which would involve a better integration of the efforts of those involved in the prescribing and use of new drugs (patients, practitioners) and better communication of the risks of drug use to both patients and physicians. In 2001, CDER renamed OPDRA the Office of Drug Safety and moved the office, along with selected other relevant programs, into a new office led by a physician with special expertise in risk assessment (see Chapter 4).

Despite such moves, many became convinced that the level of attention given to Redux, Rezulin, and other recent drug withdrawals had begun to exact a price, largely in the form of more conservative decision making in drug reviews. During 2000 and 2001, the perception of a full-blown "FDA slowdown" in drug reviews gained credibility, in part due to a downturn in new molecular entity (NME) approvals, which FDA officials claimed was related to a downturn in industry submissions and not a slowdown in FDA reviews. In fact, FDA data showed that, from 1995 to 2000, industry NME submissions had dropped 35 percent. Although the FDA continued to meet its PDUFA review goals in recent years, industry officials maintained that the agency was increasingly doing so by taking fewer positive actions (i.e., product approvals) and by stretching the review period by asking for more clarifications, data, and information through approvable and not-approvable actions.

While they initially rejected claims that CDER's NDA review performance was suffering, center officials did concede, in late 2001, that some application reviews might be suffering. In making their case

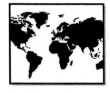

for increased funding from either user fees or congressional appropriations, CDER officials claimed that the number of review cycles necessary to approve "standard" applications seemed to be growing, something that they believed "may be due to the fact that reviewers, pressed to meet the new PDUFA II goals for drug development (e.g., meetings, special protocol assessments, and responses to clinical holds), have had less time to devote to resolving last minute problems with these standard applications in time to meet the action goal date." Without additional funding, FDA officials warned, the agency would be unable to "increase or even maintain" PDUFA performance levels.

The perceptions of FDA caution or conservatism in assessing the safety of new drugs led some companies to very publicly delay their NDA submissions so they could further characterize specific safety issues regarding their new products in what one official called "a safety-conscious FDA environment." Recent drug withdrawals along with scientific advances in the understanding of specific drug effects and their implications have almost certainly sensitized drug developers and FDA reviewers to certain adverse drug effects—perhaps liver toxicities (the most common reason for drug withdrawals) and QTc prolongation, in particular—in assessing new drugs.

Other CDER initiatives underscored the growing concern over postmarketing drug safety, and illustrated the center's desire, when possible, to address such issues in advance during the NDA review process. In late 2000, for example, CDER initiated a pilot program under which the center's drug review divisions could request a "pre-decision meeting" during which they could present a pending decision—often an NDA-related issue—to top CDER officials for their consideration and input. A year earlier, CDER had announced that its new drug review divisions and its Office of Post-Marketing Drug Risk Assessment (OPDRA) would hold "preapproval safety conferences" prior to approving applications for certain drugs, including new molecular entities. According to the center, these conferences have several primary goals, including ensuring that OPDRA is aware of any potential safety problems in drugs that are about to be approved, and providing a forum for considering the need for any special postmarketing analyses, safety studies, or other evaluations by the sponsor.

In addition to lingering questions regarding, and sensitivities over, drug safety issues, several factors seemed likely to influence the NDA review process's next phase of evolution:

The Common Technical Document. In August 2001, the ICH's "common technical document," or CTD, formally became a regulatory option to the NDA for companies seeking FDA approval of a new drug (see Chapter 7). During a "transition period" that will last until July 2003, companies will have the option of submitting original NDAs and even NDA supplements and amendments in either the CTD or conventional NDA format. In July 2003, the CTD will become the submission format "highly recommended" by the FDA. While the shift to the CTD will be more directly applicable to U.S. marketing dossiers and their development, it will also have some implications for the agency's new drug reviewers and review procedures.

Electronic NDA Reviews and Communications. A second important sea change—this one toward the electronic NDA—is having a significant effect on the new drug review process, and will ultimately dovetail with the adoption of the CTD. In recent years, CDER has continued to migrate toward an electronic NDA submission and review system (see Chapter 6), a reality that has had major implications for NDA applicants, agency reviewers, and the NDA review process itself. This migration is

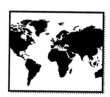

expected to accelerate going forward: Under its PDUFA II commitments, the FDA agreed to develop and implement a paperless, electronic application submission system for all applications, including NDAs and INDs, by October 2002. CDER officials made clear that their top electronic review-related priority was to make the NDA the first type of application that could be submitted entirely electronically (previously, electronic submissions had to be accompanied by paper-based applications). Following a 1997 regulation permitting the electronic-only submission of drug applications and a series of 1999 guidances informing industry on how to accomplish this for selected aspects of the NDA, electronic submissions have grown. Of the first 61 original NDAs in FY2001, for example, 35 percent were fully electronic (i.e., the archival NDA copy) and another 36 percent were mixed paper/electronic applications. In electronic NDAs, text-based documents are being submitted as PDF files, and datasets are being provided in SAS transport file format. As the FDA and industry prepared for the CTD era, both were looking ahead to the next evolutionary stage—the electronic CTD, or eCTD. Although the FDA's August 2001 draft guidance on the CTD emphasizes that the agency will release a guidance when it is prepared to accept electronic submissions in the CTD format, it also noted that industry will, in the interim, be permitted to "adapt the CTD to our current process for electronic submissions...." Meanwhile, other technological advances, including a secure e-mail system that CDER rolled out to facilitate NDA-review related sponsor/FDA regulatory communications, will likely influence the evolution of the drug review process as well.

Renewed Interest in Standardizing the NDA Review Process. In late 1999, CDER Director Janet Woodcock, M.D., re-emphasized her commitment to standardizing the NDA review process. Woodcock said that the center would attempt to standardize and improve the efficiency of the NDA review process, in part through the development and use of review "templates," in part to improve communication and to ensure that reviewers capture the most critical information in their NDA evaluations. In March 2001, CDER implemented, on a pilot basis centerwide, a standardized NDA review format, or template, for its clinical reviewers. Although the clinical review template was introduced on a pilot basis, its use is mandatory within the center and is expected to be formally implemented by early 2002. This was followed in May 2001 by a guidance detailing a standardized review format for the agency's assessments of the pharmacology/toxicology sections of NDAs and INDs. Woodcock also promised to reinvigorate CDER's Good Review Practices (GRP) initiative, which was undertaken in the mid-1990s and under which the center was in the process of developing a series of reviewer guidances that seek to provide "some level of standardization in clinical reviews of NDAs." This effort, which has languished for several years as the agency focused on meeting its user-fee goals, has been taken over by CDER's new Review Standards Staff (see discussion below), a group that is first attempting to form a consensus on the future direction of the GRP initiative. Before these recent efforts, the GRP initiative was able to produce a November 1996 draft reviewer guidance entitled, *Conducting a Clinical Safety Review of a New Product Application and Preparing a Report on the Review*—an accompanying draft on conducting an NDA's efficacy medical review was also developed and circulated internally, but has not been released by CDER. Another component of the GRP initiative was the reviewer diagram project, an attempt by various CDER medical reviewers to visualize and outline their own NDA review process. This project had produced a series of five reviewer diagrams, which appear under titles such as "NDA Review Process Overview" and "Outline for Performing an NDA Review" and which were developed by reviewers in the anti-infectives, antiviral, oncology (two diagrams), and neuropharmacological divisions.

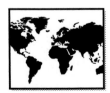

Integration of "Risk Management" into NDA Reviews. In responding to concerns regarding drug safety, CDER is integrating considerations of risk management, or risk intervention, alternatives into NDA reviews to control drug risks, center officials first claimed in early 2000. In doing so, the drug center is asking sponsors and its reviewers to consider what additional steps, aside from simply providing risk information on drug labels, can be taken to make newly approved drugs as safe as possible in the marketplace. The use of risk management in drug reviews is, in part, a function of the agency's recognition, through multiple recent product withdrawals, that labeling alone has not been sufficient to ensure the safe use of drugs in a medical system in which drugs are not always prescribed and used according to approved labeling. Risk management alternatives that CDER is evaluating increasingly in new drug reviews include restricted distribution programs, educational programs, patient package inserts, pregnancy registries, special surveillance systems, and safety-related communications. CDER's efforts in this area are now being led by its Review Standards Staff (RSS), which is attempting to create a risk-management framework from early drug development through post-marketing, and which will attempt to develop a systems-based approach for risk communication and risk intervention and for communicating risks to important audiences, including consumers and prescribers. In late 2001, CDER announced that it would form a new Drug Safety and Risk Management Advisory Subcommittee under its Advisory Committee for Pharmaceutical Science to address general drug safety and risk management issues and to consider the approval and continued marketing of specific drugs in the context of these issues.

Although significant, such factors are unlikely to affect the basic nature of drug reviews. In several ways, the NDA review is similar to the IND review. The NDA is forwarded to the same division and, most likely, many of the same reviewers who evaluated the IND for the drug. And like the IND evaluation, the NDA review involves an evaluation of key medical/clinical, nonclinical pharmacology/toxicology, and manufacturing issues. In several important ways, however, the NDA review process is unique:

- The NDA is a significantly larger and more complex document than the IND. Therefore, the NDA review absorbs far greater resources. Whereas INDs often comprise a few dozen volumes, NDAs for new molecular entities average over 200 volumes.

- The FDA's evaluation of the NDA involves a detailed assessment of the drug's clinical safety and effectiveness, while the IND review, in many cases, involves only an assessment of the drug's likely clinical effects based on preclinical animal data.

- The implications of the actions proposed in an NDA are much more substantial than those proposed in an IND. Under a newly activated IND, a drug is used in patient populations of limited size and under carefully monitored conditions. When an NDA is approved, however, a drug may be prescribed for thousands of patients who comprise a group much larger and less homogeneous than those that were involved in clinical trials. In addition, a marketed drug generally is used under significantly less carefully monitored conditions than during the clinical testing phase.

A Profile of the NDA Review Process

Several factors make efforts to profile the FDA's NDA review process somewhat challenging. While CDER traditionally has maintained guidelines on various activities, the center has offered few analyses of the NDA review process in the past. This is slowly changing, however, as the agency continues

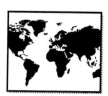

to release various internal policy guidances (i.e., MaPPs) on various aspects of the drug review process. And, as noted above, CDER's GRP initiative and related efforts to develop review "templates" for key review disciplines continue to provide important insights into the new drug review process. Meanwhile, the user-fee performance goals facing CDER have made some aspects of the review process more transparent and predictable.

Secondly, the various approaches to the NDA review by CDER's 14 drug review divisions are likely to differ in some ways. While acknowledging that CDER drug reviewers function under the same umbrella of laws and regulations, CDER Director Janet Woodcock, M.D., noted in late 1999 that the drug review process remains very much a "cottage industry," and that reviewers are "artists" who have a certain license to approach and conduct NDA reviews as they choose within this general framework.

Still, the NDA review process is sufficiently uniform across CDER's 14 new drug review divisions to permit a general analysis, such as the overview provided in the following sections.

Initial Processing of the NDA

As it does for INDs, CDER's Central Document Room (CDR) handles the initial processing of NDAs. This processing is largely administrative in nature—staffers record information on the filing, including the sponsor's name, the drug, and the application's identification number, which is assigned by the CDR. Staffers also stamp the application with a receipt date, which starts the review timeline applicable to the filing under the prescription drug user fee program (see discussion below).

CDER's Central Document Room also disassembles the various copies of the NDA for distribution to the divisions that will evaluate the application. Although the bulk of the NDA review will take place within the drug review division responsible for the product, other divisions—such as the Division of Pharmaceutical Evaluation I, II, or III (i.e., biopharmaceutics) and the Division of Biometrics I, II, or III—also receive the technical sections relevant to their reviews.

Processing Within the Drug Review Division

Following the initial processing of the NDA, CDER's Central Document Room forwards the submission to a similar document control center within the review division responsible for the application's review. After the NDA is logged in, a division staffer prepares an acknowledgement letter for the applicant. This letter informs the sponsor of the application's NDA number and date of receipt, and identifies the project manager who will be the company's FDA contact person—in many cases, the project manager assigned to a drug's IND will be assigned to the NDA as well. The project manager functions, in part, as a coordinator for the entire NDA review, ensuring that the application is distributed and is evaluated within milestones set for the NDA.

Upon receiving the NDA, the project manager performs an initial screening to ensure that the application is complete, the first and less detailed of two such screenings the application will face before the formal review process begins. If the submission is found to be seriously incomplete, the division will refuse to file the NDA, and return the submission to the applicant with a letter describing the deficiencies.

If the NDA passes this initial screening, the application's technical sections are distributed to reviewers in the primary technical review disciplines—medical/clinical, pharmacology/toxicology, chemistry,

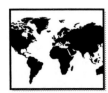

and microbiology (e.g., for anti-infective drugs). These individuals, along with consultancy reviewers (e.g., statistical and clinical biopharmacology reviewers) within other divisions, form the NDA's review team. For NDAs proposing prescription-to-OTC switches, CDER's Division of Over-the-Counter Drug Products will play a significant role in the review process as well.

Each reviewer then undertakes a more thorough, or technical, screening of the NDA, called a "completeness review" within some divisions. This evaluation ensures that sufficient data and information have been submitted in each area to justify "filing" the application—that is, initiating the formal review of the NDA.

Generally, the review team then convenes with division management in what is called a "45-Day Meeting" (so named because it takes place within 45 days of the NDA's submission) to determine whether the application should be filed or refused. If the team agrees that the application should be filed, the meeting may then be used as a review-planning session.

At this planning session, the review team assigns a review priority to the application (i.e., standard or priority), a designation that reflects the therapeutic importance of the drug and that will define the agency's timeline goal for taking formal action on the application (see discussion below). In addition, it will often set several internal review milestones that are deemed necessary for the division to meet the review goal applicable to the NDA (see discussion below). Some divisions will share these mid-review goals with the NDA's sponsor.

The FDA's Refuse-to-File Authorities

NDAs that the review team agrees, prior to the start of the formal review, are incomplete or deficient become the subject of a formal refuse-to-file (RTF) action. In such cases, the review division prepares a letter advising the applicant of the RTF decision and the deficiencies upon which it is based. The division will attempt to forward this letter within 60 days after the NDA receipt date.

For several reasons, the agency's RTF policies gained a significantly higher profile in the early 1990s. First, beginning in 1993, RTF decisions began to carry a direct financial penalty for NDA sponsors—under PDUFA, companies had to surrender a portion—25%—of the full application fee when an NDA was refused. Moreover, with new pressures to take action on NDAs within the aggressive user-fee timelines, CDER officials warned industry that the application of the RTF policy would become more stringent. In a July 1993 RTF guidance document, CDER pointed out that, "in the past, decisions to refuse to file an application generally were based on extreme deficiencies, e.g., the total omission of a needed section or the absence of any study that was even arguably an adequate and well-controlled study. More recently, applications have been refused when less extreme deficiencies existed, but when it was clear that the deficiencies were severe enough to make the application not approvable without major modification."

Several years into the prescription drug user-fee program, the agency proclaimed that industry had responded to the clarion call for higher quality submissions, and that the increased quality of NDA filings was one of the program's most significant successes. Eight years into the user-fee program, CDER's RTF rate dropped from 26% (1993) to 4% (2000). While many CDER divisions have not refused any NDAs in recent years, RTF rates can vary considerably between review units (see exhibit below).

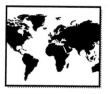

Another contributing factor to lower RTF rates may be CDER's establishment of an RTF Peer Review Committee, which meets quarterly to evaluate all of the center's RTF decisions. Divisions that issue RTFs must present and defend these decisions to the senior-level committee. In addition, applicants are given the opportunity to appear before the committee to discuss RTFs placed on their NDAs.

CDER's July 1993 RTF guidance document states that the center will exercise RTF authority under three circumstances: (1) omission of a section of the NDA required under federal regulations, or presentation of a section in so haphazard a manner as to render it incomplete on its face; (2) clear failure to include evidence of effectiveness compatible with the statute and regulations; and (3) omission of critical data, information, or analyses needed to evaluate effectiveness and safety or provide adequate directions for use. Most importantly, the document instructs CDER to continue basing RTF decisions "on omissions or inadequacies so severe as to render the application incomplete on its face. To be a basis for RTF, the omissions or inadequacies should be obvious, at least once identified, and not a matter of interpretation or judgement about the meaning of data submitted. The RTF is not an appropriate vehicle for dealing with complex and close judgments on such matters as balancing risks and benefits, magnitude of drug effect, acceptability of a plausible surrogate marker, or nuances of study design (although designs that are obviously inadequate may lead to RTF...)."

Still, CDER's review divisions have considerable discretion regarding RTF decisions. For example, the document states that "minor defects or omissions that could be repaired after the review commenced and that would not materially interfere with or delay review of the remainder of the application should not lead to RTF." Further, the RTF policy provides review divisions with several discretionary powers (e.g., the right to not employ RTFs for NDAs for critically needed new drugs).

Although certain CDER divisions had accepted incomplete applications, sometimes called "rolling NDAs," in an effort to expedite the review of high-priority products, the FDA Modernization Act of 1997 formally called on the agency to do so in specific cases. Under the legislation's "fast track" review procedure, the FDA should accept for filing and begin the review of an incomplete NDA for designated fast track product, provided that the applicant provides a schedule for the submission of information necessary to make the application complete and pays the required user fees. In most cases, the agency will accept only "complete sections" of the NDA (e.g., a complete chemistry, manufacturing and controls section) before the remaining sections are submitted. The "fast track" process applies only to drugs that have the potential to address unmet medical needs for serious and life-threatening conditions (see Chapter 15).

The Preapproval Inspection

A division's decision to file an NDA triggers a few actions, including the beginning of the primary review process (see discussion below). It also triggers a division request for a preapproval inspection of the sponsor's manufacturing facilities. During such inspections, FDA field investigators audit manufacturing-related statements and commitments made in the NDA against the sponsor's actual manufacturing practices. Specifically, the FDA has several goals in conducting these inspections:

1. To verify the accuracy and completeness of the manufacturing-related information submitted in the NDA.

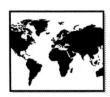

Divisional RTF Actions, 1993–2000
Percent of NDAs Refused
(# of RTF actions/# of NDA submissions)

	1993	1994	1995*	1996*	1997*	1998*	1999*	2000*
Cardio-Renal Drug Products	0% (0/11)	0% (0/8)	0% (0/11)	0% (0/9)	10% (1/10)	22% (2/9)	0% (0/9)	0% (0/7)
Neuropharmacological Drug Products	17% (1/6)	27% (3/11)	23% (3/13)	0% (0/16)	0% (0/15)	9% (2/22)	0% (0/10)	20% (3/15)
Oncologic Drug Products	–	–	0% (0/5)	10% (1/10)	0% (0/8)	9% (1/11)	8% (1/12)	0% (0/8)
Pulmonary Drug Products	–	–	20% (2/10)	14% (1/7)	0% (0/12)	0% (0/10)	0% (0/4)	0% (0/9)
Medical Imaging and Radiopharm. Drug Products	–	–	0% (0/8)	0% (0/5)	0% (0/4)	0% (0/6)	0% (0/2)	0% (0/4)
Gastrointestinal and Coagulation Drug Products	57% (4/7)	15% (2/13)	0% (0/13)	0% (0/11)	0% (0/7)	0% (0/6)	0% (0/6)	8% (1/12)
Metabolism and Endocrine Drug Products	50% (6/12)	11% (2/19)	0% (0/12)	0% (0/12)	0% (0/9)	8% (1/12)	8% (2/24)	11% (2/19)
Anti-Infective Drug Products	27% (4/15)	0% (0/8)	0% (0/12)	33% (1/3)	0% (0/11)	0% (0/6)	0% (0/5)	0% (0/6)
Antiviral Drug Products	0% (0/7)	0% (0/15)	0% (0/11)	0% (0/8)	0% (0/6)	0% (0/6)	13% (1/8)	0% (0/7)
Dermatological and Dental Drug Products	–	–	0% (0/13)	0% (0/7)	0% (0/11)	10% (1/10)	0% (0/13)	0% (0/10)
Anesthetic, Critical Care and Addiction Drug Products	–	–	0% (0/12)	0% (0/3)	0% (0/2)	0% (0/7)	0% (0/3)	0% (0/3)
Anti-Inflammatory, Analgesic and Ophthalmic Drug Products	–	–	0% (0/12)	11% (1/9)	0% (0/8)	0% (0/7)	0% (0/14)	0% (0/12)
Special Pathogens and Immunologic Drug Products+	–	–	–	0% (0/9)	0% (0/12)	0% (0/8)	0% (0/9)	0% (0/5)
Reproductive and Urologic Drug Products	–	–	0% (0/6)	7% (1/14)	0% (0/13)	0% (0/8)	0% (0/15)	0% (0/16)
Over-the-Counter Drug Products	–	–	0% (0/2)	0% (0/0)	0% (0/0)	0% (0/4)	0% (0/2)	0% (0/2)
Total**	29% (25/86)	13% (17/133)	4% (5/140)	4% (5/123)	0.8% (1/128)	5% (7/131)	3% (4/136)	4% (6/135)

* 1995, 1996, 1997, 1998, 1999, and 2000 data are fiscal year data. Data as of 4/30/98 for FY97 and 1/31/99 for FY98.

** Divisional statistics may not add to totals because of several reorganizations.

+ Division created in 1997. FY95 and FY96 figures adjusted to include drugs under this division as if it had existed as of FY95.

Source: FDA; U.S. Regulatory Reporter

Chapter 8

The NDA Review Process

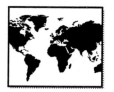

Worldwide Pharmaceutical Regulation Series

2. To evaluate the manufacturing controls for the preapproval batches upon which information provided in the NDA is based.

3. To evaluate the manufacturer's capabilities to comply with CGMPs and manufacturing-related commitments made in the NDA. In doing so, the FDA investigator will determine whether the necessary facilities, equipment, systems, and controls are functioning.

4. To collect a variety of drug samples for analysis by FDA field and CDER laboratories. These samples may be subjected to several analyses, including methods validation, methods verification, and profile sampling (i.e., taking a "fingerprint" of the actual product).

According to CDER policy, product-specific preapproval inspections generally are conducted for products: (1) that are new chemical or molecular entities; (2) that have narrow therapeutic ranges; (3) that represent the first approval for the applicant; or (4) that are sponsored by a company with a history of CGMP problems or that are manufactured in a facility that has not been the subject of a CGMP inspection over a considerable period. It is CDER's goal to have the pre-approval inspection assigned and conducted two months before the action due date applicable to an NDA. More specific guidance on CDER's preapproval inspection program is available from the center's Compliance Program Guide 7346.832.

Under a pilot CGMP-related program initiated in early 1999, CDER had been contacting drug manufacturing facilities routinely to inform them of when agency investigators would arrive for pre-approval inspections. Although the pilot program was discontinued in early 2001, FDA investigators in many district offices still have the option of providing manufacturing sites with advance notice of upcoming pre-approval inspections. If an inspection involves a new manufacturing site or a site that received a past warning letter, no such advance notice is provided.

At the conclusion of the preapproval inspection, the field office that conducted the inspection will recommend that the application be approved or that approval be withheld because of the inspection results (or because the facility was not ready). Based on preapproval inspections conducted during 1999, FDA field offices recommended that the approval of 17% of NDAs be withheld because of inspectional results. The most common reasons for recommendations to withhold approval included insufficient preparedness to commercially manufacture the drugs (31 firms), insufficient laboratory controls (22 firms), and the continued presence of previously detected GMP deviations (16 firms).

A few FDAMA provisions have implications for preapproval inspections in the context of the NDA review process. According to FDAMA, no action of a review division (e.g., NDA review) may be delayed based on the results of a preapproval inspection or other information from field personnel, or the lack of information from the field [investigators] (such as delays in conducting such an inspection), "unless the reviewing division determines that a delay is necessary to assure the marketing of a safe and effective product."

It is important to note that other types of FDA inspections that are conducted on a pre-approval basis can affect the progress, or even the outcome, of the NDA review process. Under CDER's Bioresearch Monitoring Program, agency investigators inspect clinical investigators, drug sponsors, IRBs, and others to ensure the accuracy and validity of data submitted in an NDA, and to ensure that the rights and welfare of clinical subjects were protected during clinical trials (for a complete discussion of CDER's Bioresearch Monitoring Program, see Chapter 14).

The Primary Review Process

Once the review team determines that an NDA is "fileable," the "primary" review begins. During this process, the members of the review team sift through volumes of research data, analyses, and information applicable to their reviewing expertise:

Clinical Reviewer: Evaluates the clinical data to determine if the drug is safe and effective in its proposed use(s). In determining the product's risk/benefit ratio, the clinical reviewer(s) assesses the clinical significance of the drug's therapeutic effects in relation to its possible adverse effects. As noted above, the center is in the process of developing a series of reviewer guidelines that will seek to outline both the safety and efficacy components of the clinical review. The first product of this effort was a draft reviewer guidance entitled, *Conducting a Clinical Safety Review of a New Product Application and Preparing a Report on the Review*, which stated that "the goals of a safety review are (1) to identify important adverse events that are causally related to the use of the drug, (2) to estimate incidence for those events, and (3) to identify factors that predict the occurrence of those events. If there is one principle that underlies this guidance it would be the inadequacy of an approach involving only the review of individual studies in an NDA without any attempt to integrate the findings. Consequently, this guidance focuses on approaches to organizing and integrating the findings across studies in a manner that facilitates the regulatory tasks." Also, under a component of the GRP initiative called the Reviewer Diagram Project, several CDER clinical reviewers have attempted to document and outline their individual NDA review processes to allow reviewers and managers to record and visualize the steps in the process. In mid-April 2001, CDER implemented a standardized NDA clinical review format, or template, for its clinical reviewers centerwide. This new clinical review template, which is mandatory despite being a pilot project, was expected to be formally implemented on a permanent basis by mid-2002.

Pharmacology/Toxicology Reviewer: Evaluates the entire body of nonclinical data and analyses, with a focus on the newly submitted long-term test data, to identify relevant implications for the drug's clinical safety. In May 2001, CDER implemented and released an internal review guidance entitled, *Pharmacology/Toxicology Review Format*, which provides a standardized review format for pharmacology/toxicology reviews as part of IND and NDA evaluations. Upon the release of the guidance, CDER stated that is employs a standardized format for such reviews for several reasons, including that standardization provides for unified communication among multiple audiences and that it ensures that the most important information is captured in all reviews.

Chemistry Reviewer: Evaluates commercial-stage manufacturing procedures (e.g., method of synthesis or isolation, purification process, and process controls), and the specifications and analytical methods used to assure the identity, strength, purity, and bioavailability of the drug product.

Statistical Reviewer: Evaluates the pivotal clinical data to determine if there exists statistically significant evidence of the drug's safety and effectiveness, the appropriateness of the sponsor's clinical data analyses and the assumptions under which these analyses were performed, the statistical significance

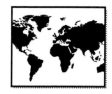

Worldwide Pharmaceutical Regulation Series

of newly submitted nonclinical data, and the implications of stability data for establishing appropriate expiration dating for the product.

Biopharmaceutics Reviewer: Evaluates pharmacokinetic and bioavailability data to establish appropriate drug dosing.

Microbiology Reviewer: For certain drug products (anti-infectives, antivirals, and special pathogen drugs), a CDER microbiologist will evaluate the drug's effects on target viruses or other microorganisms. For sterile drugs and certain non-sterile drug products (e.g., aqueous dosage forms that can support microbial growth), a microbiologist will conduct a product quality assessment.

Much of the primary review process involves reviewers' attempts to confirm and validate the sponsor's conclusion that a drug is safe and effective in its proposed use. However, it is also likely to involve a reanalysis or an extension of the analyses conducted and presented by the sponsor in the NDA. For example, the medical reviewer may seek to reanalyze a drug's effectiveness in a particular patient subpopulation not analyzed in the original submission. Similarly, the reviewer may disagree with the sponsor's assessment of evaluable patients, and seek to retest effectiveness claims based on the reviewer-defined patient populations.

There is also likely to be considerable communication between review team members during the primary review process. If a medical reviewer's reanalysis of clinical data produces results different than the sponsor's, for example, the reviewer is likely to forward this information to the statistical reviewer with a request for a reanalysis of the data. Likewise, the pharmacology reviewer may work closely with the statistical reviewer in evaluating the statistical significance of adverse drug effects in long-term animal studies (e.g., tumor rates).

From the CDER Side: The Pet Peeves of CDER Reviewers

In response to an industry request in late 1999, CDER Ombudsman Jim Morrison conducted an informal e-mail poll to determine what industry actions and behaviors most frustrate the CDER reviewers who evaluate INDs and NDAs. The complaints were then grouped into four main categories—interactions, operational and submission quality, unrealistic expectations, and "gaming the system" (i.e., efforts to subvert or misuse procedures or systems).

Interactions

- Calling very frequently regarding the status of a document or review. Actions that are perceived as overly aggressive contacts by industry representatives were easily the most common complaints noted by CDER reviewers.
- Repeatedly asking the same question in an effort to obtain a desired response (either asking the same person the question in different forms or "shopping around" in different offices for the desired response).
- Leaving a message for an FDA staffer and then calling his or her supervisor shortly thereafter complaining that calls are not being returned.
- Failing to control anger, using inappropriate and demeaning statements to staff (almost always when a manager is absent).
- Insisting on an estimate of review completion dates before anyone has looked at the submission.
- Asking for early warnings of possible problems and then demanding a meeting with the division to discuss the problems before they have had supervisory review.

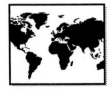

- Bypassing several levels in the supervisory chain to bring problems that could be solved at a lower level to senior management's attention.
- Contacting IND and NDA reviewers directly without going through the project manager.
- Bringing legal representatives and arguing legal issues at scientific meetings.
- Amending the agenda for a scheduled meeting at the last minute and sending in more data.

Operational and Submission Quality
- Submitting poorly organized or sloppy documents (e.g., too much redundancy, poor pagination, unnecessary data such as printouts from lab equipment, inconsistent data, and repeated mistakes).
- Ignoring advice on protocols and other input from previous meetings and correspondence.
- Not identifying the contents of an attached submission in a cover letter.
- Mixing important data with routine submissions.
- Not identifying when data have been submitted previously.

Unrealistic Expectations
- Company requests for exceptions from stated policies and procedures or for special treatment, such as expedited review or moving up in the queue. Such requests generally cite hardships, which the companies sometimes claim were brought about by past FDA actions.
- Requests from inexperienced companies that CDER, rather than an independent consultant, guide them through the entire drug development process beyond what is already available in agency guidances and from agency meetings.
- Asking for a determination when there is clearly insufficient information on which to base a decision.
- Seeking immediate answers to complex regulatory issues at meetings or on the phone.

Gaming the System
- Deviating from an agreed-upon protocol design to achieve a more favorable result (e.g., changing inclusion or exclusion criteria or using different statistical methods).
- Burying protocol changes or other key information in general correspondence and not discussing them with the review division.
- Exaggerating the consequences of failing to get whatever is being sought (e.g., claims that a company will fold if a requested accommodation is not made).
- Aiming to come as close to the "regulatory line" as possible or to do the absolute minimum work needed to fulfill regulatory requirements.
- Complaining about a competitor's behavior and then asking to do the same thing if immediate regulatory action is not forthcoming.
- Being less than forthright about safety issues with investigational or marketed drugs.
- Asking CDER to delay an action to avoid adverse publicity or postpone bad news until after a shareholders' meeting or a critical financing decision.

Source: Morrison, *News Along the Pike*, December 1999 and January 2000.

Mid-Review CDER/Sponsor Communications Invariably, the primary review results in the need for agency communication with, and the clarification of some issues or data by, the NDA sponsor. With the shortening of drug reviews, it is likely that all FDA/sponsor communication, including mid-review dialogue, has increased in recent years. Such communications may take many forms, ranging from informal telephone communications to face-to-face meetings to videoconferences.

In the interest of expediting the review process, CDER pledged, under its PDUFA II commitments, to alert sponsors to NDA deficiencies earlier in the review process. Through what are called discipline

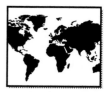

review letters, the agency "submits deficiencies to sponsors in the form of mid-review letters when each discipline has completed its initial review of the pending application," the commitments state. While some firms believe that such notifications allow them to address NDA deficiencies earlier in the review process, many agency reviewers maintain that applicants have often been alerted to mid-review NDA deficiencies in the past.

The agency outlined its use of these mid-review communications in a November 2001 guidance entitled, *Information Request and Discipline Review Letters Under the Prescription Drug User Fee Act*. The guidance outlines two forms of mid-review communications:

Discipline Review (DR) *Letter*. A new concept under PDUFA II, the DR letter is "a letter used to convey early thoughts on possible deficiencies found by a discipline review team [e.g., clinical, chemistry, pharmacology/toxicology] for its portion of the pending [NDA] at the conclusion of the discipline review. DR letters are not considered to be action letters because they do not represent a complete review of the submission and, therefore, do not stop the user fee review clock... A single DR letter may contain comments from multiple discipline reviews if it is more efficient to do so." In the guidance, the agency cautions industry about the limitations of the discipline review letters: (1) because a DR letter may be issued without input from upper supervisory levels (i.e., division or office director), the identified deficiencies ultimately may be resolved at these levels without additional applicant input or additional deficiencies may arise as a result of management input; (2) the agency is not obligated to review an applicant's response to DR letters in the review cycle in which the letter was issued, although the division may review such information if it can do so without adversely affecting its ability to meet its user-fee performance goal. Given these two limitations, applicants may want to consider the value in developing a rapid response to a DR letter rather than waiting for a formal action letter. In other words, the ultimate action letter issued on the application "may contain additional or fewer deficiencies than were provided in the previously issued discipline review letters, depending on the final review of the application and supervisory evaluation by division and/or office directors, the guidance points out.

Although the agency's guidance is not entirely clear on this point, it appears that all review disciplines involved in the NDA evaluation will be responsible for issuing discipline review letters in most cases. The guidance points out, however, that a DR letter will not be sent "if its issuance would delay or coincide with the issuance of an action letter. The absence of a DR letter for a particular discipline should not be construed to mean that the action letter will not contain any deficiencies for that discipline."

Information Request (IR) *Letters*. The information request letter, which has been used by CDER for some time, is a letter sent to an applicant during an application review to request further information or clarification that is needed or would be helpful to allow completion of the discipline review. Because an IR letter, unlike a DR letter, is issued during the discipline review and because it requests information that assists in the completion of that review, applicant responses to such a letter are usually reviewed during the review cycle in which the IR letter was issued. Applicants are expected to respond to IR letters "as quickly as possible," the guidance notes.

Although a 1999 FDA/Public Citizen's Health Research Group (HRG) legal settlement regarding the release of advisory committee meeting materials (see Chapter 10) forced the FDA to re-examine its

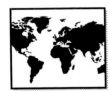

practices for sharing information with drug sponsors, CDER's review divisions are using formal discipline review letters to communicate with sponsors. At this writing, the center was developing an internal manual of policies and procedures (MaPP) for the use of both discipline review and information request letters.

FDA regulations also require other forms of sponsor communications. Specifically, sponsors must continue forwarding new safety information during the entire NDA review to ensure that reviewers have the most up-to-date information for the decision-making process. Through "safety update reports," sponsors must provide periodic updates on any new safety-related information obtained from clinical studies, animal studies, or other sources (see Chapter 7). Sponsors must submit these reports four months after the original NDA submission, following the receipt of an "approvable" letter, and after an FDA request. Usually, the agency will request a safety update within 90 to 120 days of an approval action.

Technological advances will continue to influence the nature of mid-NDA review sponsor/FDA communications in coming years. In late 1999, for example, CDER rolled out a secure e-mail system through which NDA sponsors and NDA reviewers can exchange encrypted regulatory communications electronically. CDER has been using e-mail systems on a pilot basis for a few years; in fact, CDER officials claim that the center could not have approved Pfizer's Trovan within its 12-month user-fee review goal date without the exchange of mid-review communications with Pfizer through a pilot-stage e-mail system. Center officials note that the secure e-mail system has proven particularly useful for exchanging, reviewing, and implementing revisions to proposed drug labeling during the final negotiation process that immediately precedes the formal approval.

By late 2001, an estimated 55 pharmaceutical companies—compared to just a handful in 2000—were actively forwarding regulatory documents and were communicating with the project managers and reviewers responsible for their pending NDAs through secure e-mail systems. Typical e-mail messages can range from communications necessary to schedule sponsor/division meetings to regulatory documents such as pharmacology/toxicology reports, draft clinical protocols, draft product labeling, and statistical reports, according to CDER staffers.

While e-mail communications are proving to be an increasingly popular means of supplementing or replacing telephone conversations, meetings, and faxes, they are not considered "formal communications." In other words, although a company may forward materials via e-mail, those materials cannot yet substitute for the official hardcopy submissions that are necessary for agency archiving.

Reaching an Institutional Decision on the NDA

When the technical reviews are completed, each reviewer must develop a written evaluation that presents his or her conclusions on, and recommendations regarding, the NDA. In most cases, the medical reviewer is responsible for evaluating and reconciling the conclusions of reviewers in all other scientific disciplines. The result is an action letter (see discussion below), which provides an approval or disapproval decision and the basis for that recommendation.

In reality, the reconciling of all reviewer conclusions and the development of what CDER calls an "institutional decision" on an NDA's approvability is likely to involve considerable dialogue between

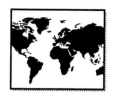

the medical reviewer and reviewers in the other disciplines, as well as each primary reviewer's supervisor, the division director and, if necessary, the office director. Since the ultimate decision hinges most directly on clinical safety, effectiveness, and risk/benefit issues, however, the medical reviewer and his or her supervisor are generally assumed to have the most influence in this process.

To address those cases in which a review team is not able to reach a consensus, CDER developed MaPP 4151.1 entitled, *Resolution of Disputes: Roles of Reviewers, Supervisors, and Management: Documenting Views and Findings and Resolving Differences* (August 1996), which states that, "the review teams' recommendations are...reviewed by discipline-specific supervisors or team leaders, the division directors, and, if necessary, the office directors. (In the case of a reviewing medical officer, a division director or deputy director reviews the primary findings.) The review process ensures that each application is considered from an array of different perspectives and concerns. The process also requires that reviewers, supervisors or team leaders, and management work together. In most cases, consensus on a drug application is usually achieved through discussion as the reviews proceed. If consensus does not occur during the review process, management ultimately must resolve the differences. In all cases, it is essential that the views of all persons involved in the review process be respected and that the official administrative record of the review reflect differences of opinion if they exist... If disagreement arises at any level of the review process and remains unresolved, the reviewing official who disagrees with the drafted conclusions or recommendations must prepare a separate document explaining: (1) the nature of the difference of opinion; (2) the reasons for the differing opinion; and (3) the recommended changes in the findings or recommendations. This document must remain in the file with the reviewer's documentation." If the division supervisors and division director are unable to resolve the scientific or regulatory dispute, it may be brought to CDER's deputy center director for review management.

Despite this policy, internal reviewer disputes in NDA reviews received considerable public attention in the late 1990s. In a December 1998 HRG reviewer survey (see discussion above), for example, several CDER medical officers claimed that there had been instances in which "inappropriate pressure" was being applied by center management and even Congress to encourage drug approvals and that, in other cases, the opinions of NDA reviewers were being suppressed. In addition, a handful of current and former CDER medical reviewers claimed in press reports that their concerns were ignored during the reviews of drugs that were later withdrawn, and that CDER management had created, during the user-fee era, a bias in favor of approving new drugs.

If there are important scientific or medical issues on which CDER reviewers would like to obtain independent advice before reaching their decision, they can bring the issues to one or more of 15 prescription drug advisory committees supporting the drug center. Consistent with the center's focus on drug safety and risk management, CDER officials told industry to expect advisory committees to be asked to consider postmarketing risk management issues in their new drug assessments prior to approval (see discussion above).

In 1998 and 1999, CDER sought advisory committee input on 40% of the new molecular entities that were eligible for committee review, according to FDA data (for a more detailed discussion of CDER's advisory committee process, see Chapter 10). For all NDAs, CDER consulted advisory committees for 10% of eligible NDAs in 1999, up from just 3% in 1998.

In 2000, CDER introduced a pilot program under which any of CDER's new drug review divisions could request an internal meeting of senior center officials to consider particularly difficult or complex regulatory decisions. Coordinated by CDER's new Review Standards Staff (RSS), the so-called "pre-decision" meeting pilot program focused largely, although not exclusively, on NDA approval decisions. During these meetings, division staff present an issue to RSS officials, CDER Director Janet Woodcock, M.D., Associate Director for Medical Policy Robert Temple, M.D., and other center officials for comment and possibly recommendations. These "internal advisory committee meetings," as CDER staffers characterize them, provide drug reviewers with a new option for obtaining additional insights and perspectives on the drug approval-related issues before them. While NDA applicants are not invited to the meetings, CDER officials claim that they are often informed when their applications are to be considered at such meetings.

In June 2001, CDER made this pilot effort a permanent program, and renamed the meetings "regulatory briefings" to reflect the fact that the meetings can be held before or following regulatory decisions. Although CDER remains fairly secretive regarding other aspects of "regulatory briefings," including possible changes in meeting format and panel membership, the center will disclose more details about the program when it releases a new manual of policies and procedures (MaPP) document that was under development at this writing.

The results of the preapproval inspection may also figure into the approval decision. When such inspections discover significant CGMP problems or other issues, the reviewing division typically will withhold approval until these are addressed and corrected (see discussion above). The division's response to such deficiencies is likely to depend on several factors, including the nature of the problem, the prognosis for the problem's correction, and the status of the NDA review.

The Formal Action on an NDA

The final channels through which an NDA must pass to obtain FDA approval will depend on issues such as the drug's novelty and importance. NDAs for NMEs and prescription-to-OTC switches, for example, need the approval of higher levels of FDA management than do marketing applications for less innovative products. Although federal regulations specify authority delegations for NDA "sign-off" powers (i.e., final approval authority), the regulations do give CDER some flexibility to delegate these powers.

Once an approval or not-approvable recommendation is reached by the reviewers and their supervisors, the decision must then be evaluated and approved by the director of the applicable drug review division. For the division director's review, the project manager assembles an "action package" containing the action letter (see discussion above), all discipline reviews, memos of meetings and teleconferences, reports on inspections, debarment certifications, patent information, all labeling, an exclusivity review, and related information supporting the reviewers' recommendation. Reviewers, their supervisors, and the division's director and deputy director then have an opportunity to examine the action package.

After conducting what is sometimes called a "secondary review," the division director may begin a dialogue with the chemistry, medical, or pharmacology reviewers or their supervisors regarding the final

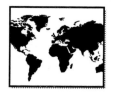

decision. Most often, the director will support the decision of the review group. For those drugs that are not considered particularly innovative or that are not seen as offering significant therapeutic advantages, the director's decision generally serves as the final FDA ruling. In this respect, the division director (or his or her deputy director) is said to have "sign-off" authority for such drugs.

According to federal regulations, applications for new molecular entities require either center-level or office-level (i.e., ODE I, II, III, IV, or V) concurrence. In most instances, however, sign-off authorities for such products have been delegated to the office level. This office level review is sometimes called the "tertiary review."

Non-NME NDAs that raise clinical issues beyond those presented by the previously approved versions of the subject drugs generally are signed off by division directors, although some office directors may opt to sign off on such applications. NDAs that propose a major new indication or the first controlled-release dosage form of a previously approved drug would be in this class of submissions.

FDA Action Letters

The FDA communicates its official decision on an NDA through what is called an "action letter." Action letters are an important element in the agency's efforts to meet its review performance goals under the user-fee program—that is, the agency must "act on" NDAs within specific time frames. CDER fulfills this requirement by issuing an action letter, which constitutes a complete action on the application and which stops the review clock for the filing.

Currently, there are three types of action letters—approval, approvable, and not-approvable—that detail CDER's decisions on NDAs. Under PDUFA II, the FDA had agreed to simplify this three-letter scheme by replacing approvable and not-approvable letters with "complete response" letters, which will detail all the application's deficiencies. CDER will have to revise its regulations before implementing this change, however, something that the center had not taken action to do at this writing.

Approval Letter When CDER sends an approval letter, the subject drug is considered approved as of the date of the letter. Generally, an applicant must submit final printed labeling before a drug is approved. However, if CDER finds that the draft labeling is acceptable or if the agency requires only minor editorial changes, the NDA may be approved based on the draft labeling. In such cases, the agency reminds the firm that marketing of the product with labeling other than that agreed to by the agency would cause the product to be viewed as misbranded (i.e., an unapproved product).

Rarely, if ever, do drug sponsors receive an approval letter for an original NDA without first receiving a request for more data (e.g., in an information request letter), a clarification of existing data or analyses, or modification of the application in its originally submitted form (e.g., product labeling). In many cases, however, such requests are made through mid-review communications that do not comprise a formal agency action on the NDAs (see discussion above).

Clearly, greater numbers of NDAs are being approved (i.e., receiving approval letters) in CDER's first formal actions on the applications during the user-fee era. After approving roughly 45% of NDAs from the FY1996 and FY1997 cohorts in the first review cycle, the agency was able to approve just 36% of

The NDA Review Process

Chapter 8

Average NME Review Times in Months, 1992-2000, by Division
(number of NME approvals in parentheses)

	1992	1993	1994	1995	1996	1997	1998	1999	2000
Division of Cardio-Renal Drug Products	42.6 (4)	30.0 (2)	36.0 (1)	21.4 (6)	14.1 (3)	12.3 (6)	12.9 (5)	13.9 (3)	*
Division of Oncology[1] Drug Products	32.3 (3)	45.7 (2)	19.2 (4)	14.0 (4)	12.0 (4)	17.7 (3)	7.4 (2)	9.1 (5)	6.3 (2)
Division of Neuropharmacological Drug Products	37.9 (3)	20.9 (5)	35.6 (3)	5.5 (1)	15.2 (7)	17.5 (5)	16.8 (5)	16.9 (3)	25.4 (3)
Division of Anesthetic, Critical Care, and Addiction Drug Products	*	*	*	11.3 (2)	13.9 (2)	*	*	12.9 (2)	24.2 (1)
Division of Gastrointestinal and Coagulation Drug Products	*	16.9 (4)	16.2 (2)	17.8 (1)	23.8 (1)	28.4 (4)	12.6 (2)	15.1 (2)	23.4 (6)
Division of Pulmonary Drug Products	*	*	*	89.3 (1)	30.7 (4)	21.2 (1)	12.0 (1)	32.0 (1)	*
Division of Antiviral Drug Products[4]	13.3 (4)	36.1 (2)	8.7 (3)	4.4 (3)	5.5 (5)	6.1 (3)	4.9 (4)	7.0 (3)	3.5 (1)
Division of Medical Imaging and Radiopharmaceutical	*	*	*	37.5 (2)	29.8 (5)	24.0 (2)	12.8 (1)	17.4 (2)	*
Division of Anti-Infective Drug Products[4]	21.1 (6)	24.9 (4)	*	25.6 (2)	14.3 (8)	15.0 (1)	*	7.8 (1)	6.0 (1)
Division of Anti-Inflammatory, Analgesic and Ophthalmic Drug Products[2]	*	*	*	15.5 (1)	11.5 (3)	24.4 (2)	9.5 (4)	5.9 (3)	9.7 (3)
Division of Metabolic and Endocrine Drug Products[3]	18.8 (2)	48.8 (2)	13.6 (2)	11.4 (4)	19.2 (7)	11.6 (7)	12.6 (4)	13.5 (5)	13.7 (4)
Division of Dermatologic and Dental Drug Products[2]	*	*	*	18.5 (1)	27.0 (3)	23.8 (1)	*	20.2 (2)	17.9 (3)
Division of Reproductive and Urologic Drug Products	*	*	*	*	30.5 (1)	12.0 (1)	12.0 (1)	6.0 (1)	25.0 (3)
Division of Special Pathogens and Immunologic Drug Products[4]	*	*	*	*	*	11.7 (3)	18.8 (1)	10.5 (2)	*

* no NME approvals during that year or division not in existence at that time

[1] Data from 1991-1994 include pulmonary drug reviews as well.

[2] In January 1996, the Division of Anti-Inflammatory, Analgesic and Dental Drug Products and the Division of Dermatologic and Ophthalmic Drug Products swapped responsibilities for dental and ophthalmic drugs. The 1996–2000 data reflect this reorganization.

[3] In 1996, the division's responsibilities for urologic and reproductive drugs were shifted to the new Division of Reproductive and Urologic Drug Products. While the 1996–2000 data reflect this change, divisional statistics for 1991 through 1995 include these products.

[4] In 1997, the Division of Anti-Infective Drug Products and the Division of Antiviral Drug Products shifted several drug categories to the new Division of Special Pathogens and Immunologic Drug Products. The 1996–2000 data reflect these changes.

Source: PAREXEL's Pharmaceutical R&D Statistical Sourcebook 2001

Worldwide Pharmaceutical Regulation Series

the FY1998 NDAs after the first review cycle, something that led many to question whether FDA's performance in this area had topped out. This decline, however, was limited to standard NDAs—CDER was able to approve fully half of the FY1998 priority NDAs in the first review cycle, a mark second only to the 67% mark that the center reached for the FY1996 priority NDA cohort.

Although CDER's first-cycle approval rate for original NDAs bounced back to the 45% mark for the FY1999 NDA cohort, most industry officials expected this rate to fall off considerably given perceptions about increasing conservatism in agency decision making. In fact, CDER approved only 38.5% of FY2000 NDAs in the first review cycle, and just 10% of the first 82 FY2001 NDAs acted on as of late 2001.

Prior to granting approval, the review division may also ask for an applicant's commitment to conduct certain drug studies following approval. Although the agency states that such postmarketing studies are not considered essential for a drug's approval, the studies provide "additional information or data that could, for example, change the prescribing information or use of the drug or provide additional assurance or verification of product quality and consistency." Under a new policy guide on such "Phase 4 commitments," the FDA and drug sponsor must agree to the specific commitments and a schedule for fulfilling these commitments prior to approval (see Chapter 11). Either prior to, or at the time of, drug approval, the applicant must submit a letter describing the Phase 4 commitments and a schedule for initiating and completing the Phase 4 studies. The approval letter should list all Phase 4 commitments and the schedule for their completion.

Approvable Letter According to federal regulations, the FDA will send the applicant "an approvable letter if the application…substantially meets the requirements [for marketing approval] and the agency believes that it can approve the application…if specific additional information or material is submitted or specific conditions (for example, certain changes in labeling) are agreed to by the applicant." Often, the FDA will use an approvable letter to request changes to the product's proposed labeling and to require the submission of safety update reports and the product's final printed labeling.

Unless otherwise specified by the FDA, the sponsor has ten days after the date of the approvable letter to do one of the following:

- Submit a resubmission (i.e., a formal response to the action letter), or acknowledge its intent to file a resubmission, to the NDA (see discussion below).

- Withdraw the application. The FDA will consider the applicant's failure to respond to an approvable letter within ten days to represent the applicant's request to withdraw the application.

- For applications involving new drugs (not including antibiotics), ask the FDA to provide the applicant an opportunity for a hearing on whether grounds exist for denying the application's approval. Sponsors would make such a request when the FDA issues an approvable letter, but specifies in the letter marketing conditions (e.g., restrictive labeling) that are unacceptable to the applicant.

- For an antibiotic, file a petition or notify the FDA of an intent to file a petition proposing the issuance, amendment, or repeal of a regulation.

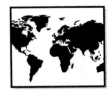

- Notify the FDA that the applicant agrees to a review period extension of a specified length so the applicant may give further consideration as to which of the previous four options it will pursue. The FDA will grant any reasonable request for an extension, and will consider the applicant's failure to respond during the extended review period to represent a request to withdraw the application.

For NDAs submitted from FY1996 through FY1999, the percentage that received approvable letters in the first review cycle was fairly consistent. Over this period, roughly a third of original NDAs accepted for review received approvable letters after the first-cycle review, although data suggest that this percentage may be higher for NDAs filed in subsequent years. In some cases, the agency will also issue approvable letters after receiving an applicant's response to an earlier not-approvable or approvable letter.

Not-Approvable Letter A not-approvable letter is forwarded to the applicant if the FDA believes that the drug application is insufficient to justify approval. The letter describes the NDA deficiencies that were the basis for the not-approvable action. Unless the FDA indicates otherwise, the sponsor must take one of the five actions specified above for approvable letters within ten days.

In general, fewer NDAs have received not-approvable letters in the user-fee era. After issuing not-approvable letters for 48 percent of FY1994 NDAs, for instance, CDER took such actions on only 24 percent of FY1995 applications, 18 percent of FY1996 NDAs, and 19 percent of FY1997 NDAs. For the FY1998 cohort, this figure jumped to 27 percent, largely because 35% of the FY1998 standard NDAs triggered not approvable actions (only 7% of the priority NDAs in the cohort met with such fates). This proved to be a one-year jump, however, as CDER took not-approvable actions on just 15% of FY1999 NDAs and 14% of FY2000 NDAs.

Applicant Responses to Approvable or Not-Approvable Letters Once the applicant has developed a complete response to all of the deficiencies and issues specified in an approvable or not-approvable letter, it should include this response in what is termed a "resubmission." Under the FDA's PDUFA II commitments, such resubmissions are now classified, and are assigned review goals, based on the information contained within them. A resubmission should include a cover letter that provides a statement indicating that the applicant considers the resubmission to represent a complete response to the action letter. In addition, the applicant has the option of offering an opinion on how the resubmission should be classified.

Under PDUFA II, all resubmissions are classified into either Class 1 or Class 2. Class 1 resubmissions are more straightforward submissions that can include the following items or any combination of these items: (1) final printed labeling; (2) draft labeling; (3) safety updates submitted in the same format, including tabulations, as the original safety submissions with new data and changes highlighted (when large amounts of new information, including important new adverse experiences not previously reported with the product, are presented in the resubmission, however, it will be considered a Class 2 resubmission); (4) stability updates to support provisional or final dating periods; (5) commitments to perform Phase 4 studies, including proposals for such studies; (6) assay validation data; (7) final release testing on the last 1 or 2 lots used to support approval; (8) a minor re-analysis of data previously submitted by the applicant (determined by the agency as fitting the Class 1 category); or (9) other minor clarifying information (determined by the agency as fitting the Class 1 category). The agency has committed to acting on 90 percent of Class 1 NDA resubmissions filed in FY2001 and FY2002 within 2 months.

At this writing, CDER appeared to be exceeding its Class 1 resubmission goals, even for earlier fiscal year cohorts to which less-aggressive review goals applied. All of the 17 FY1999 Class 1 resubmissions filed, for example, were reviewed within 2 months. Fourteen of the resubmissions triggered approval actions, while the remaining three triggered approvable actions.

A Class 2 resubmission is a resubmission that includes any item not identified above for Class 1 resubmissions, including any item that would warrant presentation to an advisory committee or any issue that would warrant a re-inspection of a manufacturing facility. For all years covered by PDUFA II (FY1998-FY2002), CDER committed to reviewing 90 percent of Class 2 resubmissions within 6 months.

Of the 47 FY1999 Class 2 resubmissions, the FDA was able to approve 22 in the first review cycle. Another 22 triggered approvable actions, while the remaining 3 produced not-approvable actions.

According to an April 1998 guidance entitled, *Classifying Resubmissions in Response to Action Letters*, the agency will forward an acknowledgement letter to the applicant within 14 days of a resubmission's receipt. Assuming that the agency finds the resubmission to be complete, the acknowledgement letter will reveal the classification of the resubmission and specify the review performance goal for the application.

Final Printed Labeling

Generally, labeling is the final major consideration in a drug's approval. Not until an NDA is virtually approved, or is judged to be "approvable," does labeling become the primary focus of the drug approval process.

There are several practical reasons why labeling concerns are left until late in the drug review process. First, it is impossible to develop labeling with accurate accounts of indications, warnings, contraindications, and specific use instructions without conclusions drawn from pivotal clinical study data. Also, FDA reviewers will not invest significant time in evaluating proposed labeling until they are reasonably convinced that a drug is safe and effective for its proposed use, and that the drug's NDA is nearing approval.

Labeling often becomes a principal concern once the agency issues an approvable letter, which, among other things, requests that the applicant forward its final printed labeling (i.e., all the labeling to appear on or to accompany a drug's package or container). At this point, only the labeling and possibly some minor deficiencies in an NDA stand between a drug and its approval.

Perhaps because of this, CDER officials began moving toward the electronic submission of the complete package insert during 2000 in an effort to speed what can be a lengthy labeling negotiation process. Ultimately, the center hopes to permit labeling submissions to be made, and related negotiations to be conducted, through the Internet. In January 2000, CDER Director Janet Woodcock, M.D., claimed that the center would reduce, to one to two weeks, the review of NDA labeling supplements as a quid pro quo for companies submitting labeling changes electronically, although she noted that the center would consider requiring electronic submissions. Today, CDER officials claim that companies are submitting draft labeling and proposed labeling changes electronically, although they have not released any data to indicate how frequently e-labeling submissions are being made.

Draft Package Labeling Drug sponsors first propose labeling for a new pharmaceutical through what is called draft package labeling. Generally, draft labeling is submitted as part of the original NDA.

The specific labeling requirements facing a drug in its finished package form will depend on whether it is proposed for use as a prescription or as an over-the-counter (OTC) medicine. Principally because of dispensing differences, FDA labeling requirements for OTC and prescription drugs differ significantly.

Prescription Drug Labeling According to federal regulations, prescription drug labeling must be "informative and accurate…, contain a summary of the essential scientific information needed for the safe and effective use of the drug…," and "be based, whenever possible, on data derived from human experience." In enforcing these and other requirements, the FDA has authority over the format and types of information that appear: (1) on the immediate drug container (i.e., manufacturer name, general brand name, lot number, etc.); and (2) on the outer carton in which the drug is shipped to physicians, hospitals, pharmacies, and other prescription drug dispensers.

A primary element in prescription drug labeling is the package insert. Drug manufacturers use prescription drug package inserts to meet the requirement that the physician or pharmacist be provided with the essential information needed to ensure the safe and effective use of the drug. Since the large body of information needed to satisfy this requirement cannot reasonably be placed on a prescription product's immediate container or package, manufacturers include it on a package insert. Such inserts generally comprise several sections, including the following:

- a product description section describing the drug's dosage form, route of administration, ingredients, and therapeutic/pharmacologic effect;
- a clinical pharmacology section describing the action of the drug in humans and, if pertinent, its activity and effectiveness in animal and *in vitro* tests;
- an indications and usage section describing specific safety conditions and identifying indications supported by evidence of clinical effectiveness;
- a contraindications section;
- a warnings section describing potential safety hazards and steps to be taken if reactions occur;
- a precautions section discussing drug interactions and possible side effects in specific population groups such as pregnant women;
- an adverse reactions section;
- a drug abuse and dependence section, including a discussion of possible abuses and physical or psychological dependencies;
- an overdose section identifying specific signs, symptoms, complications, and laboratory findings that are associated with overdosage (this section might also specify

the amount of the drug in a single dosage likely to cause overdosage symptoms and/or a life-threatening situation);

- a dosage and administration section identifying the recommended usual dose, safe upper dosage limit, and dosage modifications for children and the elderly; and
- a section describing how the drug is supplied (i.e., the drug's dosage form, strength, and unit availability).

Based on its perceptions of the package insert's limited effectiveness in conveying important risk-related information to physicians and patients, the FDA issued a long-awaited proposed regulation that would require a new and simplified format for the package insert. The proposed rule called for the package inserts of new and recently approved drugs to include a new introductory "Highlights of Prescribing Information" section featuring the most important and most commonly referred-to prescribing information in bulleted format, as well as an index to prescribing information. The agency also proposed that the labeling of all new molecular entities approved for less than three years contain an inverted black triangle "to serve as a signal for increased vigilance and reporting of suspected adverse reactions…and to help ensure that drugs are used with particular care during their initial years of marketing." The proposed regulation is designed to streamline what are now viewed as requirements that have led to an overly complicated drug label, and to upgrade the useability of the package insert by requiring companies to place the most important drug- and risk-related information at the beginning of the label.

A June 2000 draft guidance also sought to focus labeling-development efforts on key risk-related information. Entitled *Content and Format of the Adverse Reactions Section of Labeling for Human Prescription Drugs and Biologics*, the draft guidance emphasized the need for sponsors to focus the label's adverse reactions section on drug safety information that is important to prescribing decisions and to observing, monitoring, and advising patients. The common format recommended in the guidance divides the adverse reactions section into two subsections: (1) a new "overview" subsection that highlights the adverse reactions that are most serious and most commonly occurring, and those that most frequently result in clinical interventions; and (2) a "discussion" subsection that addresses in greater detail the significance of adverse reaction data obtained from the clinical trials. The guidance also recommends that subjective and nonspecific terms, such as "well tolerated," "rare," "infrequent," and "frequent," should be avoided, since they have no precise meaning and can, therefore, be misleading.

A July 2001 draft guidance entitled, *Guidance for Industry: Clinical Studies Section of Labeling for Prescription Drugs and Biologics*, attempts to better focus a drug's labeling on key clinical studies. In focusing on a drug's effectiveness for its approved indication, the clinical studies section of drug labeling should include information on clinical studies that provide primary support for effectiveness or important information on the limitations of effectiveness, or other clinical studies that contribute important efficacy data not provided by these primary support studies, the draft guidance states. Generally, studies that imply effectiveness for unapproved indications, active control studies that imply comparative efficacy or safety claims not supported by substantial evidence, and studies that are not adequate and well controlled should not be included in the labeling's clinical studies section, the FDA states.

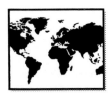

These efforts to revise the package insert are just the latest in a series of recent regulatory and legislative initiatives to upgrade drug labeling. Under an August 1997 final rule, the FDA requires that prescription drug labeling provide information on product use in elderly patients (i.e., patients aged 65 and older). A "Geriatric use" subsection within a label's "Precautions" section must now describe what is known about the effects of a drug in the elderly and list any limitations, hazards, or monitoring needs associated with geriatric use. The agency instituted a staggered "priority implementation" program, under which sponsors of certain approved drugs (e.g., psychotropics, NSAIDs, anticoagulants) that were more likely to cause problems in the elderly had to submit revised labeling earlier (i.e., by August 1998). NDAs submitted after August 27, 1998, must include a "Geriatric Use" subsection in the proposed labeling for the product. While the agency "encourages further study of drug effects in the elderly" through this regulation, the agency makes clear that the new labeling requirements are designed to specify a place and format for available information and not to require additional clinical studies on geriatric uses. In October 2001, the FDA released an industry guidance document entitled, *Content and Format for Geriatric Labeling*.

Under the FDA Modernization Act of 1997, Congress made some modifications to prescription drug labeling requirements. Most importantly, the legislation required that the "Rx only" symbol replace the previous mandatory statement—"Caution: Federal law prohibits dispensing without a prescription." In a July 1998 guidance entitled, *Implementation of Section 126 of the Food and Drug Administration Modernization Act of 1997—Elimination of Certain Labeling Requirements*, the FDA published a revised implementation schedule for this change. Sponsors submitting NDAs after September 19, 1998, are required to submit, in their applications, labels and labeling that comply with the new requirements.

Although the information on many package inserts is reprinted in publications such as the *Physician's Desk Reference for Prescription Drugs*, consumers are generally not given this information directly when the prescription drug is dispensed. Under a cooperative public/private program launched in January 1997, however, industry and pharmacists and other health-care professionals will work to provide consumers with more prescription drug information. The plan calls for "useful drug information" to reach 75 percent of patients by the year 2000 and 95 percent of patients by 2006.

Meanwhile, industry is actively working to replace the current system of paper-based product package inserts for providing current drug information to pharmacies and patients. PhRMA was working with technology vendors to use electronic media, including the Internet, in developing a paperless drug labeling system that industry hoped to implement fully by year-end 2002.

OTC Drug Labeling OTC labeling requirements are, with regard to content at least, similar to those for prescription pharmaceuticals. Information regarding active ingredients, dosage and administration, indication, drug action, warnings, precautions, drug interaction, and overdosage must be provided.

However, because OTC products are self-prescribed, and because their use often does not involve the guidance of a physician or pharmacist, OTC drug labeling must be structured differently. Much of the essential information provided to a pharmacist or physician through the package insert of a prescription drug must be detailed on the outer package of the OTC product's container. In fact, all of the information that will allow the consumer to select and use the OTC product safely and effectively

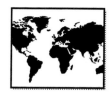

must appear on the outer package. This information must be presented in a manner suitable for the comprehension of the lay public.

Due to what it perceived as consumer difficulties in understanding OTC product labeling information, the FDA implemented a March 1999 regulation to establish new, consumer-friendly format and content requirements for OTC drug labels. The regulation requires that the information provided in OTC drug labeling include standardized headings, be presented in a specified order, and meet minimum type size, type style, and graphics requirements.

The FDA's Review of Draft Labeling When it becomes apparent that an NDA will be approved, agency reviewers evaluate the draft package labeling on at least two levels. First, the draft labeling is reviewed for its consistency with the regulatory requirements for prescription or OTC drugs. Each important element of the proposed labeling (i.e., indications, use instructions, warnings, etc.) is then evaluated in view of conclusions drawn from nonclinical and clinical testing. All claims, instructions, and precautions must be based upon, and accurately reflect, the findings of the key test results, preferably from clinical studies. It might also be affected by CDER's increasing focus on "getting labeling right" when a product is first introduced (i.e., because prescribers tend not to pay as much attention to postapproval label modifications).

If the FDA has major reservations about the draft labeling, the agency will usually forward to the sponsor a letter detailing its suggestions for revised labeling. In some cases, FDA reviewers themselves may revise a portion of the labeling, and instruct the sponsor to include the revision in the final printed labeling. Agency comments can relate to virtually any aspect of the proposed drug labeling, including the drug indications, general wording, the labeling format, and the warnings/precautions.

The labeling "negotiation process," through which a drug's final approved labeling is agreed upon, can consume several weeks or several months. The length and complexity of the process will depend upon several factors, including the nature and number of the FDA's comments and the degree to which the applicant is agreeable to making recommended revisions. It might also be affected by CDER's increasing focus on "getting labeling right" when a product is first introduced (i.e., because prescribers tend not to pay as much attention to postapproval label modifications).

In some cases, the sponsor will have to submit several revisions of its labeling before the FDA finds an acceptable version. Disagreements over labeling content, wording, and design are generally resolvable through either mail and telephone correspondence or through FDA-sponsor meetings.

Sponsor Rights During the NDA Review Process

Over the past decade, legislative and regulatory initiatives affected several aspects of NDA sponsors' rights during the review of their applications. Companies should be aware of these rights and the courses of action available to them should these rights be violated. Sponsor rights during the NDA review process fall into roughly four categories: (1) the right to a timely review; (2) the right to request meetings or conferences with the FDA; (3) the right to protest if the sponsor believes its rights are violated; and (4) the right to confidentiality.

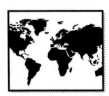

CDER NDA Review Goals, FY1998–FY2002

Original NDA and Efficacy Supplement Submission Cohort	Standard NDAs	Priority NDAs
FY1998	90% in 12 mo.	90% in 6 mo.
FY1999	30% in 10 mo. 90% in 12 mo.	90% in 6 mo.
FY2000	50% in 10 mo. 90% in 12 mo.	90% in 6 mo.
FY2001	70% in 10 mo. 90% in 12 mo.	90% in 6 mo.
FY2002	90% in 10 mo.	90% in 6 mo.

The Right to a Timely Review Under the Prescription Drug User Fee Act of 1992, PDUFA reauthorizing legislation passed in late 1997, and FDA/industry agreements associated with PDUFA II, the federal government has redefined the timeframes applicable to drug application reviews. For years previous to PDUFA, CDER had operated under legal requirements mandating that the agency review and act on NDAs within 180 days of their submission. Most often, however, the 180-day time frame has been called a "phantom" requirement that CDER used as a goal or target, but seldom as a strictly enforced rule.

Agreements associated with PDUFA I and II established a new series of drug review targets for the FDA, while the laws themselves provided the means—specifically, revenues derived from user fees—through which the agency could restaff and retool itself to meet these deadlines. Under PDUFA II, the FDA implemented a series of new five-year review performance goals, beginning with NDAs submitted in FY1998 (October 1, 1997 through September 30, 1998). Although the six-month review timeframe applicable to FY1997 priority NDAs will remain in place during all five years of PDUFA II, CDER will be required to review increasing percentages of standard NDAs within ten months over this term (see table below).

Because of different review performance goals applicable to standard and priority applications, the agency introduced detailed criteria for classifying priority original and supplemental submissions (see Chapter 9):

Priority Application. A priority application is for a product that, if approved, "would be a significant improvement compared to marketed products [approved (if such is required), including non-'drug' products/therapies] in the treatment, diagnosis, or prevention of a disease. Improvement can be demonstrated by, for example: (1) evidence of increased effectiveness in the treatment, prevention, or diagnosis of disease; (2) elimination or substantial reduction of a treatment-limiting drug reaction; (3) documented enhancement of patient compliance; or (4) evidence of safety and effectiveness of a new subpopulation."

Standard Application. All applications not qualifying as priority are classified as standard submissions.

Editor's Note: Although it has no significance in a drug's review priority, each drug also receives a chemical rating, which represents the product's chemical novelty. These ratings may be one of the following: Type 1-new molecular entity; Type 2-new ester, new salt, or other noncovalent derivative; Type 3-new formulation; Type 4-new combination; Type 5-new manufacturer; Type 6-new indication; or

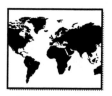

Type 7-drug already marketed but without an approved NDA. CDER is currently revising its policy on assigning chemical ratings. Also, in cases in which a drug's conventional therapeutic rating is considered inadequate to identify a product's defining characteristics, the agency may assign a "special situation" rating, such as Type AA for AIDS drugs or Type V for designated orphan drugs. Like the chemical rating, these ratings have no direct effect on a product's review priority.

The applicable review timelines can be extended if the sponsor submits a "major" amendment to the original application during the review process. A major amendment involves the submission of a large amount of new, previously unreviewed data (e.g., new clinical or animal studies) or any submission that significantly affects the review process (e.g., a reanalysis involving multiple reviewing disciplines). When major amendments are submitted within three months of an application's action due date, the FDA can extend the review time frames by three months.

In reviewing data on new drug approvals over the past decade, it remains difficult to see lasting trends in the FDA's assignment of priority status to new drugs. After granting priority status to fully half of the NMEs approved from 1990 to 1994, CDER granted the designation to only 32 percent of the NMEs

Key Drug Submission and Approval Statistics, 1991–2000

	1991	1992	1993	1994	1995	1996	1997	1998	1999	2000
NDA Submissions	112	100	86	133	140+	123+	128+	131+	136+	135+
NDA Approvals	63	91	70	62	82	131	121	90	83	98
Avg. Review Time for All Original NDAs (in months)	25.7	26.3	24.1	26	22.7	21.6	17.6	12.8	13.5	15.0
Avg. FDA Review Time for Original NDAs*	–	–	–	21.5	18.8	17.1	14.9	11.6	11.7	12.7
Median Review Time for All Original NDAs (in months)	21.4	20.0	20.8	19	16.5	15.4	14.4	12.0	12.0	11.2
Median FDA Review Time for Original NDAs*	–	–	–	15.8	15.3	14.8	12.2	12.0	11.8	10.9
NME Approvals	30	26	25	22	28	53	39	30	35	27
Avg. Review Time for NMEs (in months)	30.3	29.9	26.5	19.7	19.2	17.8	16.2	11.7	12.6	17.6
Avg. FDA Review Time for NMEs*	–	–	–	21.2	17.4	15.8	14.3	10.7	10.9	13.4
Median Review Time for NMEs (in Months)	22.2	22.6	21.0	17.5	15.9	14.3	13.4	12.0	11.6	15.6
Median. FDA Review Time for NMEs*	–	–	–	15.3	15.2	12.0	12.8	11.9	10.0	13.9
IND Submissions	2,116	2,576	2,323	2,156	1,566	1,419	1,996	2,419	1,763	1,815
Commercial IND Submissions	374	370	382	345	358	412	437	498	440	424

+ fiscal year data; *excludes sponsor time

Source: U.S. Regulatory Reporter, 2001

approved during both 1995 and 1996. In 1997, only 23 percent of approved NMEs were priority products, what was easily the lowest percentage since at least 1985. In both 1998 and 1999, about 53 percent of the approved NMEs had priority designations. Only a third of new drugs approved in 2000 were priority products, however. For NDAs overall (i.e., for NMEs and non-NMEs), priority designations were granted to 27 percent, 39 percent, and 32 percent of applications in FY1997, FY1998, and FY1999, respectively.

Throughout the PDUFA I years and in the first years of PDUFA II, the FDA reported that it exceeded its review performance goals for NDA reviews. In a December 2000 performance report to Congress, for example, the agency declared that it had met the review targets for 100 percent of the original FY1999 NDA submissions, surpassing the performance goal applicable to that cohort. CDER's PDUFA II agreements called on the center to act on 90% of priority NDAs within 6 months, and to review 30% of standard NDAs within 10 months and 90% within 12 months.

In fulfilling its user-fee goals, CDER has produced significant reductions in average and median NDA review times, even if these measures have risen somewhat more recently. In 1999, for example, the center improved its median NME approval time for the seventh consecutive year, clearing 30 NMEs in a median of 11.6 months (see table below). In 2000, however, this trend was broken as CDER's median NME review time rose to 15.6 months, still well under the pre-PDUFA marks. The center's average NME review time rose for the second consecutive year in 2000, to 15 months.

What is also striking about the transformation of CDER's drug approval process under the user-fee program is the number of drugs obtaining rapid drug reviews. In both 1998 and 1999, for instance, 60 percent of the NMEs (39 of 65) were approved in 12 months or less, and a quarter (16 of 65) were approved in 6 months or less. Just 41 percent of the new drugs cleared in 2000 obtained approval in 12 months or less.

The Right to Meetings Given their importance in the drug development and review process, agency/sponsor meetings were the subject of several industry and CDER initiatives in the mid-1990s. In early 1996, for example, CDER released a policy document outlining the center's procedures for scheduling and conducting formal meetings with sponsors. Through FDA/industry agreements associated with PDUFA's reauthorization, the agency agreed to implement a new meetings-management system under which CDER would adopt new standards for scheduling and holding sponsor meetings.

CDER communicates openly with sponsors about scientific, medical, and procedural issues that arise during the NDA review process. These exchanges may take the form of telephone or video conferences, letters, or face-to-face meetings, whichever is the most appropriate to discuss and resolve the relevant issue.

All sponsors have the right to at least one, and possibly several, conferences with the FDA during and after the NDA review. While other forms of correspondence will occur routinely throughout the NDA review, the sponsor must make a formal written request before CDER will grant and schedule a conference.

The number of meetings to which a sponsor is entitled may depend upon the subject drug and the priority given to it by the FDA. Under regulations codified in 1985, the agency claimed to have made

FDA-sponsor conferences more accessible to all applicants. Conferences relevant to the NDA review process include the following:

The 90-Day Conference. Approximately 90 days after it receives an NDA, CDER provides sponsors of certain drugs an opportunity to meet with officials and drug reviewers. Generally, such meetings are available only to sponsors of either NMEs or major new indications of currently marketed drugs. The purpose of the conference is to inform an applicant about the general progress and status of its NDA, and to advise the company of deficiencies that have been identified but not yet communicated. However, the 90-day conference is not mandatory, and sponsors may choose not to request such a meeting. Also, the conference may be either a telephone or face-to-face meeting.

The End-of-Review Conference. The end-of-review conference is offered to all applicants after CDER has issued either an approvable or not-approvable letter for an NDA. During this meeting, FDA officials discuss what further steps the sponsor must take before the application can be approved.

Other Meetings. Sponsors may request additional meetings to discuss scientific, medical, and other issues that arise during the review process. Because of already heavy demands for its time, however, CDER is likely to grant conferences only for more important issues. For resolving less significant issues, the agency will probably suggest communication by telephone or letter.

Under the FDA's new meetings-management system, a review division should notify the sponsor of the meeting date within 14 calendar days of receiving the formal meeting request. The agency will be called upon to meet this goal for increasing numbers of meeting requests—90% in FY2001 and FY2002.

Agreements under PDUFA II classify FDA/sponsor meetings during NDA reviews as Type C meetings, meaning that the FDA should ensure that the meetings take place within 75 calendar days of the agency's receipt of formal meeting requests. The agency must meet these goals for 90% of meetings requests in FY2001 and FY2002 (for a more detailed profile of CDER's new meetings-management system, see Chapter 5).

Applicants seeking to schedule a meeting with CDER should consult two documents: a 1996 CDER policy document entitled, *Formal Meetings Between CDER and CDER's External Constituents* (MaPP 4512.1), and a February 2000 industry guidance entitled, *Formal Meetings with Sponsors and Applicants for PDUFA Products*.

The Right to Protest and Appeal FDA Actions/Decisions Although recent regulatory initiatives have done much to make the FDA and sponsors "partners" in drug development, the NDA review process can, in some cases, result in disputes based on scientific or other issues. Agency regulations permit any "interested person"—which includes a sponsor or applicant—to obtain a formal review of any agency decision by raising the matter with the supervisor of the employee who made the decision at issue.

Dispute resolution has become a fairly visible issue over the past several years. In fact, CDER has undertaken several related initiatives on the subject:

- Under PDUFA II, the FDA has established a two-tier appeals process for resolving scientific agency/sponsor disputes (see discussion below).

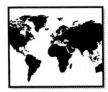

- In February 2000, CDER released an industry guidance entitled, *Formal Dispute Resolution: Appeals Above the Division Level* to provide guidance for resolving scientific and procedural disputes that cannot be resolved at the division level, and to describe procedures for formally appealing decisions that cause such disputes.

- In a November 18, 1998, revised regulation, the FDA explicitly stated that a sponsor, applicant, or manufacturer of a drug may request a review of a scientific controversy by an appropriate advisory committee. Since the agency still retains the discretion as to whether advisory committee input will be sought on such issues, the amended regulation calls for the agency to inform the requestor, in writing, of the reasons for a denial of a request for advisory committee review (see Chapter 10).

- In 1996, CDER Director Janet Woodcock pledged to include, in all of the center's action letters, instructions on how sponsors can dispute FDA decisions.

- In 1995, CDER established the CDER ombudsman function, which is designed to provide a mechanism through which sponsors and others can "seek solutions to problematic interactions and suggest better ways for [the center] to do its work." In virtually all cases, however, interactions with the CDER ombudsman are considered informal and, therefore, are not subject to the dispute resolution policies and goals set out for formal dispute resolution efforts.

Despite CDER's implementation of formal dispute resolution mechanisms, it is important to note that, for many firms, resolving issues through informal means remains the preferred route. Many center officials expect most firms, particularly larger and more experienced firms, to attempt to address and resolve disputes through less formal means, in part because formalizing the process can lengthen and complicate it. According to CDER officials, one of the more common informal ways that companies seek to address disputes is to request a meeting with a review division and to request that the relevant office director (i.e., ODE I, II, III, IV, or V) be present at the meeting to offer senior management input on the issue.

Traditionally, CDER has had a fairly sophisticated process for helping sponsors settle disputes. The process through which a particular dispute is resolved may depend upon whether the problem is procedural/administrative or scientific/medical in nature.

Administrative and Procedural Disputes. Administrative and procedural disputes may involve problems such as sponsor difficulties in scheduling FDA meetings and obtaining timely agency responses to inquiries. The sponsor may also believe that the agency is not following procedures consistent with current laws or regulations. When such problems arise, the FDA recommends that a sponsor first contact the project manager who is handling its application. Most project managers are experts in the NDA review process, and are likely to have the most complete information about the status of a pending application. Because of this and because project managers work very closely with NDA reviewers, they can resolve many procedural or administrative problems if the agency is at fault.

Scientific and Medical Disputes. The FDA believes that the 90-day and end-of-review conferences as well as various other FDA-sponsor communications provide adequate vehicles for addressing and resolving scientific and medical disputes. The agency recognizes, however, that there are exceptions. When the sponsor believes that conferences have proven inadequate, it may request a meeting with the

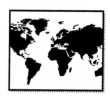

management of the appropriate reviewing division. At that time, the applicant may suggest that the FDA seek the advice of outside experts, such as consultants and other agency advisors. The sponsor may also invite its own consultant when such a meeting is granted.

If a specially scheduled meeting fails to resolve a dispute, the applicant or the agency may propose that the scientific/medical issue be referred to one of the FDA's standing advisory committees, which consist largely of non-FDA medical experts (see Chapter 10). The committee will review the issue and make recommendations. The FDA can then follow these recommendations or take its own course of action.

Formal Dispute Resolution Under FDA regulations and policies, a sponsor should first attempt to address an NDA- or supplemental NDA-related scientific or procedural issue at the review division level. If division-level formal or informal mechanisms fail to resolve the issue, the sponsor can request that the division reconsider the issue after the company gives the division an opportunity to review any materials on which the sponsor intends to rely in an appeal to the next level.

Issues that are unresolvable at the review-division level (i.e., after a formal request for reconsideration) should then be appealed at the office level (i.e., ODE I, II, etc.). If necessary, the sponsor can then appeal to the deputy center director and then to the center director.

According to CDER's February 2000 guidance, the applicant should request formal dispute resolution at the office or center level by submitting a written request and supporting documentation to the center's formal dispute resolution project manager (DRPM). The DRPM will forward the request to the appropriate CDER official, who will provide a response after reviewing the materials and the administrative record. That response may represent any one of several outcomes, including a decision on the matter, a decision to seek input from an advisory committee or other internal or external experts, or a request for more information from the sponsor. If the agency denies the appeal, its written response should identify the reasons for the denial and any actions that the sponsor might take to address the specific issue.

The agency's response (i.e., via letter or telephone) to a sponsor appeal regarding a user-fee product should occur within 30 calendar days of the DRPM's receipt of the formal request. According to its user-fee goals, CDER is expected to provide such responses within this timeframe for at least 90% of the written appeals received in FY2001 and FY2002.

The Right To Confidentiality Given the quantity of competitively sensitive data and information submitted in NDAs, confidentiality issues are of great importance to drug sponsors. Both the FDA and the federal government have policies and procedures designed to protect from public disclosure certain types of information submitted in NDAs.

The degree of protection (from public disclosure) afforded to information and data submitted in an NDA depends on a few factors, including the nature of the information or data and the application's status (i.e., under review, approvable, or approved).

Under current laws and regulations, the agency may not, at any time either during the NDA review or after approval, publicly disclose or release any information or test data that qualify as trade secret or commercial or financial information. According to FDA regulations, a trade secret "may consist of any commercially valuable plan, formula, process, or device that is used for the making, preparing, compounding, or processing of trade commodities and that can be said to be the end product of either innovation or substantial effort." The regulations also emphasize that "there must be a direct relationship between the trade secret and the productive process."

Commercial or financial information considered privileged or confidential means "valuable data or information which is used in one's business and is of a type customarily held in strict confidence or regarded as privileged and not disclosed to any member of the public" by the company to which it belongs.

Under certain circumstances, the FDA does have the authority to disclose confidential commercial information to foreign regulatory agencies and to certain international organizations. It is important to note, however, that the regulations that authorize such exchanges also include several safeguards to prevent unauthorized disclosures, and that virtually all disclosures of confidential commercial information have occurred with the sponsor's consent. The situations under which the agency would consider disclosing confidential commercial information without the sponsor's consent generally involve cases in which obtaining the sponsor's consent might adversely affect or compromise an enforcement action (see discussion below).

Confidentiality Prior to Approval In general, the FDA will not publicly disclose the existence of an NDA before it issues an approvable letter for the application, unless the NDA's existence has been previously publicly disclosed or acknowledged (e.g., by the sponsor or other lawful manner). Once an approvable letter has been issued, the FDA can disclose the NDA's existence, which the agency does in a monthly listing of applications that have reached the approvable stage.

If an unapproved NDA's existence has not been publicly disclosed or acknowledged, no data or information contained within it is available for public disclosure until an approval letter is issued (see discussion below). If, however, the pending NDA's existence has been publicly disclosed or acknowledged, the FDA commissioner may, at his or her discretion, "disclose a summary of selected portions of the safety and effectiveness data that are appropriate for public consideration of a specific pending issue" (e.g., for consideration at an open session of an advisory committee meeting).

Confidentiality Following Approval Once the agency issues an approvable letter, the NDA's existence and certain non-confidential data within it can be publicly disclosed by the agency. Unless an applicant can show that "extraordinary circumstances" exist, the following information will become immediately available for public disclosure:

- a "disclosable review package," sometimes called an "approval package" and previously termed a "summary basis of approval" document, that provides information on the results of each aspect of the NDA review (e.g., medical, pharmacology, and chemistry review);

- a protocol for a test or study, unless it is shown to fall within the definition of trade secret or confidential commercial information;

- adverse reaction reports, product experience reports, consumer complaints, and other similar data and information after certain confidential information is deleted (information that would identify the subject or any physician or institution);

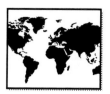

- a list of all active ingredients and any inactive ingredients previously disclosed to the public; and
- an assay method or other analytical method, unless it serves no regulatory or compliance purpose and is shown to fall within the definition of trade secret or confidential commercial information.

The Sharing of NDA Review-Related Materials Among Drug Regulators With international harmonization efforts, and more importantly the regulator-to-regulator relationships that are deepening as part of these efforts, the limited amount of information sharing done on the part of regulators is certain to increase in coming years. The subject of marketing dossier-related information sharing received considerable attention when it was revealed that Novartis had requested that the FDA share certain review-related information with another regulator evaluating its new drug Gleevec, apparently in an effort to speed the drug's availability in that foreign country.

Although the FDA has a long history of entering into cooperative agreements to share or exchange specific types of information and documents with foreign regulators, the nature and sensitivity of the data and information contained in NDAs and review documents called for somewhat different exchange standards. The current regulatory framework relevant to NDA review-related information sharing took shape largely the early 1990s, when new regulations provided the agency with greater powers to disclose confidential commercial information found in NDAs—otherwise called "nonpublic drug safety, effectiveness, and quality information"—to foreign regulatory agencies.

To permit such NDA review-related disclosures, CDER will ask for the sponsor's permission to provide the requested NDA and review-related information to a foreign regulator that has requested the information. For the foreign regulator, the FDA will seek a confidentiality commitment—assuming one does not already exist with that country—as well as a copy of the country's regulations that provide the foreign regulator with the authority or ability to maintain the confidentiality of the information that the FDA will provide. Currently, the FDA is known to have general confidentiality agreements with three countries—Canada, Australia, and Japan—but is actively seeking such agreements with selected other countries.

The Novartis request was, at least at the time it was made, thought to be unique, essentially because it had been largely—if not exclusively—foreign governments, and not drug manufacturers, that had requested review-related information and documents from the FDA in previous cases. At this writing, however, it was unclear whether such information sharing with foreign governments speeded or even affected foreign approvals.

CHAPTER 9

The FDA's Priority Review Policy

Given the workload-to-staffing disparity that has often characterized the FDA during its history and the corresponding disparity in the therapeutic significance of new medicines under review, it is not surprising that the agency has evolved a system under which marketing applications for new drugs could be prioritized based on their implications for the public health. Traditionally, CDER has employed a relatively straightforward drug classification system to assist its reviewers in prioritizing NDA reviews. Although the system has been revamped to some degree under the FDA's user-fee program, it continues to permit the agency to allocate its resources to what are perceived to be the most important NDAs, independent of such factors as the chronological order of the submissions.

Essentially, the FDA's priority review policy is important because it puts public health before something that is also critical to any government regulatory agency: the absolute need to act impartially and to adopt procedures, policies, and practices that reinforce its impartiality to those that it serves and to which it answers. Without such a policy, the practical realities of reviewing and approving applications based on any criterion other than their dates of submission would be far more difficult for an agency whose every move can be scrutinized by Congress, industry, the media, and the public.

While some have argued that CDER's drug classification system was not significant in the past, the prescription drug user fee program has placed greater emphasis on a drug's "therapeutic rating," which CDER generally assigns upon an NDA's submission. Under CDER commitments made as part of PDUFA II, a drug's therapeutic rating—either priority or standard—determines the center's review goal for the product's NDA. Throughout the life of PDUFA II (October 1, 1997 through September 30, 2002), the center must review and take action on 90 percent of priority drugs within 6 months. CDER's goals for standard NDAs shift during the PDUFA II years, although the agency is expected to review 90% of all standard applications submitted in FY2002 within 10 months.

Over the last several years, the implications that a priority designation had for a drug's review time were unmistakable. On average, priority new molecular entities (NME) cleared in 2000 gained FDA approval more than 15 months faster than their standard counterparts (see discussion below). There were other benefits for products with the prized priority designation: In recent years, CDER has been far more likely to approve priority NDAs at the conclusion of the first review cycle (i.e., rather than taking an approvable or not-approvable action).

Such realities raised the stakes for industry, which craved the priority designation even more than it had in the past. Company officials reported pursuing fast track designation, which offers benefits for

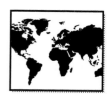

Worldwide Pharmaceutical Regulation Series

certain drugs that fulfill unmet medical needs, not because of the benefits flowing directly from the designation, but because they believed that such designations could help them obtain for their drugs a review status that is more likely to lead to rapid product approval—priority review status.

The great rewards (i.e., earlier approval) associated with priority designation also raised the profile of the designation system under user-fee program. Critics charged that the FDA's criteria for priority designation was too broad, and that it should be revised to ensure that only genuinely innovative therapies gain the top review status. Others went further, calling for the criteria to be revised to include only drugs for severe and life-threatening illnesses and conditions for which no current treatments are available. It was unclear whether such views would carry significant weight during the PDUFA reauthorization process to be undertaken in 2002.

CDER NDA Review Goals, FY1998–FY2002

Original NDA and Efficacy Supplement Submission Cohort	Standard NDAs	Priority NDAs
FY1998	90% in 12 mo.	90% in 6 mo.
FY1999	30% in 10 mo. 90% in 12 mo.	90% in 6 mo.
FY2000	50% in 10 mo. 90% in 12 mo.	90% in 6 mo.
FY2001	70% in 10 mo. 90% in 12 mo.	90% in 6 mo.
FY2002	90% in 10 mo.	90% in 6 mo.

In the mid-1990s, CDER decided to replace its existing policy guide on the drug classification system—1992's Staff Manual Guide 4820.3—with a pair of policy documents. The first of these, an April 1996 guidance entitled, *Priority Review Policy* (MaPP 6020.3), addresses the assignment of a drug's therapeutic rating. Although the agency has been planning to release a second policy document to address issues relating to a drug's chemical rating, that document had not been published as of this writing.

Therapeutic Rating

While the existing alphanumeric classification system generally comprises two primary elements—a chemical rating and a therapeutic rating (e.g., 1P)—it is the therapeutic rating that determines a drug's review priority. According to MaPP 6020.3, all original NDAs and effectiveness supplements are to be given a therapeutic rating "based on an estimate of [the drug's] therapeutic, preventative or diagnostic value." The document adds that "the priority determination does not take into consideration any information or estimate of price and is based on conditions and information available at the time the application is filed. It is not intended to predict a drug's ultimate value or its eventual place in the market."

This estimate of therapeutic, preventative or diagnostic value must be considered in the context of CDER's definition of a "priority" product.

Priority Drugs Under CDER policy, a priority drug is one that "if approved, would be a significant improvement compared to marketed products [approved (if such is required), including non-'drug' products/therapies] in the treatment, diagnosis, or prevention of a disease. Improvement can be demonstrated by, for example: (1) evidence of increased effectiveness in treatment, prevention, or diagnosis of disease; (2) elimination or substantial reduction of a treatment-limiting drug reaction; (3) documented enhancement of patient compliance; or (4) evidence of safety and effectiveness of a new subpopulation."

Standard Drugs Under the FDA's user-fee program, drugs that do not qualify as priority products (P) are classified as standard therapies (S).

Special Situation Drugs The FDA may consider the conventional priority or standard rating code to be inadequate to properly identify a product's defining characteristics. In such cases, a review division may assign a drug one or more "special situation" ratings in addition to the "P" or "S" rating:

Type AA-AIDS Drug: "The drug is indicated for the treatment of AIDS or HIV-related disease."

Type E-Subpart E Drug: "The drug was developed and/or evaluated under the special procedures for drugs intended to treat life-threatening and severely debilitating illnesses" (see Chapter 15).

Type F-Fraud Policy Applies: "Substantive review of the application is deferred pending the outcome of a validity assessment of the submitted data as provided for by Compliance Policy Guide 7150.09. This code remains in the system throughout the audit and after when (a) the data are found to be not valid and a not approvable letter is issued or (b) the applicant withdraws the application before the audit is completed or after the audit is completed (data found to be not valid) but before a not approvable letter is issued."

Type G-Data Validated: "A validity assessment was performed on the application as provided for by CPG 7150.09, and the questions regarding the reliability of the data were satisfactorily resolved."

Type N-Non-Prescription Drug: "The drug has product labeling that provides for non-prescription (over-the-counter [OTC]) marketing. Applications will be labeled with an N designator whether all indications, or only some, are non-prescription."

Type V-Designated Orphan Drug: "The drug has officially received orphan designation...at the request of its sponsor/applicant" (see Chapter 13).

Assigning the Therapeutic Rating Because of a priority classification's significance, drug sponsors will often engage review division staff in classification-related discussions well before the NDA is submitted. Depending on clinical trial results, some sponsors may attempt to explore with a division its chances of obtaining a priority classification as early as the IND phase, while others may wait until later in the process (e.g., the pre-NDA meeting). Given that there is no formal process through which sponsors seek priority designations, different companies are likely to employ various practices in proposing such designations for their products.

The FDA's Priority Review Policy

Chapter 9

CDER's Priority Review Policy (MaPP 6020.3) puts the responsibility for assigning a drug's priority classification on the relevant medical team leader within the division evaluating the product. The team leader is to make the decision "after consulting, as needed, with the reviewing medical officer, supervisory chemist, pharmacologist, microbiologist and new drug division director."

Since the priority classification determines the review timeline applicable to an NDA, MaPP 6020.3 states that "the review priority should be determined and assigned at the 45-day meeting if the application is to be filed." The document is clear in establishing that, although a drug may be classified down from a priority to a standard product during the NDA review, the initial classification is locked in during the initial 6- or 12-month review cycle.

"The final review classification of a new drug may change from [priority] to [standard] during the course of the review of a marketing application (NDA), either because of the approval of other agents or because of availability of new data; however, the review priority classification assigned at the time of filing will not change during the first review cycle and the user fee time frame of the original review cycle will be that based on the original priority." If the reviewing medical officer or team leader wishes to change a drug's classification following the first review cycle, he or she must recommend the change "justified on the basis of, for example, new information in an IND or NDA, medical literature, advisory committee opinions or approval of a pharmacologically similar drug." The division director is responsible for approving the recommended change. MaPP 6020.3 makes no reference to the possibility of applications being upgraded from standard to priority during the initial review cycle.

Chemical Novelty Rating

The numeric element in CDER's priority classification code represents the chemical novelty of a drug product's active ingredient. This rating, which has no implications for the drug's review priority, indicates to FDA chemistry reviewers whether the active ingredient is new or is related to compounds already on the market.

Until CDER releases a new MaPP for assigning chemical novelty ratings, policy guide 4820.3 will remain in effect. According to this document, a drug is to be assigned one of the following seven chemical ratings:

Type 1-New Molecular Entity: "A drug for which the active moiety (present as the unmodified base [parent] compound, or an ester or a salt, clathrate, or other noncovalent derivative of the base [parent] compound) has not been previously approved or marketed in the United States for use in a drug product, either as a single ingredient or as part of a combination product or as part of a mixture of stereoisomers.

"The active moiety in a drug is the molecule or ion, excluding those appended portions of the molecule that cause the drug to be an ester, salt (including a salt with hydrogen or coordination bonds) or other noncovalent derivative (such as a complex, chelate, or clathrate) of the molecule, responsible for the physiological or [pharmacological] action of the drug substance. The active moiety is the entire molecule or ion, not the 'active site.'

"Ordinarily, an ester is not considered an active moiety as most ester linkages are rapidly broken, with the de-esterified molecule circulating in the blood. However, there can be exceptions to this where a

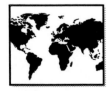

stable ester is the active moiety, the de-esterified molecule being inert; an example of this is organic nitrates, where the nitrate esters are the active moieties. The organic base molecules (glycerol, isosorbide) are inert."

Type 2-New Ester, New Salt, or Other Noncovalent Derivative: "A drug for which the active moiety has been previously approved or marketed in the United States but for which the particular ester, or salt, clathrate, or other noncovalent derivative, [of] the unmodified base (parent) compound has not yet been approved or marketed in the United States, either as a single ingredient, part of a combination product, or part of a mixture of stereoisomers."

Type 3-New Formulation: "A new dosage form or formulation, including a new strength, where the drug has already been approved or marketed in the United States by the same or another manufacturer. The indication may be the same as that of the already marketed drug product or may be new.

"A drug with changes in its inactive ingredients such that clinical studies (as opposed to bioequivalence studies) are required is considered to be a Type 3 drug. A drug previously approved or marketed only as a part of a combination (either a manufactured combination or a naturally occurring mixture) or a mixture of stereoisomers will also be considered a Type 3 drug. A combination product all of whose components have previously been approved or marketed together in combination with another drug will also be considered to be a Type 3 drug.

"A change in the strength of one or more drugs in a previously approved or marketed combination is considered to be a new formulation, not a new combination."

Type 4-New Combination: "A drug product containing two or more active moieties that have not been previously approved or marketed together in a drug product by any manufacturer in the United States. The new product may be a physical or a chemical (ester or non-covalent) combination of two or more active moieties. A new physical combination containing one or more active moieties that have not been previously approved or marketed is considered to be a Type 1,4 drug.

"A chemical combination of two or more active moieties previously approved or marketed as a physical combination is considered to be a Type 1 drug if the chemical bond is a non-ester covalent bond. If the two moieties are linked by an ester bond, the drug is considered a Type 4 drug if the moieties have not been previously marketed or approved as a physical combination, and a Type 2 drug if the combination has been previously marketed or approved."

Type 5-New Manufacturer: "A drug product that duplicates a drug product (same active moiety, same salt, same formulation [i.e., differences not sufficient to cause the product to be a Type 3; may require bioequivalency testing, including bioequivalence tests with clinical endpoints, but not clinical studies], or same combination) already approved or marketed in the United States by another firm. This category also includes NDAs for duplicate products where clinical studies were needed because of marketing exclusivity held by the original applicant."

Type 6-New Indication: "A drug product that duplicates a drug product (same active moiety, same salt, same formulation, or same combination) already approved or marketed in the U.S. by the same or another firm except that it provides for a new indication."

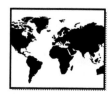

Type 7-Drug Already Marketed But Without An Approved NDA: "The application is the first NDA for a drug product containing one or more drugs marketed at the time of application or in the past without an approved NDA. Includes (a) first post-1962 application for products marketed prior to 1938, and (b) first application for DESI-related products first marketed between 1938 and 1962 without an NDA. The indication may be the same as, or different from, the already marketed drug product."

CDER's Prioritization Policy At Work

It is difficult to know precisely how CDER's drug review divisions implement the drug classification system on a day-to-day basis. According to MaPP 6020.3, "a 'priority' designation is intended to direct overall attention and resources to the evaluation of applications for products that have the potential for providing significant preventative or diagnostic therapeutic advance as compared to 'standard' applications.

"The review priority classification determines the overall approach to setting review priorities and user fee review time frames but is not intended to preclude work on all other projects. It does not imply that staff working on a priority application cannot work on other projects, such as 30-day safety reviews of a newly submitted investigational new drug application (IND), preparation for end-of-phase 2 conferences, etc. Certain ad hoc special assignments may also take precedence. The supervisor is to advise the reviewer and team leader when an ad hoc assignment is to take precedence."

Although CDER's priority review policy and the user-fee review goals are designed to focus resources on important new drugs, the user fee timelines also offer important assurances for non-priority products. While CDER must concentrate reviewing resources on priority products, for example, it cannot do so to the point that it is unable to meet the 12-month review goal for standard applications. In addition, since priority classifications are made independently by each of CDER's 14 review divisions, drugs are prioritized within each therapeutic area, ensuring that products in high-priority and high-profile areas such as AIDS and cancer do not compete for resources against drugs in lower-profile therapeutic areas. This policy does not prevent the agency, however, from giving more staffing resources to certain divisions (e.g., AIDS) based on workload and the significance of the therapeutic area, something that has come under scrutiny in the past.

The Impact of CDER's Priority Review Policy

Assessing the true impact of CDER's priority review policy—and its ability to promote faster approvals for high-priority products—is difficult because there are a variety of factors that affect the speed with which drugs are reviewed. While it is true that the agency's review goal for high-priority products is shorter compared to that for other products, for example, it might also be true that sponsors and reviewers may tend to invest more time early on in an important product's development and pre-NDA period, an investment that will often result in speedier reviews.

Whatever the factors, however, it is clear that CDER is reviewing and approving priority drugs more quickly than standard products. CDER's average review times for priority and standard new molecular entities (NME) approved in 2000 were 7.4 months and 22.7 months, respectively (see exhibit below). Over the past five years, the priority-versus-standard product review gap has varied consider-

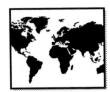

ably, from 4.8 months in 1998 to 15.3 months in 2000. The general perception, based on historical review time trends and the comments of FDA officials, is that this review gap is likely to continue widening in the future.

Not surprisingly given their shorter approval times, priority products are significantly more likely to be approved in CDER's first review cycle (i.e., an approval rather than an approvable or not-approvable action). While CDER approved 63.1% (19 of 31) of the priority NDAs submitted during FY1999 (October 1998-September 1999), it approved just 40% (38 of 95) of the standard NDAs in the FY1999 cohort.

Priority/Standard NME Review Gap, 1995-2000
(in months)

	Mean Review Time for Priority NMEs	Mean Review Time for Standard NMEs	Gap
2000	7.4	22.7	15.3
1999	8.8	16.9	8.1
1998	9.5	14.3	4.8
1997	9.5	18.2	8.8
1996	13.7	19.7	6
1995	10.1	23.6	13.5

Source: PAREXEL's Pharmaceutical R&D Statistical Sourcebook 2001

Patterns in Priority/Standard Designations for New Drugs

Given the value of priority review status, it is not surprising that industry has watched trends in the FDA's assignment of priority designations quite closely. There have been no lasting trends in priority/standard designations since the user-fee era began.

During the 1980s and early 1990s, roughly half of all NMEs approved by CDER were priority products. As the user-fee era matured, however, the prevalence of priority designations for new product approvals declined markedly. After rising during the first years of the user-fee program (from 42% in 1992 to 52% in 1993 and 59% in 1994), the percentage of approved NMEs with priority designations began a several-year decline. In both 1995 and 1996, less than one in three NMEs was granted priority status. Less than 25% of NMEs approved in 1997 received priority designations, the lowest level in at least 15 years.

At the time, some observers speculated that the decline in priority designations might have represented a conscious or subconscious effort by CDER's review divisions to limit the number of drugs for which they had to meet the more demanding 6-month review goal. In other words, at a time when obtaining a priority classification for a new drug meant the most to drug applicants (i.e., in terms of a shortened review), such designations were becoming more elusive than ever.

Through its 1998 and 1999 NME approvals, however, CDER appeared to have answered this charge. More than half—or 54% (35 of 65)—of CDER's 1998 and 1999 NME approvals were for priority

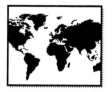

The FDA's Priority Review Policy

Chapter 9

products. For all NDAs (i.e., including NME and non-NME submissions), 32% of the NDAs filed in FY1999 received priority designation, down from 39% in FY1998.

CDER's 2000 NME approvals once again showed a decline in priority designations. Priority NMEs comprised only a third of the new drugs approved during the year.

Of the 98 total original NDAs (NMEs and non-NMEs) approved in 2000, 20 were for priority products, according to the FDA. CDER approved these NDAs in a median of 6 months.

NMEs Approved Based on Therapeutic Potential, 1985–2000

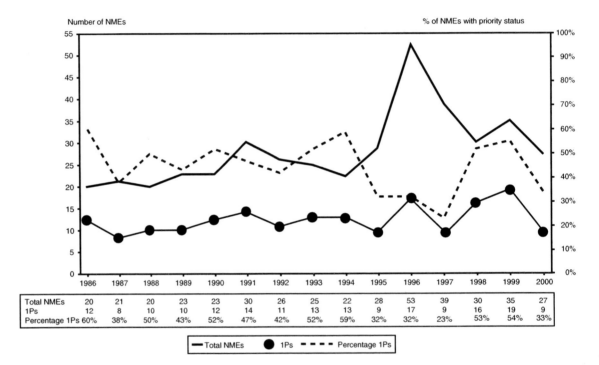

	1986	1987	1988	1989	1990	1991	1992	1993	1994	1995	1996	1997	1998	1999	2000
Total NMEs	20	21	20	23	23	30	26	25	22	28	53	39	30	35	27
1Ps	12	8	10	10	12	14	11	13	13	9	17	9	16	19	9
Percentage 1Ps	60%	38%	50%	43%	52%	47%	42%	52%	59%	32%	32%	23%	53%	54%	33%

Source: PAREXEL's Pharmaceutical R&D Statistical Sourcebook 2001

New Drug Approval in the United States

CHAPTER 10

Advisory Committees and the Drug Approval Process

While it employs a larger contingent of medical, scientific, and drug development specialists than any drug regulatory agency in the world, the FDA does not necessarily conduct its new drug reviews in a vacuum free from all outside input. Throughout the review process, CDER's 14 new drug review divisions have access to independent prescription drug advisory committees whose purpose is to provide advice and added perspective on technical and medical issues related to the safety, effectiveness, testing, labeling, and use of new and approved drugs.

Today, CDER has access to 15 prescription drug advisory committees (see listing below) comprised largely of leading scientists, most of whom are active researchers with academic appointments. In addition, CDER has three other advisory panels—the Pharmacy Compounding Committee, the Nonprescription Drugs Advisory Committee, and the Advisory Committee for Pharmaceutical Science—that can also become involved in prescription drug issues.

CDER's advisory committees, which are regulated under the Federal Advisory Committee Act of 1972 along with all other government advisory committees, convene periodically to discuss issues that CDER believes to be of major importance to public health. Since 1964, CDER's new drug review divisions have looked to the advisory committees for recommendations on issues such as the approvability of specific drugs, the adequacy of drug development approaches (e.g., evaluating new guidelines or study design issues), and the status of certain marketed drugs. According to the agency, committee discussions of such issues bring more diverse input to the decision-making process, provide access to technical expertise that may not be available within the agency, and open FDA decision-making procedures to broader scrutiny.

Perhaps surprisingly for a program that is generally perceived to work reasonably successfully, CDER's advisory committee program was the subject of various reform initiatives throughout the 1990s. During the early 1990s, CDER faced growing pressure to standardize committee processes. In response to a series of Institute of Medicine (IOM) recommendations in 1991, CDER revised its existing advisory committee procedures and detailed them in a document entitled, *Policy and Guidance Handbook for FDA Advisory Committees* (1994). The handbook represented the agency's first real attempt to establish criteria for identifying intellectual bias and for granting conflict-of-interest waivers for committee members (see discussion below). The agency has adopted many of the IOM's recommendations,

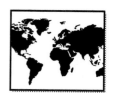

Worldwide Pharmaceutical Regulation Series

Advisory Committees and the Drug Approval Process

Chapter 10

including a system for advance scheduling of committee meetings and a policy that sponsors will "generally" receive questions to be posed to advisory committees prior to the meeting.

More recently, the advisory committee process has seen change due to significant legislative initiatives, legal proceedings and regulatory developments:

- Reflective of CDER's increasing focus on drug safety and risk management issues, the center announced that it had formed a new Drug Safety and Risk Management Advisory Subcommittee under its Advisory Committee for Pharmaceutical Science. The panel, which CDER hoped would begin meeting in early 2002, will address general drug safety and risk management issues facing the center, as well as safety/risk management issues relevant to specific drugs.

- The Food and Drug Administration Modernization Act of 1997 (FDAMA) introduced several important reforms to the advisory committee process, including a handful of reforms that affect the drug review process directly. Under FDAMA, CDER must either take action within 90 days of a committee recommendation (e.g., on a drug's approval) or specify why such an action has not been taken. To date, CDER officials report that the center has not had any problem meeting this new requirement. In addition, a committee must now meet within 60 days of the date on which a subject is ready for its review. FDAMA also includes new provisions on committee membership, conflict-of-interest issues, and training (see discussions below). To provide guidance on FDAMA's impact on the advisory committee process, CDER has released a guidance for industry entitled, *Advisory Committees: Implementing Section 120 of the Food and Drug Administration Modernization Act of 1997* (October 1998).

- Under a legal settlement associated with a Public Citizen's Health Research Group (HRG) lawsuit against the FDA, CDER agreed to provide the public, in advance or at the time of certain committee meetings, with access to materials provided to advisory committee members. This settlement applies directly to meetings (beginning with those on January 1, 2000) at which pending product approval issues will be discussed (e.g., NDAs for new drugs, prescription-to-OTC switches, ANDAs for generic drugs), but not to "post-approval and non-approval issue-oriented advisory committee meetings," including those that will involve the discussion of guidance documents, product classification/re-classification, post-approval adverse drug events, product withdrawal, and post-approval monitoring programs. To minimize the time involved in complying with these disclosure requirements, CDER used a December 1999 draft guidance to "strongly encourage" sponsors to submit advisory committee background packages (i.e., background information packages that sponsors provide in advance of committee meetings) that may be disclosed in their entirety (i.e., that do not contain any information that the sponsor asserts is exempt from disclosure because it is trade secret or confidential or because it would constitute an unwarranted invasion of personal privacy) and to submit an electronic version of the package. Under the draft guidance, a sponsor can submit a fully releasable submission 22 business days prior to the committee meeting, but must submit a partially releasable package (i.e., a package that must be redacted by CDER) 48 days before a meeting. Submitting a partially releasable package for a priority review product has other significant implications for the sponsor: "Such a submission will be

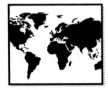

considered an agreement by the sponsor to extend by 2 months the review time for the review cycle in which the advisory committee will be held," the agency states in its draft guidance. The December 1999 draft guidance establishes that several types of information in such packages will be considered disclosable in most cases, including summary tables of safety and effectiveness data, summaries of adverse drug reaction data, and clinical and preclinical protocols.

- In a July 1998 direct final rule that ultimately would be withdrawn, CDER amended its regulations governing the review of agency decisions by inserting a statement to establish that drug sponsors may request the review of a "scientific controversy" by an appropriate scientific advisory committee. The FDA was required to make this change under the provisions of FDAMA. Several weeks after releasing this final rule, the agency was forced to withdraw the rule when the Pharmaceutical Research and Manufacturers of America (PhRMA) responded that the final rule did not "fulfill the mandate" of FDAMA because it relied largely on existing mechanisms and that it did not establish new procedures for dispute resolution (the agency is required to withdraw direct final rules automatically when they trigger significant adverse comments within the comment period). In response to an earlier FDA draft guidance on dispute resolution, PhRMA held that the FDA should not be able to deny sponsors' requests for advisory committee review of scientific disputes unless it can present "compelling" reasons for such a denial. In late 1999, CDER officials speculated that the role of advisory committees in the dispute resolution process is likely to be minor, pointing out that disputed issues are likely to have been addressed by the time that the agency can coordinate and convene a committee meeting to address it. Still, in a February 2000 guidance document entitled, *Formal Dispute Resolution: Appeals Above the Division Level*, CDER does provide a mechanism through which sponsors can seek committee review of a disputed issue.

- As it did at the beginning of the 1990s, CDER again faced pressure to standardize its use of advisory committees at the close of the decade. In February 1999 comments to the agency, PhRMA asserted that "only novel products or issues or scientific controversies that cannot be resolved between FDA and the sponsor should be referred for advisory committee review." Citing the "significant variability" in the use of advisory committees by various divisions, PhRMA emphasized that the committees should not be used to simply confirm, or rubber stamp, existing CDER decisions or FDA/sponsor agreements.

Although it is not thought to have significant implications for the center's advisory committee program, a January 2002 reorganization shifted CDER's Advisors and Consultants Staff, the unit that manages the program, from the old Office or Review Management to the center's new Office of Executive Programs.

Largely because advisory committee recommendations often have major medical and financial implications, the public profile of the committees has risen dramatically since the late 1980s. Although committee recommendations are not binding on the FDA, these recommendations are seen by the financial community and the pharmaceutical industry as forerunners of agency decisions on products. As a result, committee meetings receive considerable attention not just from the companies whose products are being considered, but from financial analysts and the trade press as well.

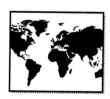

Advisory Committees and the Drug Approval Process

Chapter 10

So rarely does a CDER action contradict a committee recommendation that it makes significant news when one does. In August 1999, CDER's Division of Antiviral Drug Products approved Glaxo Wellcome's influenza treatment Relenza despite an earlier committee recommendation against approval. Specifically to address this seeming contradiction, Division of Antiviral Drug Products Director Heidi Jolson, M.D., authored a memo pointing out that Glaxo Wellcome had addressed the advisory committee's concerns regarding post-treatment symptom fluctuation by submitting new analyses, adequate labeling, and Phase IV study commitments.

The advisory committee system and its role in the drug approval process have been the target of criticism in recent years. CDER received some criticism in the late 1990s for approving a few drugs (later withdrawn) when certain advisory committee members disagreed on the drugs' approvability. In a December 1999 issue of the *Journal of the American Medical Association*, FDA officials defended the agency's actions by stating that critics who complain that certain advisory committee members disagreed with FDA's decision to approve products that were later withdrawn are, in effect, arguing "for approving a product only when there is unanimity or...for the suppression of dissent."

A November 2000 FDA "lessons learned" report on CDER's experience with Rezulin, an approved diabetes therapy whose 1997 approval and March 2000 withdrawal due to liver toxicity created considerable controversy, cited several problems with the center's pre-approval and postmarketing processes, including the advisory committee process. The clinical biases of advisory committee members and the committee's lack of expertise in risk management were factors in the pre- and post-marketing assessment of Rezulin, CDER staffers interviewed for the report stated. The "ability [of the advisory committee evaluating Rezulin] to fully grasp the many highly complex scientific and regulatory issues surrounding the approval and eventual withdrawal" of Rezulin could have been improved by the addition of experts in epidemiology and hepatology, or by the formation of a "safety advisory committee," the report noted. One CDER interviewee even claimed that the advisory committee's composition and the selection of public speakers were intentionally biased in Rezulin's favor.

Although CDER's advisory committee program is four decades old, the significant evolution in the center's drug review process has had several implications for the program. For example, even though advisory committee meetings have been more common in recent years, the environment for committee use is now more complex. Tight drug review timelines under the agency's user-fee program, for example, have made it difficult to schedule and hold advisory committee meetings in some cases.

One division, the Division of Neuropharmacological Drug Products, even announced in the mid-1990s its intention to forego, whenever possible, bringing new drugs to an advisory committee. According to this policy, which was a direct response to user-fee timelines, the division announced its intention to seek committee input only when a drug presents a particularly difficult issue or question. Some CDER officials claimed at the time that this is not necessarily a new policy, and pointed out that only 55 percent of new drugs approved in 1995 were reviewed by an advisory committee.

More recent CDER disclosures provide detailed and telling statistics on trends in advisory committee use. CDER sought advisory committee review on 40%—19 of 39—of the NMEs eligible for such review during 1999. Although this is consistent with the percentage of NMEs that were brought before

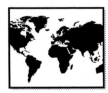

CDER's Prescription Drug Advisory Committees

Division of Gastrointestinal and Coagulation Drug Products
- Gastrointestinal Drugs Advisory Committee

Division of Antiviral Drug Products
- Antiviral Drugs Advisory Committee

Division of Cardio-Renal Drug Products
- Cardiovascular and Renal Drugs Advisory Committee

Division of Neuropharmacological Drug Products
- Peripheral and Central Nervous System Drugs Advisory Committee
- Psychopharmacologic Drugs Advisory Committee

Division of Oncologic Drug Products
- Oncologic Drugs Advisory Committee

Division of Pulmonary Drug Products
- Pulmonary-Allergy Drugs Advisory Committee

Division of Medical Imaging, Surgical, and Dental Drug Products
- Medical Imaging Drugs Advisory Committee

Division of Anti-Infective Drug Products
- Anti-Infective Drugs Advisory Committee

Division of Special Pathogens and Immunologic Drug Products
- Anti-Infective Drugs Advisory Committee
- Antiviral Drugs Advisory Committee

Division of Metabolism and Endocrine Drug Products
- Endocrinologic and Metabolic Drugs Advisory Committee

Division of Reproductive and Urologic Drug Products
- Advisory Committee for Reproductive Health Products

Division of Anesthetic, Critical Care, and Addiction Drug Products
- Drug Abuse Advisory Committee
- Anesthetic and Life Support Drugs Advisory Committee

Division of Anti-Inflammatory, Analgesic and Ophthalmic Drug Products
- Arthritis Advisory Committee
- Dermatologic and Ophthalmic Drugs Advisory Committee

Division of Dermatologic and Dental Drug Products
- Dermatologic and Ophthalmic Drugs Advisory Committee

Source: FDA

advisory committees in 1998 (39%), CDER also points out that the proportion of all NDAs brought to advisory committees more than tripled, from 3% to 10%, between in 1998 and 1999. In response to congressional inquiries regarding whether earlier advisory committee advice would maximize the value of committee deliberations, the drug center pointed out that the number of INDs brought

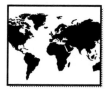

before committees decreased from 3% in 1998 to 1% in 1999 (as of late 1999), and that the quantity of INDs and the availability of committee members would make increases in this area difficult.

In FY2001, CDER held 30 prescription drug advisory committee meetings, a significant drop from previous years. Although the reasons for the downturn are not clear, it could be related to the drop in industry NDA submissions for new drugs in recent years.

A Look at Committee Membership

The nature of an advisory committee's membership is a function of several factors, including the panel's charter and the technical expertise necessary to evaluate the issues likely to come before the panel. Membership comprises primarily physicians, although qualified experts in such disciplines as epidemiology, nursing, biostatistics, pharmacology, toxicology, and psychology are also included. A technically qualified, consumer-nominated member may be designated as a voting member of a committee as well.

Nominated by professional or consumer organizations, other committee members, private individuals, or FDA staffers, advisors must be judged to be broadly trained and experienced, of established professional reputation and personal integrity, and committed to the public interest. Although the agency seeks balance in terms of gender, race, and geographic location, technical competence is the overriding consideration in selecting members. Because members serve four-year terms and are likely to address a wide variety of issues during these periods, perhaps the ideal committee members are those who have recognized accomplishments and leadership within their fields and demonstrated abilities and interests in issues outside their specialties.

Although FDAMA includes provisions regarding membership requirements for newly formed advisory committees (i.e., new panels formed under FDAMA), it does not require existing committees to comply with the new provisions. In its October 1998 guidance document, however, FDA establishes that, to further the goals of the statutory amendments, it intends to modify current advisory committee membership on a meeting-by-meeting basis and to recharter committees when necessary to reflect the FDAMA provisions. Further, in late 2001, CDER was completing paperwork to add an "industry representative" to each of its advisory committees.

Under FDAMA, an advisory committee comprises two types of members: (1) core members, who are appointed by the FDA commissioner or his or her designee based on their scientific or technical expertise and who serve for the duration of the committee or until the terms of appointment expire, they resign, or they are removed by the commissioner or the designee; and (2) ad hoc members, who are called upon to supplement the core membership on an ad hoc basis so that the committee considering an issue includes a consumer/patient representative, an industry representative, and at least two representatives who are specialists with expertise in the particular disease or condition for which the drug is proposed. Provided that their participation is not blocked by conflict of interest laws or regulations (see discussion below), core members will be voting members at committee meetings. The ad hoc committee members who represent consumer/patient interests and who have expertise in the drug indication under evaluation will be voting members only when they possess the requisite scientific or technical expertise and when their participation is not prevented by conflict of interest considerations.

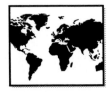

In late 2001, CDER was completing the paperwork to add industry representatives to existing committees, something that FDAMA requires only for newly formed committees. CDER officials point out that the industry representatives, who will not be considered voting committee members, are being added in the spirit of FDAMA.

The FDA has several standards for ensuring the independence and objectivity of its advisory committees. First, no FDA employees may serve as voting committee members. Under FDAMA, no person who is a full-time government employee and who is engaged in the administration of the Food, Drug and Cosmetic Act may be a voting member. The FDA does, however, appoint an employee as an executive secretary for each committee. Although not a panel member, the executive secretary is the agency's liaison to the committee, and is responsible for all administrative planning and preparation for meetings. Within CDER, this executive secretary is generally a staffer within the center's Advisors and Consultants Staff.

The agency's dialogue with advisors is an aspect of the committee process that has remained controversial over the years. Some critics argue that agency staffers influence the views of advisors during such exchanges, an argument that top agency staffers openly reject. According to an internal CDER guide on policies and practices for center discussions with committee members, "it is never appropriate for either applicants or agency staff to lobby or negotiate with committee members about positions or conclusions the advisory committee should adopt on issues about to come before them. It is, however, appropriate for agency staff and corporate sponsors to provide members with background information on the issues at hand, and during meetings, to discuss the data and their own interpretation of the data with the whole committee."

Finally, the agency has stringent financial conflict-of-interest standards for its members. As mentioned, FDAMA has introduced several new administrative conflict of interest provisions, and the agency updated its *Policy and Guidance Handbook for* FDA *Advisory Committees* in mid-2000 to more fully address conflict-of-interest criteria. Committee members are screened for such conflicts when they are nominated. Unless a waiver is obtained, a committee member may not vote on any matter relevant to a clinical investigation or drug approval if the member or his or her immediate family (i.e., spouse and minor children) stands to gain financially from the ultimate recommendation. In addition, appointed members must file a statement disclosing their financial interests prior to each meeting.

Since many leading clinicians and scientists in academia work closely with product sponsors and since at least two members of an advisory committee must be knowledgeable about the disease that a product under committee review is intended to treat, conflict-of-interest concerns can be a severely limiting factor for the agency in maintaining the committee program. Individuals who have affiliations or investments that might present conflict-of-interest problems may be appointed to committees based on their qualifications, however. On a case-by-case basis, the agency will consider waivers to allow the participation of such advisors in committee deliberations.

Under FDAMA provisions, waivers may be granted if the member's participation is necessary to afford the committee essential expertise. A waiver may not be granted if a committee is to consider the member's own scientific work, however (i.e., the committee member's work as a principal investigator or as a major participant in the studies to be considered). In less clear-cut situations, the decision on whether to exclude, or seek a waiver for, a committee member will involve the weighing of the extent of the financial interest against the agency's need for the member's expertise.

In June 2000 hearings, the FDA's waiver process came under fire from certain members of Congress. The agency, for example, was questioned why a committee member had obtained a waiver to vote on, and participate in discussions of, a vaccine product when that member had received an annual $75,000 grant from the sponsor and had served as a principal investigator in studies for a directly competitive product. FDA officials countered that the member's involvement in the product's development was not relevant to the issue being discussed at the committee meeting, and that she was an expert in the areas in which the agency most needed expertise. The officials also emphasized that vaccine expertise is rare, and that committee members are permitted to participate when their expertise is considered more critical than the relevant conflict of interest. Members of Congress also criticized the FDA and other agencies for permitting committee members who are not allowed to vote on an issue due to conflict of interest issues to participate in committee discussions and, therefore, to influence the votes of other panel members.

Committee members are paid for their time, and are reimbursed at the standard federal rate for travel, food, and lodging costs. Because of this cost structure, the advisory committee program is seen as a cost-efficient vehicle for obtaining input from many of the country's most knowledgeable, talented, and experienced scientists and clinicians.

When CDER Uses Advisory Committees

As stated, the advent of the prescription drug user fee program has complicated CDER's use of advisory committees in some ways. Further, given the limited number of advisory committee meetings, CDER must be careful to select for panel consideration issues with major implications for the public health.

As an internal FDA policy document points out, "advisory committees are composed of committed but busy leading scientists, most of whom are active researchers with academic appointments. Participation in FDA deliberations does not free them of their other obligations. As meetings are usually 2 days long, occur 2 to 5 times per year, and involve substantial pre-meeting preparation, it is clear that, for many committee members, current meeting schedules represent a substantial commitment. Therefore, we must select issues for discussion in ways that maximize the valuable contribution of our advisors as a public health resource, as well as make efficient use of the agency's staff's time preparing for and participating in such meetings."

Various FDA and CDER documents have attempted to identify the broad range of issues that may be considered by the committees, and general rules for selecting the most significant issues. Although this range includes general drug development issues (e.g., guidelines, study designs), emerging issues regarding marketed drugs (e.g., adverse reactions, labeling), and CDER's management of the drug evaluation process, the most important in the context of this discussion is committee deliberation on the approvability of specific drugs.

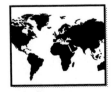

The FDA's 1994 advisory committee handbook made no important changes to the criteria that the agency uses in selecting drugs and issues. According to the handbook, CDER attempts to select topics for advisory committee presentations as follows:

- "Applications for approval of the first entity in a pharmacological class will routinely be presented as well as any other new chemical entity whose evaluation poses special problems or raises issues of broader interest."

- "New drugs that are expected to have a major therapeutic impact, whether or not they are [new chemical entities] will ordinarily be presented. Similarly, major new uses of marketed drugs will ordinarily be presented to advisory committees."

- "Applications for initial Rx to OTC switches of a drug will routinely be presented to an advisory committee...."

- Major safety concerns involving marketed drugs will "usually be presented" to advisory committees.

- Clinical guidelines "will routinely be presented" to the relevant committee for consideration before being adopted.

- At least once annually, a new drug review division will be selected to present a "program review on important and controversial drugs under development and applications for NCEs that are pending."

The process for selecting issues often involves several steps. To identify potential topics for committee meetings, the executive secretary for each advisory committee periodically meets with the director of the drug review division that the committee serves. These topics may be discussed during internal staff meetings.

It is important to note that CDER is not the only body involved in setting committee agendas. For example, a drug sponsor may request that a pending issue involving its product be brought before a committee. Likewise, committee members themselves may request that certain issues of interest be considered.

Agenda items agreed to within CDER are then discussed with the committee chairperson to obtain his or her advice on the ones that should be selected and how best to present the issues. Meeting agendas agreed to during this process are then published in the *Federal Register*.

In considering the data on a new drug or a significant new use of an already approved drug, the committee might evaluate any of several issues, depending on the nature of the questions posed to it. These issues can include:

- the adequacy of the design and conduct of studies intended to provide substantial evidence of effectiveness;

- the data supporting the proposed dose and dosing schedule;

- critical studies;

- the appropriateness of surrogate endpoints for particular situations;

- the safety data base;

- the need for additional studies or special surveillance after marketing;
- the need to limit indications to a particular subset of the overall potential treatment population;
- the overall risk/benefit relationship of the new agent;
- the need for special labeling features, such as boxed warnings, limitations on use, monitoring requirements, or patient package inserts;
- the appropriateness of proposed prescription-to-OTC switches; and
- the primary review of selected portions of NDAs.

How Advisory Committees Function

CDER officials are quick to point out that each advisory committee has its own personality and its own unique relationship with the review division that it serves. The committee's personality and method of functioning are influenced largely by the committee's chairperson. As noted above, the chairperson has input on which issues are selected for committee deliberation and the presentation of these issues.

Although the product of the advisory committee process is generally a recommendation discussed and issued during a committee meeting, the process is considerably more involved. In many respects, periodic committee meetings represent the final stage of a lengthier and more complex process.

One of the fundamental principles of this process is that advisors be given sufficient information to allow them to provide informed recommendations during meetings (see discussion below). According to CDER's policy guide on committee discussions, "it is essential that the advisory committee collectively receive input from the agency regarding the staff's review of the data that will be presented to the committee. This provides committee members with the agency's expert analysis of the validity and organization of the data offered by sponsors, an analysis to which the agency usually brings more resources, expertise and experience than are available to the committee. It is also important that the committee have access to the agency's evaluation of the sponsor's data analyses, including the agency's evaluation of statistical techniques used, analysis of design issues, and assessment of the results of studies. Without such information, the committee may fail to address issues that will be critical to the agency's reasoning when it formulates a final decision on the issue." Sponsors often provide "additional data, sometimes with additional documentation to focus discussion or assist an identified committee member serving as a primary or secondary reviewer of the drug."

Because they often play important roles during committee meetings, sponsors must also be informed of meeting agendas. "Every effort should be made to be sure the sponsor understands the issues that will be raised for discussion by agency reviewers. There are many ways to do this, including deficiency letters to sponsors, pre-meetings between the sponsor and agency in anticipation of any advisory committee discussions (it is useful to offer the sponsor an opportunity for such a meeting), and communicating to the sponsor any questions to be posed to the committee in advance of the meeting."

Committee Meeting Scheduling and Practices FDAMA introduced several new requirements for CDER's scheduling of advisory committee meetings. Specifically, FDAMA establishes that CDER must schedule advisory committee meetings so that a matter can be presented to a committee within 60 calendar days of its being considered "ready for review"—that is, when the center and sponsor have completed all preparatory work for its presentation at such a meeting. Because of the busy schedules of committee members, the law encourages CDER to schedule committee meetings on an annual basis based on anticipated and pending drug applications to fulfill this daunting requirement.

So committee members can appropriately prepare for a meeting, a review division assembles an information package and forwards it (through the CDER executive secretary for the committee) to the committee members before the scheduled meeting. Under practices adopted as a result of the HRG settlement, the agency now forwards this CDER background package to the committee members at least 18 business days before the meeting (the agency must send a redacted version of this package to the sponsor at least 14 business days before the meeting). Under these same practices, the agency must also send a sponsor-prepared background package (assuming the sponsor has submitted one in time) to the committee members at least 21 business days prior to the meeting. Advisory committee members have responded positively to the new practices, claiming that such information is now provided on a much more predictable basis (i.e., previously, it might be forwarded a month to a day in advance of a meeting, according to FDA staffers). Committee members also report that the pre-meeting information packages are now smaller and more focused.

Among the unfortunate outcomes of the HRG settlement are new restrictions that, in certain cases, will be placed on sponsor and advisory committee member access to the questions that CDER will pose at committee meetings. This is a complicated—and seemingly unintended—outcome of the detailed post-settlement timelines that have been established for the processing and release of committee materials. As noted, the newly established timetable requires CDER to get its background package to the advisory committee members at least 18 business days in advance of a committee meeting. In most cases, however, one of the important items that comprise the CDER background package—CDER's list of final questions to the committee—is not ready by this time. When a CDER review division is unable to finalize its questions by this deadline and to send the questions as part of the CDER background package, the new and highly structured timetable does not permit the agency to forward its questions to the committee—and therefore make them available to the sponsor—until the morning of the day before the committee meeting (i.e., when all the releasable meeting-related materials are provided to the public). To the degree that the drug sponsor is unable to glean the precise wording and focus of the division's questions from informal discussions with CDER staff and from reviewing other elements of CDER's background package (i.e., CDER must send a copy of its background package at least 14 business days in advance of a meeting), this can be a significant hurdle for a sponsor's efforts to prepare for a committee meeting. Requesting a meeting with a review division close to a committee's meeting date may be one way for an applicant to address this challenge.

In some cases, the FDA will post "issues for discussion" (not the final questions) on its web site 24 hours before a meeting. Further, CDER has established an FDA Advisory Committees and Information Line (800-741-8138) to provide information on upcoming meetings.

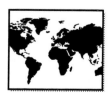

Rarely, if ever, do committee members review an entire NDA or IND, although some committee chairpersons are encouraged to appoint a "committee reviewer"—a committee member who would either become involved in the evaluation of an application or would receive more detailed information on an application and make a separate report to the full committee. While a few divisions—the Division of Oncologic Drug Products, in particular—like to involve a single advisory committee member early in the development and review process, the considerable work involved in coordinating such activities is likely to prevent more divisions from adopting such practices.

Generally, a majority of voting committee members comprises a quorum (i.e., the number of members that must be present to hold a meeting). Under existing regulations, however, CDER may specify in a particular advisory committee charter that a quorum is less than the majority of total current voting members. In some cases, such as when a committee comprises two diverse groups of experts (e.g., the Dermatologic and Ophthalmic Drugs Advisory Committee), the subgroup of committee members with expertise relevant to the issue under discussion is sufficient to represent a quorum.

Committee meetings, during which issues are discussed and recommendations are voted upon, are attended by committee members, key personnel from the relevant drug review division(s), and often representatives from the drug firm whose product is under discussion. A meeting will generally consist of two or more of the following segments:

- Open Public Hearing. Every advisory committee meeting includes an open hearing (at least an hour in duration), during which any interested person may present data, information, or oral or written views that are relevant to the advisory committee's agenda or other work.

- Open Committee Discussion. With limited exceptions, advisory committees are required to conduct their discussions of pending matters in open sessions. Although access to open discussions is not restricted, no public participation is permitted during this segment without the consent of the committee chairperson. External consultants and the drug sponsor may be asked, or may request the opportunity, to present data to the committee. Typically, sponsor and FDA presentations consume much of the time allocated to open committee discussions.

- Closed Presentation of Data. Data and information that are prohibited from public disclosure are presented to the advisory committee in a closed portion of the meeting. This policy applies to discussions involving information considered to be trade secrets by the sponsor, and the disclosure of personal information about clinical subjects. Only key FDA staffers, advisory committee members, agency consultants, and drug sponsors attend this segment of a meeting. This allows the sponsor to present and discuss sensitive information, such as manufacturing processes, without concern that competitors will gain access to the information.

- Closed Committee Deliberations. Committees may also choose to discuss issues in a closed session, in which attendance is limited to agency staff, committee members, and individuals invited by the committee chairperson. Such sessions are generally reserved for the discussion of existing internal documents whose premature disclosure might significantly impede proposed agency action.

Advisory committees are asked to make their recommendations as specific as possible, and to address key questions posed by the FDA. Depending on the nature of the question being considered, the committee may vote on an issue by a show of hands or a more in-depth discussion of individual member recommendations and the rationales for them.

FDAMA introduced a new provision under which CDER will be required, within 90 calendar days of a committee's recommendation, to notify the sponsor or applicant of the "status of FDA's decision on the matter." If CDER has not reached a decision by this point, it should provide an indication of the reasons that a determination has not been reached.

How Influential Are CDER's Advisory Committees?

There is no real measure of advisory committee influence in the drug review process. Although committee recommendations are not binding on the FDA, there are few instances in which agency decisions contradict these recommendations. According to FDA statistics from 1975 to mid-1978, the agency followed 98.7 percent of advisory committee recommendations.

Still, it remains difficult to gauge whether committee decisions direct or simply support FDA decisions. As stated above, some critics of the process even suggest that FDA officials direct committee recommendations during pre-meeting communications. Others claim that, all too often, the agency convenes committees to simply confirm conclusions that agency reviewers have already made.

It is also difficult to determine whether the agency would have reached the identical decision had the division not consulted an advisory committee. In fact, CDER's advisory committee policy guide acknowledges that a division may seek committee recommendations on a drug for which the division has already reached "a strong conclusion as to approvability."

In all likelihood, the influence of committee recommendations differs from case to case. Some FDA officials claim that the degrees of committee influence are best portrayed through several scenarios:

Scenario #1: The review division is faced with a particularly complex technical issue on which it has not reached a decision. This might also include situations in which the advisory committee has expertise not available within the agency, or situations in which a drug's approval represents a "close call" given the risk/benefit profile of the product. In such situations, advisory committees are likely to have the most influence on FDA decision making.

Scenario #2: The review division has reached a preliminary decision, but wants advice on specific issues. For example, the division may have decided to approve a certain drug, but wants committee input on issues such as appropriate dosing, labeling, or the need for follow-up studies.

Scenario #3: The review division has made a decision, but would be more comfortable if an independent review supported the initial determination. For example, the FDA may have reached a not-approvable decision on an NDA, but may decide to bring the decision before an advisory committee to permit the sponsor to present its case to an outside review body. Although the division is open to reconsider its decision if so advised by the committee, recommendations offered in this context may be less likely to affect agency decision making.

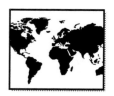

What Sponsors Should Know About Advisory Committees

Given the importance of advisory committee meetings, drug sponsors have much to gain by studying a committee before making a presentation to it. This is particularly important given the dynamic nature of the advisory committee process and the fundamental differences between the panels themselves.

Today, researching advisory committees is much easier than it has been in the past. Another outgrowth of the HRG settlement is that the agency is making considerably more committee-related information available, particularly through its website. Meeting background materials, transcripts, agendas, and agency questions are now accessible, as are the presentation materials prepared and submitted by other sponsors for committee meetings. In the future, CDER hopes to post the curriculum vitae of each advisory committee member on its website as well.

The advisory committee meeting process, sponsor approaches to and preparations for committee meetings, and commercial services designed to support sponsors in preparing for such meetings are all far more sophisticated than they were even a few years ago. Although detailed discussions on the technical and content-related issues important in preparing for committee meetings cannot be presented here, several essential principles remain as relevant as they have in the past:

- Learn as much as possible about the committee members, particularly the chairperson. Each member's particular areas of expertise and interest are also extremely important. Some experts advise obtaining each member's curriculum vitae and research papers to gain insights about their interests, and to help anticipate possible concerns and questions.

- Gain a full understanding of the relevant issues as the review division views them. Division reviewers set the committee's agenda, and frame and phrase the specific questions to which the committee must respond.

- Learn how the committee functions, how meetings are conducted, how the committee reaches its decisions, and how much it values solicited and unsolicited input from the sponsor, clinical investigators, statisticians, outside consultants, and others.

- Research what topics are on the committee's agenda. This will affect the amount of time a drug sponsor will be given to present its case. For example, the Oncology Drugs Advisory Committee is known to move quickly through agenda topics, and to address two or more products at a single meeting. CDER provides agenda-related materials to all companies scheduled to participate in an upcoming meeting.

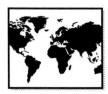

CHAPTER 11

Beyond Approval: Drug Manufacturer Regulatory Responsibilities

When a new drug obtains FDA approval, it enters another stage of the product life cycle to which different regulatory standards apply. But considering the fundamental differences between general marketing and comparatively tightly controlled clinical testing, the premarketing and postapproval responsibilities facing drug companies are remarkably similar in many respects.

Just as the sponsor must ensure that its drug is produced according to accepted manufacturing standards during clinical testing, the company must provide similar assurances when the product is marketed to the general public. Similarly, as the FDA calls upon sponsors to submit important test data during a drug's development, the agency also requires sponsors to report any postmarketing data or information that might cause the FDA to reassess a drug's safety and effectiveness.

In addition to abiding by the conditions of use (e.g., labeling, manufacturing commitments) detailed in its approved application and any subsequent supplements, an NDA holder must fulfill several postapproval responsibilities in both product reporting and manufacturing. Most postmarketing requirements fall into one of four broad areas:

- General Reporting Requirements;
- Adverse Drug Experience (AE) Reporting Requirements;
- Current Good Manufacturing Practice (CGMP); and
- Phase 4 Clinical Study Commitments.

Like virtually all other aspects of drug regulation in the late 1990s, the FDA's postmarketing requirements have been affected by FDAMA, international harmonization initiatives, and an increasing focus on drug safety. The quickening pace of drug approvals combined with the public attention garnered by safety-related drug withdrawals in the United States in recent years, for example, has moved CDER to focus more intently on postmarketing drug surveillance, which the drug center has done through its Office of Post Marketing Drug Disk Assessment (OPDRA). In early 2002, CDER moved OPDRA directly under a new CDER deputy director with expertise in epidemiology and risk assessment, and renamed the unit the Office of Drug Safety. Meanwhile, CDER continues to tweak its regulations to standardize its premarketing and postmarketing AE reporting requirements, and to harmonize these requirements with international standards.

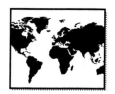

Beyond Approval: Drug Manufacturer Regulatory Responsibilities

Chapter 11

General Reporting Requirements

According to federal regulations, sponsors of approved NDAs must develop and submit to the FDA several different types of reports and materials—field alert reports, annual reports, advertising/promotional labeling specimens, and "special" reports. Taken together with AE reports, these submissions allow the FDA to monitor the distribution and effects of the drug. The reports also alert the FDA to information that might represent grounds for regulatory action (e.g., product recall).

Field Alert Reports Federal regulations require NDA holders to report, within three working days of receipt, any information:

- "…concerning any incident that causes the drug product or its labeling to be mistaken for, or applied to, another article."

- "…concerning any bacteriological contamination, or any significant chemical, physical, or other change or deterioration in the distributed drug product, or any failure of one or more distributed batches of the drug product to meet the specifications established for it in the application."

Companies may provide this information by telephone or other rapid means to the FDA district office responsible for the reporting manufacturing facility, assuming that the initial notification is followed by a prompt written follow-up report. The written report should be plainly marked "NDA-Field Alert Report."

Annual Reports The annual report plays several important roles in the FDA's monitoring of a marketed drug's safety and quality. First, the report provides the FDA with a convenient summary of new research data, distribution information, and labeling changes. Also, the annual submission is the vehicle through which manufacturers must report certain types of information that need not be provided in any other mandatory filing.

Annual reports must be filed with the FDA drug review division responsible for evaluating and approving a subject drug's NDA. These reports must be submitted each year within 60 days of the anniversary date of the drug's approval, and must be accompanied by a completed *Transmittal of Periodic Reports for Drugs for Human Use* form (Form FDA-2252).

Annual reports must include the following types of information "that the applicant received or otherwise obtained during the annual reporting interval which ends on the anniversary date [of the drug's approval]:"

Summary of New Information. A brief summary of "significant" new information obtained during the previous year that might affect the safety, effectiveness, or labeling of the drug product. Also, the sponsor must detail any action that it has taken or is planning to take in response to this new information (e.g., submitting a labeling supplement, adding a warning to the labeling, or initiating a new study). Under regulations that went into effect in April 1999, the agency also requires that this summary "briefly state" whether labeling supplements for pediatric use have been submitted, and whether new studies have been initiated in the pediatric population to support appropriate labeling for the pediatric population (see Chapter 16). When possible, the applicant should also provide an estimate of

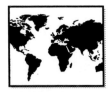

patient exposure to the drug product, with special reference to the pediatric population (neonates, infants, children, and adolescents), including dosage form.

Distribution Data. Information on the quantity of the product distributed, and the amounts forwarded to drug distributors. This section must provide the National Drug Code (NDC) number, the total number of dosage units of each strength or potency distributed (e.g., 100,000/5 milligram tablets, 50,000/10 milliliter vials), and the quantities distributed for domestic and foreign use.

Labeling. Labeling information and samples, including currently used professional labeling, patient brochures or package inserts (if any), a representative sample of the package labels, and a summary of product labeling changes implemented since the last report. If the manufacturer implemented no labeling changes, this should be stated in the report. In late 2000, CDER officials revealed that they are developing a proposed regulation that will require drug manufacturers to alert the agency whenever labeling changes are made for drugs in foreign countries. It is uncertain what mechanism the agency will require manufacturers to use in communicating these labeling changes (i.e., annual report or special filing).

Chemistry, Manufacturing, and Controls Changes. Information on chemistry, manufacturing, and controls (CMC) changes, including reports of any new experiences, investigations, studies, or tests involving chemical, physical, or other properties of the drug, that may affect the FDA's previous conclusions on the product. The report should also provide a full description of all implemented manufacturing and controls changes that did not require a supplemental application (see Chapter 12). Under a new "risk based CMC review" initiative, CDER planned to streamline supplemental filing and annual report requirements for approved products for which reduced post-marketing reporting requirements would be unlikely to result in product quality problems. Due to what the FDA viewed as the "wide variability" of CMC sections submitted in annual reports, the agency published a 1994 guidance entitled, *Guidance for Industry: Format and Content for the* CMC *Section of an Annual Report.*

Nonclinical Laboratory Studies. Information from nonclinical laboratory studies, including copies of unpublished reports, summaries of published reports of new toxicological findings in animal studies, and *in vivo* studies conducted or otherwise obtained by the sponsor relating to the product's ingredients. The agency may also request copes of published reports.

Clinical Data. Published clinical trials on the drug (or abstracts of them), including: trials on safety and effectiveness; studies on new uses; biopharmaceutic, pharmacokinetic, and clinical pharmacology studies; and reports of clinical experiences pertinent to safety (e.g., epidemiologic studies) conducted or obtained by the sponsor. Also needed are summaries of completed unpublished clinical trials—a study is considered completed one year after its conclusion—or pre-publication manuscripts developed or obtained by the applicant. Supporting information should not be reported. Review articles, papers describing the use of the drug product in medical practice, papers and abstracts in which the drug is used as a research tool, promotional articles, press clippings, and papers that do not contain tabulations or summaries of original data should not be reported. Consistent with its pediatric initiative, the FDA now requires that this section of the annual report also include an analysis of available safety and efficacy data in the pediatric population and changes proposed in the labeling based on this information. It must also include an assessment of data needed to ensure appropriate labeling for the pediatric population.

Postmarketing Study Status Report. A statement on the current status of any postmarketing studies performed by, or on behalf of, the applicant, including those that the sponsor agreed to conduct as part of the drug's approval (see section below on Phase 4 commitments). This statement must also include whether postmarketing clinical studies in pediatric populations were required or agreed to, and if so, the status of these studies (e.g., to be initiated, ongoing, completed, completed and results submitted to the NDA).

Under FDAMA and an October 2000 implementing regulation, CDER revised its requirements for the postmarketing study status report in the NDA annual report. According to current requirements, each annual report to an approved NDA must include "a status report of each postmarketing study of the drug product concerning clinical safety, clinical efficacy, clinical pharmacology, and nonclinical toxicology that is required by FDA (e.g., accelerated approval clinical benefit studies, pediatric studies) or that the applicant has committed, in writing, to conduct either at the time of approval of an application for the drug product or a supplement to an application, or after approval of the application or a supplement." An applicant must report on the status of such postmarketing studies each year until the FDA notifies the company, in writing, that the agency concurs with the company's determination that the study commitment has been fulfilled or that the study is either no longer feasible or would no longer provide useful information (see discussion on Phase 4 clinical studies below).

According to the FDA's April 2001 draft guidance entitled, *Reports on the Status of Postmarketing Studies—Implementation of Section 130 of the Food and Drug Administration Modernization Act of 1997*, postmarketing status reports submitted in annual reports should be accompanied by Form FDA-2252 (Transmittal of Annual Reports for Drugs for Human Use). The cover letter should clearly identify the submission as an Annual Report on Postmarketing Studies. It is important to note that, although sponsors must continue to report on other types of postmarketing studies (e.g., product stability studies, product dissolution studies, the development of an improved potency assay) in the annual report, these reports are not subject to the same FDAMA provisions as those identified above (i.e., required or agreed to).

According to the draft guidance, a sponsor may characterize the status of its Phase 4 study in any one of five ways: pending (study has not begun, but the projected date for patient accrual has not passed); ongoing (the study is proceeding, but is behind the original schedule); terminated (the study was ended before completion, the company does not intend to complete the study as originally designed, and the company has not yet submitted a final study report to the FDA); or submitted (the study has been concluded or terminated and the company has submitted a study report to the FDA and is awaiting the agency's advice as to whether the study commitment has been met).

Other Reports Federal regulations state that sponsors must be prepared to file other reports, including:

Advertisements and Promotional Labeling. NDA holders must "submit specimens of mailing pieces and any other labeling or advertising devised for promotion of the drug product at the time of initial dissemination of the labeling and at the time of initial publication of the advertisement for a prescription drug product. Mailing pieces and labeling that are designed to contain samples of a drug product are required to be complete, except that the sample of the drug product may be omitted. Each submission is required to be accompanied by a completed transmittal Form FDA-2253 (Transmittal of

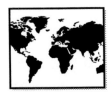

Advertisements and Promotional Labeling for Drugs for Human Use) and is required to include a copy of the product's current professional labeling."

The agency has different standards for the submission of advertisements and promotional labeling approved under its accelerated approval program (see Chapter 15). Under this program, a sponsor must submit these materials (i.e., for evaluation during the NDA review process) for any advertising and labeling that the company plans to disseminate within 120 days of a drug's approval. For advertising and promotional labeling that the firm hopes to disseminate after this 120-day period, the sponsor must submit the materials at least 30 days prior to the intended date of initial dissemination or publication. To describe the process for reviewing promotional materials for drugs approved under the accelerated review program, CDER released a March 1999 draft industry guidance entitled, *Accelerated Approval Products—Submission of Promotional Materials*.

Advertising and promotional labeling are among the submissions that CDER is including in its electronic submissions initiative. According to a February 2001 draft guidance entitled, *Providing Regulatory Submissions in Electronic Format—Prescription Drug Advertising and Promotional Labeling*, CDER states that applicants that decide to submit advertisements and promotional labeling in electronic format should file the entire submission electronically.

Special Reports. The FDA may request that the applicant submit any of the reports profiled above at times different than those required under federal regulations.

Report on Withdrawal of Approved Drug Product From Sale. Within 15 working days of withdrawing an approved drug product from the market, the applicant must submit, on Form FDA 2657 (Drug Product Listing), the following information: (1) the National Drug Code number; (2) the identity of the drug product by established name and proprietary name; (3) the NDA number; and (4) the date of the drug's withdrawal. The agency requests, but does not require, that applicants also indicate the reasons for the withdrawal.

Adverse Drug Experience Reporting Requirements

Following a drug's approval, NDA holders must continue to collect, analyze, and submit data on adverse drug experiences (AE) so that the company and the FDA can continually reassess the product's risk/benefit relationship and the conditions under which it should be used. Perhaps more than any other aspect of FDA regulation, the agency's AE reporting standards have been in transition throughout the past decade. This transition has been driven by several factors, including international harmonization efforts, continuing FDA efforts to transition to the electronic submission of regulatory filings and, during the late 1990s, an increased focus on drug safety.

At this writing, CDER's postmarketing AE reporting program and requirements had been, or stood to be, affected by several developments, including the following:

- In the late 1990s, CDER began to take steps toward what some in the center called a "revitalized pharmacovigilance program," an effort that has continued along with an increasing focus on risk management in recent years. Specifically, the drug center transitioned its former Division of Pharmacovigilance and Epidemiology into a

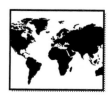

new Office of Post-marketing Drug Risk Assessment (OPDRA). Facing new demands from the increasing number of drug approvals, various international initiatives, and new analytical and surveillance tools associated with the center's emerging electronic AE reporting system (see discussion below), CDER's "imperative to have an outstanding system of post-marketing drug risk surveillance, assessment, and management is all the greater," center officials said in their announcement of OPDRA's founding. In addition to spearheading CDER's postmarketing surveillance and assessment efforts, OPDRA was made responsible for tracking safety-related Phase 4 study commitments as well (see discussion below). In an early 2002 reorganization, OPDRA was renamed the Office of Drug Safety, and was moved under a new Office of Pharmacoepidemiology and Statistical Science (OPSS). The new OPSS is to be led by Paul Seligman, M.D., who joined CDER in mid-2001 as a senior advisor on risk management.

- Since late 1997, the FDA has been planning to re-propose changes to its periodic postmarketing AE reporting requirements first put forward in a 1994 omnibus proposed rule (see discussion below). The agency decided to develop a re-proposal to incorporate standards included in the ICH guidance entitled, E2C *Clinical Safety Data Management: Periodic Safety Update Reports*. Among other provisions, the proposed rule will establish new timeframes for periodic postmarketing AE reports (see discussion below), will mandate a new format for periodic reports called product safety update reports (PSUR), and will ask sponsors for information on off-label drug use. CDER officials have added that the proposed rule will seek to shift the responsibility for "active analysis of safety data" from the agency to sponsors, and will attempt to evolve periodic reports from "essentially data dumps" to thoughtful and complete summaries of adverse experiences. This reproposal, which will also have implications for the use and meaning of AE-related terms and the content of periodic postmarketing AE reports, remained in the final stages of the federal government's review and approval process in early 2002.

- As the FDA and the pharmaceutical industry began discussions over reauthorizing the prescription drug user fee program, which will expire in October 2002, the agency was seeking additional user fees and or congressional appropriations to upgrade its postmarketing surveillance activities. In the years leading up to these discussions, FDA officials made clear their desire to have the user fee program include the full product lifecycle, in particular to obtain new fees to upgrade the postmarketing surveillance area in the same way that existing fees had improved the new drug review process. A December 1999 Department of Health and Human Services report had claimed that the FDA's existing funding for handling adverse drug reaction reports would not be sufficient in the face of anticipated increases in the number of drug approvals. Although the report claimed that existing funding was sufficient for the current workload, it stated that "as more drugs are approved for marketing, the agency will have to step up its monitoring responsibilities and more resources will likely be needed." In response to the report, the FDA conceded that additional funding would allow the agency to develop new tools to assess the scope of the adverse drug reaction problem, expand its pharmacoepidemiological and methodological research, become more proactive in collecting AEs, and expand its use of product registries and sentinel surveillance sites.

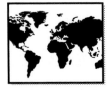

- In October 2001, CDER upgraded its ability to monitor the use of marketed drugs by gaining access to three commercial databases containing "non-patient-identifiable" information on the actual use of marketed prescription drugs in adults and children. The agency hopes to use the information to "determine the public health significance" of the reports it obtains through its adverse event reporting system, published information, and other data sources. The information from the databases will permit the agency to examine the duration of treatment for medications and to learn which combinations of medicines are being prescribed.

- A spate of three safety-related drug withdrawals within a nine-month period from late 1997 to mid-1998 sparked public and congressional concern over whether new user-fee-related review deadlines were adversely affecting the quality of CDER's premarketing reviews, and whether CDER's postmarketing surveillance capabilities were adequate to monitor adverse effects associated with the growing number of new drugs reaching the market each year. In part a response to these concerns, then-FDA Commissioner Jane Henney, M.D., established a task force to evaluate the existing system for managing the risks of FDA-approved medical products, focusing on the FDA's role in the process, including postmarketing surveillance and risk assessment programs. Although the task force concluded that CDER's current program is "good at rapidly detecting most unexpected serious adverse events that occur during the postmarketing period," it recommended that CDER "rapidly complete" its system for the electronic submission of AEs (see discussion below), and that it consider increasing its access to outside data sources, such as broad-based health information databases (see discussion above). The speed and efficiency of the FDA's drug approval process was clearly creating new challenges for the agency's postmarketing surveillance efforts: Because the United States is now the first country in which so many new drugs are reaching the market, the FDA no longer has the opportunity to monitor drug use and effects in other countries before approving the new medicines.

- In recent years, CDER continued to migrate slowly toward a system for the electronic submission of adverse experiences. During 1997, a new system called the Adverse Event Reporting System (AERS) replaced the FDA's Spontaneous Reporting System (SRS) database for adverse event reports. According to the agency, AERS enables the agency to receive adverse experience reports from pharmaceutical companies by electronic submissions, "transmitted data base to data base through standardized pathways." Under the AERS system, most of the content (e.g., narratives and fields other than medical history and laboratory data) from paper-based reports are full-text entered and are scanned by the agency upon their receipt. In addition, the AERS system utilizes MedDRA (the Medical Dictionary for Regulatory Activities), which was developed by ICH. Currently, manufacturers are encouraged to code reports prior to their electronic submission. AERS is designed to provide a "paperless" means for FDA postmarketing safety evaluators to screen individual reports, and to provide new tools for the enhanced surveillance of drug safety. Today, CDER continues to accept electronic expedited (15-day) AE reports from selected sponsors under program that began as a pilot effort in 1998 (see discussion below). When CDER released a May 2001 draft industry guidance entitled, *Providing Regulatory Submissions in Electronic Format—Postmarketing Expedited Safety*

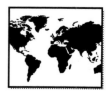

Reports, CDER brought this pilot program into its "production phase," under which these reports are accepted in a completely electronic format (see discussion below). In a November 1999 advanced notice of proposed rulemaking, however, CDER announced its plans to issue a proposed rule that would require industry to submit electronic versions of postmarketing expedited individual case safety reports and individual case safety reports contained in periodic AE reports. The agency claims that such requirements, which will apply only to postmarketing AE reports and will provide a waiver process for small companies, will help to harmonize the reporting of postmarketing safety information worldwide and expedite the detection of safety problems.

- An October 1997 final rule that became effective in April 1998 implemented a variety of changes designed to standardize the FDA's own pre- and postmarketing AE reporting regulations and harmonize the agency's requirements with international standards. Specifically, the rule redefined many of the terms crucial to AE reporting, recast the reporting timeframes for expedited pre- and postmarketing AE reports, and codified the use of the MedWatch Form (FDA Form 3500A) for AE reports (see discussion below).

Key Definitions Relevant to Adverse Drug Experience Reporting The adverse drug experience (AE) reporting area has very much its own language. In fact, reporting requirements are directly linked to criteria outlined in the definitions of several terms that appear in federal regulations: "adverse drug experience," "unexpected adverse drug experience," "life-threatening," "serious adverse drug experience," and "disability."

Adverse Drug Experience. An adverse experience is defined as "any adverse event associated with the use of a drug in humans, whether or not considered drug related, including the following: an adverse event occurring in the course of the use of a drug product in professional practice; an adverse event occurring from drug overdose whether accidental or intentional; an adverse event occurring from drug abuse; an adverse event occurring from drug withdrawal; and any failure of expected pharmacological action." To promote consistency with international terminology, the FDA plans to issue, in 2002, a proposal to eliminate the term "adverse drug experience" from its regulations and replace it with the ICH-accepted term, "adverse drug reaction." The agency will also propose to adopt the ICH's definition for adverse drug reaction, which FDA officials claim will not have a significant effect on the types of AEs that are reported to the agency.

Unexpected Adverse Drug Experience. An "unexpected" event is any adverse drug experience "that is not listed in the current labeling for the drug product. This includes events that may be symptomatically and pathophysiologically related to an event listed in the labeling, but differ from the event because of greater severity or specificity. For example, under this definition, hepatic necrosis would be unexpected (by virtue of greater severity) if the labeling only referred to elevated hepatic enzymes or hepatitis. Similarly, cerebral thromboembolism and cerebral vasculitis would be unexpected (by virtue of greater specificity) if the labeling only listed cerebral vascular accidents. 'Unexpected,' as used in this definition, refers to an adverse drug experience that has not been previously observed (i.e., included in the labeling) rather than from the perspective of such experience not being anticipated from the pharmacological properties of the pharmaceutical product."

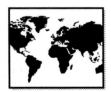

Serious Adverse Drug Experience. A "serious adverse drug experience" is "any adverse drug experience occurring at any dose that results in any of the following outcomes: Death, a life-threatening adverse drug experience, inpatient hospitalization or prolongation of existing hospitalization, a persistent or significant disability/incapacity, or a congenital anomaly/birth defect. Important medical events that may not result in death, be life-threatening, or require hospitalization may be considered a serious adverse drug experience when, based upon appropriate medical judgement, they may jeopardize the patient or subject and may require medical or surgical intervention to prevent one of the outcomes listed in this definition. Examples of such medical events include allergic bronchospasm requiring intensive treatment in an emergency room or at home, blood dyscrasias or convulsions that do not result in inpatient hospitalization, or the development of drug dependency or drug abuse."

Life-Threatening Adverse Drug Experience. A "life-threatening" AE is "any adverse drug experience that places the patient, in the view of the initial reporter, at immediate risk of death from the adverse drug experience as it occurred, i.e., it does not include an adverse drug experience that, had it occurred in a more severe form, might have caused death."

Disability. The term "disability," which is important because it is used in the definition of serious AE, is defined as "a substantial disruption of a person's ability to conduct normal life functions." For clarification, the FDA adds that "only a persistent or significant disability or incapacity is intended... Thus, disability is not intended to include experiences of relatively minor medical significance such as headache, nausea, vomiting, diarrhea, influenza, and accidental trauma (e.g., sprained ankle)."

Adverse Drug Experience Reporting Requirements NDA holders and certain "nonapplicants" (any person whose name appears on the drug product's label as a manufacturer, packer, or distributor) have AE reporting responsibilities. To avoid unnecessary duplication of reporting, however, federal regulations permit "nonapplicants" to meet their reporting requirements by submitting all serious AE reports directly to the applicant rather than to the FDA.

Under federal regulations, NDA holders and relevant nonapplicants must develop and implement written procedures for the surveillance, receipt, evaluation, and reporting of postmarketing adverse drug experiences. Further, NDA holders must promptly review all adverse drug experience information obtained or otherwise received by the applicant from any source, foreign or domestic, including information derived from commercial marketing experience, postmarketing clinical investigations, postmarketing epidemiological/surveillance studies, reports in the scientific literature, and unpublished scientific papers.

Given the degree of recent and continuing evolution in the postmarketing safety reporting area, none of CDER's existing guidance documents fully captures current requirements. In March 2001, however, CDER released a draft guidance entitled, *Postmarketing Safety Reporting for Human Drugs and Biological Products, Including Vaccines.* When finalized, this guidance will replace CDER's two existing guidances: *Postmarketing Reporting of Adverse Drug Experiences* (March 1992) and *Postmarketing Adverse Experience Reporting for Human Drug and Licensed Biological Products: Clarification of What to Report* (August 1997). CDER concedes, however, that even the newer draft guidance will have to be revised to reflect all of the pending changes in the safety reporting area.

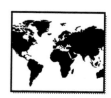

The agency requires NDA holders to make two types of postmarketing AE reports when necessary: 15-day alert reports, sometimes called postmarketing expedited safety reports, and periodic adverse experience reports. In June 1997, the FDA eliminated the requirement that companies also make "expedited 15-day increased frequency reports" to alert the FDA to any significant increases in the frequency of reports on AEs that are both serious and expected and reports of therapeutic failures.

15-Day Alert Reports. NDA holders and relevant nonapplicants must report each postmarketing AE "that is both serious and unexpected, whether foreign or domestic, as soon as possible, but in no case later than 15 calendar days of initial receipt of the information by the applicant" or nonapplicant. These reports are sometimes called "expedited postmarketing reports."

Unless the FDA's MedWatch Program agrees to an alternative format, FDA Form 3500A must be completed and submitted for each report of an adverse drug experience. Foreign events may be submitted either on an FDA Form 3500A, or, if preferred, on a CIOMS I form. Applicants and relevant nonapplicants may use the CIOMS I form without prior FDA approval. Such companies can also use an alternative reporting format, such as a computer-generated FDA Form 3500A or computer-generated tape or tabular listing, provided that the content is equivalent to that found in the FDA Form 3500A and that CDER's MedWatch office agrees to the alternative in advance. Each completed FDA Form 3500A should refer only to an individual patient or a single attached publication.

Consistent with CDER's August 1997 guidance entitled, *Postmarketing Adverse Experience Reporting for Human Drugs and Licensed Biological Products: Clarification of What to Report*, applicants and relevant nonapplicants are expected to have access to certain information before making postmarketing AE reports. To reduce or eliminate incomplete reports, CDER recommends that, at a minimum, an AE report, including both 15-day alert and periodic reports (see discussion below), provide the following "four basic elements:" an identifiable patient (even if not precisely identified by name and date of birth); an identifiable reporter; a suspect drug product; and an adverse event or fatal outcome.

15-day alert reports based on information in the scientific literature must be accompanied by a copy of the published article. The alert reporting requirements for serious, unexpected AEs "apply only to reports found in scientific and medical journals either as case reports or as the result of a formal clinical trial."

Unless the applicant or nonapplicant concludes that there is a reasonable possibility that the drug caused the adverse experience, the firm is not required to submit a 15-day alert report for an AE obtained from a postmarketing study (whether or not conducted under an IND). Applicants and relevant nonapplicants must separate and clearly mark alert reports for AEs that are derived from postmarketing studies and those that are being reported spontaneously.

One of the FDA's goals in the October 1997 final rule, which became effective in April 1998, was to more clearly delineate relevant requirements following the submission of an initial 15-day alert report. Applicants and relevant nonapplicants must "promptly" investigate each AE that is the subject of a 15-day alert report, and submit follow-up reports within 15 calendar days of receipt of the new information or as requested by the FDA. If additional information is not obtainable, a company should maintain records of its unsuccessful attempts to obtain the information. As before, the 15-day

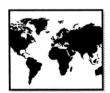

alert reports and follow-ups to them must be submitted under separate cover and may not be included, except for summary or tabular purposes, in a periodic report (see discussion below).

CDER and the Electronic Submission of Expedited AE Reports After its eNDA efforts, CDER's electronic submissions program for postmarketing adverse experiences (AE)—at least in terms of 15-day expedited reports—is easily its second most advanced. Following the release of the ICH's subsequently modified guidance entitled, *E2B Data Elements for Transmission of Individual Case Safety Reports* in early 1998, a CDER/Pharmaceutical Research and Manufacturers of America (PhRMA) working group agreed to initiate a pilot program for the electronic submission of postmarketing expedited AE reports. While there was some initial discussion regarding whether CDER's pilot program should focus on postmarketing expedited or periodic reports, expedited reports won out largely because these documents provide the center with the all-important first "signals" of potential health problems. An estimated 15 to 20 pharmaceutical companies were members of the working group and participated in the pilot program at various times.

Other advances within the center—largely AERS— had set the stage for the pilot program. For the pilot program, CDER developed a three-step process that remains relevant for any company seeking to submit electronic postmarketing expedited AE reports to AERS today:

Pilot Phase: In the pilot phase, the manufacturer forwards a proposed AE report in SGML format to CDER, which runs the report against its "test" database. This process continues iteratively until both CDER and the manufacturer are satisfied that the report meets all the edit criteria of the SGML specification.

Pilot Production Phase: Once the pilot phase is complete, the manufacturer then begins to submit electronic expedited reports on a routine basis, but also forwards an identical paper-based version of each electronic report in parallel.

Production Phase: The formal availability of the so-called production phase began in May 2001, when CDER added postmarketing AE reports to the e-submissions public docket and then published a draft guidance entitled, *Postmarketing Expedited Safety Reports*. In this phase, CDER accepts the reports electronically without any accompanying paper version. According to the draft guidance, the individual case safety report (ICSR) component of the expedited report can be forwarded on either physical media (i.e., floppy disk, CD-ROM, or digital tape), or through the agency's electronic data interchange (EDI) gateway. CDER prefers that companies use the EDI gateway "because this allows the most efficient processing of the reports." For now, the second element of the expedited report—the ICSR attachments (e.g., published articles, autopsy/death certificates) must be submitted on physical media because they are generally in binary files, which the EDI gateway does not accept. CDER expects to be able to accept the ICSR attachments through the EDI gateway within a few months, however.

At this writing, there was just one company—GlaxoSmithkline—in the full production phase, according to CDER officials. Another four companies are said to be in the pilot production stage, and are submitting electronic postmarketing AE reports on a routine basis along with paper-based versions. Several other companies are understood to be in the pilot phase and in the process of advancing to the pilot production stage.

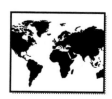

CDER has already revealed its intentions to require electronic reporting of expedited AE reports. In a November 1999 advanced notice of proposed rulemaking, CDER announced its plans to issue a proposed rule that would require industry to submit electronic versions of postmarketing expedited ICSRs and ICSRs contained in periodic AE reports using ICH-recommended standardized medical terminology, data elements, and electronic submission standards (see discussion below). The agency claims that such requirements, for which there would be a waiver for smaller companies, would help to harmonize the reporting of postmarketing safety information internationally, and would expedite the detection of drug safety problems.

Periodic Adverse Drug Experience Reports. Periodic reports must be submitted, in duplicate, quarterly for the first three years following a drug's approval in the United States, and annually thereafter. The quarterly reports must be submitted within 30 days of the close of each quarter (i.e., the first quarter beginning on an application's U.S. approval date). Annual reports must be filed within 60 days of the anniversary date of the application's U.S. approval.

A periodic report must contain each of the following components:

- A copy of FDA Form 3500A for each AE not reported as a 15-day alert report, with an index consisting of a line listing of the applicant's patient identification number and adverse reaction terms.

- A narrative summary and analysis of the information in the periodic report, and an analysis of the 15-day alert reports submitted during the reporting period.

- A narrative discussion of actions taken since the last report because of adverse drug experiences (e.g., labeling changes or studies initiated).

In its August 1997 clarification of postmarketing AE reporting requirements, the FDA encouraged manufacturers to request waivers from the requirement that an FDA Form 3500A be submitted for postmarketing AEs that are both nonserious and labeled. In making waiver requests, companies are asked to certify that complete (i.e., including the four basic informational elements) individual case safety reports of nonserious and labeled AEs will be maintained in corporate safety files. The companies should also agree, following an FDA request, that they will submit one or more of these AE reports to the agency within five calendar days of receiving the request. The FDA reminds companies that it will continue to expect, in periodic reports, a history by body system of all AE terms and counts of occurrences for nonserious and labeled AEs. This waiver process, which the agency is planning to incorporate into its postmarketing reporting regulations, is covered in a November 1999 MaPP entitled, *Granting Waivers Under 21 CFR 314.90 for Postmarketing Safety Reporting Requirements Under 21 CFR 314.80* (MaPP 6004.1).

FDA regulations point out that, unlike 15-day reporting standards, periodic reporting requirements are not applicable to adverse drug experiences encountered in postmarketing studies (whether or not conducted under an IND), reports in the scientific literature, or foreign marketing experience. Periodic reporting requirements also do not apply to manufacturers of human use prescription drugs without approved NDAs, which are covered under FDA regulations at 21 CFR 310.305.

Under a waiver process implemented following the release of the ICH guidance entitled, E2C *Clinical Safety Data Management: Periodic Safety Update Reports*, CDER first permitted companies to file their peri-

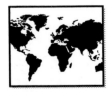

od reports in a new format—the periodic safety update report (PSUR)—that was advocated in the E2C guidance and that CDER proposed to require under its 1994 omnibus proposed rule (see discussion below). Although few companies have opted to submit periodic reports in the PSUR format, more are now pursuing waivers in response to CDER's encouragement.

At its discretion, the FDA may require an applicant to submit periodic reports at intervals different than those specified above. Upon its approval of a supplement for a major new indication for an already approved drug, for instance, the agency may reestablish a quarterly reporting interval for the product.

Federal regulations state that follow-up information on AEs reported in a periodic report may be provided in the subsequent periodic report.

e-Submissions for Periodic Postmarketing AE Reports As noted above, CDER had discussed undertaking a pilot program for the electronic submission of periodic postmarketing AE reports, but until late 2001, had not taken formal steps to permit or encourage such filings. In November 2001, CDER announced that postmarketing periodic individual case safety reports may be submitted electronically without accompanying paper-based copies.

In at least one earlier case, CDER had accepted periodic postmarketing reports electronically. In a fairly recent circumstance, a sponsor running a patient registry had an estimated 2,000 reports for which it was unsure whether postmarketing periodic AE reporting requirements applied. Because CDER was interested in seeing the reports but did not want to enter the reports manually, it agreed to accept the reports electronically.

CDER officials point out, in fact, that transitioning periodic AE reports to the electronic reporting system will be helped by the fact that they are similar to expedited reports in so many respects. The periodic reports comprise the individual case reports that are submitted with, and are formatted exactly as they are in, the expedited reports, as well as an analysis component that will appear, to the AERS system, much like the attachments now submitted with the expedited reports.

Pending Revisions to the FDA's Postmarketing AE Reporting Requirements In October 1994, the FDA first proposed to revamp its periodic postmarketing AE reporting requirements to conform to a CIOMS II Working Group's proposal. Among its other provisions, the proposal called for a new format for periodic reports called a periodic safety update report (PSUR). Specifically, the agency's October 1994 proposed rule called for the following:

- A six-month periodic reporting cycle throughout a product's life. Currently, the agency requires quarterly periodic reports for the first three years following U.S. approval, and then annual reports thereafter.

- Submission of the periodic report within 45 days of the date on which the product was first licensed anywhere in the world. This is referred to as the international birth date. In the upcoming omnibus proposed rule, however, the FDA plans to be as consistent as possible with the ICH's E2C guidance (see discussion below), which requires that PSURs be submitted within 60 days of a product's international birth date.

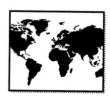

- An international core data sheet containing all relevant safety information. The core data sheet enables an applicant to produce a periodic report acceptable to all participating countries. This core data sheet differs from the FDA-approved product labeling. The U.S. labeling will remain the document of reference when determining if an event is "unlabeled" for purposes of expedited (15-day) reporting.
- A report format that is based on CIOMS II and that includes information on patient exposure and worldwide regulatory decisions concerning marketing, regulatory, or manufacturer actions taken for safety reasons.

In October 1997, the FDA announced its decision to repropose the elements of the October 1994 proposal that were relevant to periodic postmarketing AE reporting. This proposed rule, which the FDA hoped to release by 2002 (see discussion above), will be revised to make it consistent with the provisions of the ICH's May 1997 E2C *Clinical Safety Data Management: Periodic Safety Update Reports for Marketed Drugs*. In addition to the previously proposed changes specified above, the proposal is also expected to include a variety of other provisions designed to increase the quality of postmarketing AE reports beyond the provisions specified in the ICH guidance.

The pending proposed rule is also expected to revise what was a controversial element of the agency's original 1994 proposal—to require six-month AE reports throughout a product's life. To remain consistent with ICH requirements, however, the FDA is certain to propose a revised reporting time frame that is also based on six-month reporting intervals.

The agency is also planning to propose additional amendments to its expedited safety reporting regulations. Some, but not all, of these proposals will be based on standards in the ICH's March 1995 E2A *Clinical Data Safety Data Management: Definitions and Standards for Expedited Reporting*.

At this writing, CDER is also developing a proposed regulation on postmarketing AE reporting requirements for over-the-counter (OTC) drug products and, as noted above, a proposed regulation to require the electronic submission of postmarketing safety reports.

Current Good Manufacturing Practice (CGMP)

Since 1962, federal drug law has mandated that firms producing drugs for administration to humans operate under standards called Current Good Manufacturing Practice (CGMP). The statutory requirement calls for all drugs—including drug products (i.e., finished dosage forms) and drug components (i.e., bulk ingredients)—to be made in conformance with CGMP to ensure that the substances meet legal requirements of safety, and that they have the identity, strength, quality, and purity that they purport or are represented to possess.

In the late 1970s, the FDA had envisioned several different sets of CGMPs, with separate standards for finished dosage forms, bulk ingredients, and other classes of products. To date, however, the FDA has published only one broadly applicable CGMP regulation, which is relevant to finished dosage forms. Since establishing CGMP requirements, the FDA has exhibited a preference for a "general regulatory approach," and for supplementing this approach with additional specificity when necessary. In its most recent effort to add specificity to its CGMP requirements, the agency proposed to clarify

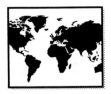

certain manufacturing, quality control and documentation requirements and to update requirements for process and methods validation (see discussion below).

The agency states that its CGMP regulations are based on "fundamental concepts of quality assurance: (1) Quality, safety, and effectiveness must be designed and built into a product; (2) quality cannot be inspected or tested into a finished product; and (3) each step of the manufacturing process must be controlled to maximize the likelihood that the finished product will be acceptable."

It is worth noting that the applicability of CGMP requirements is not restricted to approved drug products. As the FDA establishes in its *Guideline on the Preparation of Investigational New Drug Products (Human and Animal)* (March 1991), experimental drugs used in clinical testing are subject to certain CGMP requirements as well.

Similar to other key regulatory standards, CGMP standards in the United States, Japan, and the European Union have been a topic area under the ICH harmonization initiative. Most recently, the ICH steering committees released an August 2001 final guideline entitled, Q7A *Good Manufacturing Practice for Active Pharmaceutical Ingredients* (API). Intended to ensure the manufacturing of APIs "under an appropriate system for managing quality," the guideline provides CGMP-related recommendations in several areas, including quality management, production and in-process controls, validation, change control, and clinical trial APIs. In March 1998, the FDA had released its own related draft guidance entitled, *Manufacturing, Processing, or Holding Active Pharmaceutical Ingredients*.

The FDA's CGMP regulations seek to ensure the quality of drugs by setting minimum standards for all drug manufacturing facilities. The regulations establish standards in ten separate areas:

- organization and personnel;
- buildings and facilities;
- equipment;
- control of components and drug product containers and closures;
- production and process controls;
- packaging and labeling controls;
- holding and distribution;
- laboratory controls;
- records and reports; and
- returned and salvaged drug products.

Organization and Personnel One of the most important CGMP requirements addresses a facility's quality control unit, which each manufacturing facility must have to ensure compliance with CGMP. According to federal regulations, the quality control unit assumes "the responsibility and authority to approve or reject all components, drug product containers, closures, in-process materials, packaging materials, labeling, and drug products and the authority to review production records to ensure that no errors have occurred or, if errors have occurred, that they have been fully investigated." In addi-

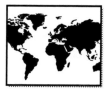

tion, the one-or-more-person quality control unit is responsible for approving or rejecting all procedures or specifications affecting the identity, strength, quality, and purity of the drug product.

Obviously, the professionals responsible for performing, supervising, or consulting on the manufacture, processing, packing, or holding of a drug must be adequate in number, free from any illness that may endanger the product, and sufficiently qualified by education, training, and experience to carry out their respective tasks. Facility staff must be trained not only in their specific tasks, but in CGMP as well. The facility must document this training.

Buildings and Facilities CGMP building and facility requirements are designed to ensure that any structures used to manufacture, process, pack, or hold a drug are of a suitable size, construction, and location to allow proper cleaning, maintenance, and operation. These requirements call for the separation of several plant operations (e.g., control and laboratory operations, packaging and labeling operations) to reduce the possibility of cross-contamination and other mishaps. Specific requirements for lighting, ventilation, heating and cooling systems, plumbing, sanitation, and maintenance are also provided.

Equipment CGMP equipment requirements are generally concerned with equipment design, size, location, and maintenance. To ensure that drug product attributes are not adversely affected, surfaces that contact components, in-process materials, or drug products must not be reactive, additive, or absorptive. Lubricants and other substances required for equipment operations must not cause product contamination.

At predetermined intervals, all utensils and equipment must be cleaned, maintained, and sanitized according to specific written procedures. Filters and automatic, mechanical, and electronic equipment (including computers) face special validation requirements.

Components and Drug Product Container and Closure Controls A facility must maintain detailed written procedures for the receipt, identification, storage, handling, sampling, testing, and approval/rejection of components and drug product containers and closures. Upon receipt, these materials must be inspected visually for appropriate labeling and contents, container damage, broken seals, and contamination. Before use, samples from each lot of components must be drawn, and the components tested for identity and conformity with purity, strength, and quality specifications. Drug product containers and closures must be tested for conformance to applicable written requirements.

Production and Process Controls Manufacturing facilities must maintain written procedures for production and process controls designed to ensure that the drug products have the identity, strength, quality, and purity they claim or are represented to possess. Special CGMP requirements exist for the charge-in of components, yield calculations, the identification of compounding and storage containers, processing lines, and the major equipment used in the production of drug batches, the sampling and testing of in-process materials and drug products, and the limiting of production times.

Packaging and Labeling Controls All packaging and labeling materials must be sampled, examined, or tested before their use. Documented procedures must be established for the receipt, identification, storage, handling, sampling, examination, and testing of labeling and packaging materials. CGMP regulations also specify requirements for labeling issuances and accountability, packaging and labeling operations control and inspection, tamper-resistant packaging for OTC drugs, drug product inspection, and expiration dating.

To reduce the frequency of drug product mislabeling, the FDA revised the CGMP labeling control regulations in 1993. Specifically, the revision defined the term "gang-printed labeling," specified conditions for the use of gang-printed or cut labeling, and exempted manufacturers that employ certain automated inspection systems from labeling reconciliation requirements. The agency has delayed the implementation of some elements of this regulation (i.e., those provisions applicable to labeling other than immediate container labels) until it can finalize a related regulation proposed in July 1997. The proposed regulation would amend CGMP packaging and labeling control provisions by limiting the application of special control procedures for the use of cut labeling to immediate container labels, individual unit cartons, or multiunit cartons containing immediate containers that are not packaged in individual unit cartons. The FDA also proposed to permit the use of any automated technique that physically prevents incorrect labeling from being processed by labeling and packaging equipment when cut labeling is used.

Holding and Distribution Requirements Facilities must maintain detailed written procedures describing the warehousing operations (including quarantine and special storage procedures) and distribution methods in use for a drug product. To expedite the process of locating products in case of a recall, facilities must maintain records relating to the distribution of products. In most cases, facilities should implement the "first in, first out" (FIFO) principle in storing and distributing the product.

Laboratory Controls Each organizational unit within a firm is required to maintain procedures for control mechanisms. These procedures and mechanisms, such as specifications, standards, sampling plans, and test procedures, are designed to ensure that components, drug product containers, closures, in-process materials, labeling, and drug products conform to appropriate standards of identity, strength, quality, and purity. Laboratory controls, which must be reviewed and approved by the quality control unit, include: (1) the determination, through documented sampling and testing procedures, that each shipment lot of components, drug product containers, closures, and labeling conforms to relevant specifications; (2) the determination, through sampling and testing procedures, that in-process materials conform to written specifications; (3) the determination that the laboratory is complying with written descriptions of drug product sampling procedures and specifications; and (4) the determination that instruments, apparatus, gauges, and recording devices have been calibrated at suitable intervals according to written procedures that provide specific directions, schedules, limits for accuracy and precision, and provisions for remedial action in the event accuracy and/or precision limits are not met.

A written program must be designed for stability testing studies. The results of these tests are used to determine appropriate storage conditions and expiration dates for each drug. Reserve samples of drug substances and drug products must be retained for specific intervals.

Also included in the laboratory controls subpart of the CGMP regulations are requirements for: (1) the sampling, testing, and release for distribution of drug product batches; (2) special testing for sterile, pyrogen-free, ophthalmic, and controlled-release drugs, reserve sample retention, laboratory test animals; and (3) testing for penicillin contamination.

In September 1998, CDER released a draft industry guidance entitled, *Investigating Out of Specification (OOS) Test Results for Pharmaceutical Production*. The draft guidance, which defines OOS results as "all suspect results that fall outside the specifications or acceptance criteria established in NDAs, official compendia, or by the manufacturer," provides CDER's thinking on how manufacturers should evaluate suspect, or out of specification, test results in the manufacture and laboratory testing of active pharmaceutical ingredients, excipients, and other components. The draft guidance applies to laboratory testing during the manufacture of active pharmaceutical ingredients, excipients, and other components as well as the testing of the finished product to the extent that GMP requirements apply.

Records and Reports Appropriately approved and checked master records must be maintained to assure uniformity between product batches. The facility must prepare batch records for each batch of product. Facilities must retain records for all drug components, drug product containers, closures, and labeling for at least one year after the expiration date of the drug product for which they were used. Certain OTC drugs do not require expiration dating because they meet specific exemption criteria. For these drugs, records must be kept for three years after distribution of the last lot of drug product incorporating the component or using the container, closure, or labeling. CGMP regulations also specify requirements for master and batch production records, laboratory records, distribution records, and complaint files.

The agency's March 1997 electronic signatures and electronic records rule (21 CFR Part 11) had significant implications for production, standard operating procedure, laboratory, quality, and all other GMP and non-GMP records and documents that CDER regulations require industry to maintain or submit. Provided that certain standards were met, Part 11 gave industry, for the first time, the authority to use electronic records and electronic signatures in lieu of paper-based records and signatures, respectively. The agency's goal in Part 11 was to permit the use of electronic records and signatures while establishing standards that would minimize opportunities for readily falsifying electronic records and to maximize the chances for detecting such falsifications.

It is important to note that, although the earliest push for electronic records and signatures was in the CGMP area (i.e., full handwritten signatures for master and batch production records), Part 11 is applicable to every FDA recordkeeping requirement across all of the agency's program areas. The agency's enforcement policy regarding Part 11 is detailed in Compliance Policy Guide 160.850 (May 1999), which establishes that legacy systems are not exempt from the rule (although the agency recognizes that some of these systems may take longer to be in compliance with some of the rule's technical provisions), and that the agency will examine, on a case-by-case basis, the nature, extent, and impact of deviations from Part 11 and will take action when necessary. It is important to note that Part 11, which took effect in August 1997, simply permits, rather than requires, companies to employ electronic records and signatures in lieu of paper-based records and signatures, respectively.

Returned and Salvaged Drug Products Any returned drug products must be identified and held. A manufacturer must destroy such products if there is any doubt about their safety, identity, strength, quality, or purity, but may reprocess the products if the resultant drug can meet applicable standards,

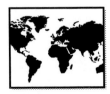

specifications, and characteristics. Reprocessing must be conducted according to written and company-approved procedures. Drugs subjected to improper storage, including extremes in temperature, humidity, smoke, fumes, pressure, age, radiation due to natural disasters, fires, accidents, or equipment failures may not be salvaged and returned to the marketplace.

Expected Changes to CGMP For several reasons, including rapid technological change, industry misunderstanding of certain CGMP requirements, and serious validation deficiencies at some firms, the FDA proposed to clarify and amend certain CGMP requirements in mid-1996. The proposed rule, which had not been finalized at this writing, would do the following:

- Define and Clarify Process Validation and Methods Validation Requirements. Because the agency continued to find a few firms that did not validate and that did not revalidate their manufacturing processes when necessary, the agency proposed to specify in the CGMP regulations "the nature and extent of validation that are necessary to ensure that the resulting products have the identity, strength, quality and purity characteristics that they purport to possess."

- Dedicated Production Processes for Certain Drugs. For certain substances that pose a serious threat of contamination (i.e., substances to which humans or animals show a particular sensitivity even at extremely low levels), the FDA has proposed requiring dedicated production facilities and equipment.

- Clarify Requirements for Testing and Investigation of Discrepancies/Failures. After finding that some firms are not conducting adequate testing and are not adequately evaluating test discrepancies or investigating failures, the FDA has proposed to clarify related CGMP requirements, to amend procedures for component testing, calculation of yield, and blend testing, and to specify procedures for out-of-specification results.

- Quality Control. The proposed rule would make the quality control unit responsible for reviewing changes in the product, process, equipment, or personnel, and for determining if and when revalidation is required.

Although CDER had hoped to finalize this regulation by January 2001, its release was delayed due, in part, to blend uniformity issues, according to center officials. At this writing, the center continued to review the several hundred comments forwarded in response to the proposed rule.

The Enforcement of CGMP While some critics have claimed that CGMP provisions are too general and difficult to enforce, the FDA has an active program designed to ensure manufacturer compliance. Enforcement responsibilities fall mainly on the FDA's district offices located throughout the United States. These offices monitor the industry by inspecting each drug manufacturing facility within their regions at least once every two years.

When a foreign or domestic inspection is completed, the manufacturer is alerted to any detected CGMP violations. Minor violations are generally handled by the FDA's district offices, which provide the manufacturer a period of time within which to address the detected violations. For major violations, the district office files a report with FDA headquarters, which reviews the case and decides on the appropriate regulatory action.

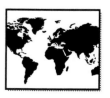

Beyond Approval: Drug Manufacturer Regulatory Responsibilities

Chapter 11

In early 2002, CDER hoped to fully implement a systems-based GMP inspectional approach that it had been using on a pilot basis in several districts. While the existing inspection approach focuses on products, the systems-based approach focuses on the assessment of six manufacturer systems: quality; production; laboratory controls; facilities and equipment; materials; and packaging and labeling. Based on specific criteria and assessments, CDER inspectors can choose to assess specific combinations of these systems, although an assessment of the quality systems will always be required. In analyzing data from the pilot program, CDER officials found that the systems-based approach improved inspectional efficiency and reduced mean inspection time by 12 hours.

In recent years, FDA inspections have tended to focus on failure investigations, microbiological issues, and stability. Laboratory controls, in particular the handling of out-of-specification results, remains the most problematic CGMP area for industry, according to CDER officials.

Traditionally, CGMP inspections have been conducted on an unannounced basis—that is, the facility to be inspected generally was not given advance notice by the FDA field office. The CGMP inspector arrived at the plant and, after the presentation of credentials and a notice of inspection, is given immediate access to the building.

In early 2001, CDER announced that it would not extend a pilot program under which the agency was conducting pre-announced manufacturing inspections. Under the program, CDER provided, for the first time, notification of an upcoming inspection (at least five days before the scheduled inspection), formal notification to drug manufacturers of positive inspection results, and annotated FDA-483 forms—the forms on which problems discovered during inspections are noted. CDER decided to implement the pilot program after preannounced inspections in the medical device area produced a 70 percent time savings over unannounced inspections.

Although CDER decided not to extend the pilot program, it is allowing FDA district offices to continue to conduct pre-announced inspections at their own discretion. In addition, the agency will leave to the districts' discretion whether they will continue the practice of annotating FDA-483s.

The use of announced inspections has long been the modus operandi for inspections of non-U.S. drug manufacturers. For foreign manufacturing facilities, the FDA makes only CGMP inspections that are pre-arranged with the manufacturers a few months in advance. The most frequent subjects of foreign CGMP inspections are bulk active pharmaceutical ingredient manufacturers.

In recent years, the FDA's international surveillance activities have increased considerably. With greater funding for foreign inspections, the FDA had significantly increased its inspectional activities targeted at foreign manufacturing facilities during the mid-1990s. In mid-1997, the FDA and European Union (EU) regulators established a mutual recognition agreement (MRA) under which they would exchange and generally accept each other's drug and medical device CGMP inspections without necessitating reinspections. The MRA, which was ratified in the United States and Europe, begins with a three-year transitional period (December 1999-December 2002), during which the regulators were to establish the equivalence of their preapproval and postapproval GCMP inspections and determine the essential information that must be present in CGMP inspection reports to facilitate their mutual acceptance by the participating regulatory agencies.

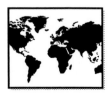

Due to resource issues and competing priorities, the transitional period stands to last far more than three years. In late 2001, the FDA was still in the process of conducting its equivalency evaluation in its first EU country—the United Kingdom—which it hopes to complete by early 2002. The agency will use the same process to assess the inspectional systems of all other EU countries, a process that will involve an evaluation of systems on paper, a visit to the regulatory authority's office to evaluate and audit inspectional systems, and then accompanying the regulatory authority on actual manufacturing inspections.

Phase 4 Commitments

Sponsor commitments made at the time of a drug's approval may also become, in effect, postmarketing requirements. For example, a sponsor may agree, at the time of approval, to conduct additional testing on a drug to further discern the product's safety/effectiveness or effects in specific subpopulations. Often called "Phase 4 commitments," these commitments—and sponsors' progress in fulfilling them—are actively tracked by the FDA following approval (see discussion below).

Although the agency can pursue Phase 4 commitments for any drug, the FDA's 1993 regulations on accelerated approval (Subpart H) codified its authority to require postapproval studies under the Subpart H program. These regulations established that the FDA can require Phase 4 studies when it approves an application on the basis of a surrogate endpoint or on the basis of an effect on a clinical endpoint other than survival or irreversible morbidity. Since this time, the Phase 4 study requirement has been extended to other products, including those approved under the FDA's new "fast track" product approval system (see Chapter 15).

CDER's enforcement of industry's Phase 4 commitments came under fire in mid-2000 following the Public Citizens Health Research Group's (HRG) release of a study disclosing that less than one in five sponsors of NMEs approved in the early 1990s had fulfilled relevant Phase 4 study commitments. CDER officials countered, however, that the HRG's report revealed that the center's tracking system had failed to indicate that many of the Phase IV commitments had been fulfilled and that the non-compliance rates were exaggerated because the center's database includes many Phase 4 studies that are not being conducted under formal commitments.

Recent drug approval trends—most importantly, the fact that so many new drugs are being approved so rapidly—have also led to an increasing focus on postmarketing studies and surveillance and on whether industry was fulfilling its Phase 4 study commitments. Under the FDA Modernization Act of 1997, for example, sponsors that are required, or that commit, to conduct Phase 4 studies as part of an NDA approval must provide, within their NDA annual reports, yearly updates on the status of the postmarketing studies (see discussion above). In addition, CDER's Office of Post Marketing Drug Risk Assessment (OPDRA) now has a unit responsible for tracking all Phase 4 study commitments.

For required or agreed-to studies, FDAMA also requires sponsors to submit postmarketing study protocols. Typically, protocols for required studies (e.g., accelerated approval clinical benefit studies) should be submitted prior to an NDA's approval, while it is general FDA practice to ask sponsors to submit protocols for other postmarketing studies (e.g., agreed-to studies) within three months of the date of the postmarketing study commitment. All study protocols should include the sponsor's proposed schedule for the completion of patient enrollment (or initiation of an animal study, if applicable), completion of the study, and the submission of a final report to the FDA.

When a postmarketing study is completed, the sponsor should submit the final report as a separate submission to the NDA with a form FDA 356h and a cover letter. The final study report should describe the study and its results, and should explain how the study fulfills the Phase 4 requirement or commitment. Otherwise, the report should explain why the study was unable to fulfill the requirement or commitment. After reviewing the final report, the FDA will determine whether or not the sponsor has fulfilled the requirement/commitment. If the agency concludes that the study commitment has been met or that the study is either no longer feasible or would no longer provide useful information, the commitment will be considered satisfied and the sponsor will no longer be required to report on the study's status in the annual report. In other cases, the agency could determine that a new study and study commitment are necessary.

Under FDAMA, CDER is also required to make publicly available certain information that sponsors submit in their annual Phase 4 status reports for required and agreed-to studies. FDAMA establishes that information in these reports should be made available to the extent necessary "to identify the applicant or to establish the status of the study including the reasons, if any, for failure to conduct, complete, and report the study." In its final rule implementing this aspect of FDAMA, CDER states that such information would include the Phase 4 study protocol, patient accrual rates, reports of unexpected suspected adverse drug reactions, and study results, but would not include trade secrets or information considered important to preserve personal privacy. FDAMA also requires the FDA to publish an annual report in the *Federal Register* on the status of Phase 4 studies. CDER has announced that it will establish a web site that will provide certain information about Phase 4 studies and their status.

Because differing policies within the center's review divisions made tracking Phase 4 commitments unmanageable in the past, CDER used an October 1996 MaPP entitled, *Procedures for Tracking and Reviewing Phase 4 Commitments* (MaPP 6010.2) to standardize the manner in which these commitments are sought, implemented, and tracked. MaPP 6010.2 states that CDER's policy regarding Phase 4 commitments will be based on the following requirements:

- Phase 4 commitments and a schedule for fulfillment of those commitments should be agreed upon with the applicant prior to the approval of an application.

- The agency's approval letter should list all Phase 4 commitments and the schedule for completing each commitment.

- Relevant information regarding Phase 4 study commitments also should be documented in the administrative record. These might include, for example, study objectives, research designs, reporting frequency, and study report formats for clinical studies or test methodology, frequency of testing, and method of data analysis for chemistry commitments. If these details are not determined at the time of approval, this should be noted and a schedule for resolving the issues should be described in the approval letter.

- A Phase 4 tracking system linked to the Centerwide Oracle-based Management Information System (COMIS) will be used to monitor the status of Phase 4 commitments.

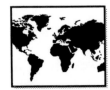

Just prior to, or at the time of, NDA approval, a division's project manager (i.e., consumer safety officer) will be responsible for assuring "that the applicant of the pending NDA submits a letter of commitment describing any Phase 4 studies they agree to conduct after approval of the application and the schedule for initiation and completion of those studies and submission of the study results," MaPP 6010.2 states.

For applications that receive accelerated reviews (Subpart H), the division must assure at this time that the Phase 4 study protocols are evaluated for their ability to meet the stated objectives and commitments. Phase 4 protocols for other applications may be submitted following approval, after which CDER must review the protocols "promptly (usually within 30 days)."

At least annually, a division's project manager must evaluate the status of outstanding voluntary Phase 4 commitments and, at least twice annually, must evaluate the status of outstanding Subpart H Phase 4 commitments. "For overdue outstanding commitments (some studies may be time-sensitive and need closer scrutiny), [the project manager must] generate what is called a 'Dunner Letter,'" which is a notification to the sponsor that it has failed to respond to a Phase 4 commitment. Editor's note: "dunner" is a generic term used to refer to a letter that is not an action letter (i.e., approval, approvable, or not-approvable). MaPP 6010.2 does not address compliance actions beyond the issuance of dunner letters.

CHAPTER 12

The Supplemental NDA and Postapproval Changes to Marketed Drugs

Following a drug's approval, the NDA holder can access and "supplement" the application's data to seek FDA authorization to market variations of the drug beyond those provided for in the approved NDA. Supplemental NDAs (SNDA) are submitted to the FDA when a firm wants to change an approved drug (e.g., dosage form, strength), its specifications, its manufacturing processes, its indication, or certain elements of its labeling. Federal regulations require that "the applicant...notify the Food and Drug Administration about each change in each condition established in an approved application beyond the variations already provided for in the application."

In practice, SNDAs are submitted to obtain regulatory authorization for a wide variety of modifications to approved drugs. These include proposed changes to an approved drug's manufacturing and control methods (manufacturing supplement), dosage form or route of administration, indication (efficacy supplement), ingredients or strength, dosage schedule, labeling, and container and closure system.

Perhaps more than any other aspect of FDA drug regulation, requirements for SNDAs were reshaped almost continually by regulatory reform initiatives in the mid- and late 1990s. While these reforms did not affect the nature or function of the supplemental NDA, they fundamentally changed the situations in which such submissions are needed, and provided detailed clarifications regarding the data and information that they must include.

Recent History of Regulatory Reform and SNDAs The most significant regulatory reforms affecting SNDAs address the review and approval of manufacturing changes. In early 1995, the FDA promised to issue a guidance document that would "reduce the number of manufacturing changes that require preapproval by FDA." The agency fulfilled this commitment by publishing a November 1995 guideline that established submission requirements for a variety of postapproval manufacturing and drug composition changes to immediate release solid oral dosage form drugs (see discussion below). Specifically, the guideline exempted more types of manufacturing process, site, equipment, and formulation changes from the requirement for FDA approval prior to implementation. This guideline has since been followed by other guidances applicable to other dosage forms.

Worldwide Pharmaceutical Regulation Series

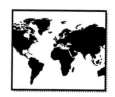

In March 1997, following months of industry/FDA negotiations and agency efforts to find ways to encourage drug companies to develop and submit SNDAs for new uses of approved drugs, the agency unveiled what it called the New Use Initiative. The goal of this initiative was "to speed up the development of new and supplemental uses of medications by using all available data to determine the effectiveness of drugs and biological products."

Essentially, the agency's New Use Initiative comprised two guidances that clarified efficacy data requirements for new and supplemental uses. The guidances establish that the FDA is willing to accept efficacy data from a variety of different sources (i.e., not just from two pivotal trials) as the basis for approving supplemental uses (see discussion below).

These initiatives were followed, in November 1997, by a series of reforms brought by the FDA Modernization Act of 1997 (FDAMA). The reforms, which did not formally take effect until late 1999 and which in many ways mirrored the initiatives discussed above, were intended to streamline SNDAs for manufacturing changes, new indications, and other types of postapproval modifications.

With regard to manufacturing changes, the FDA reform legislation provides that a company must submit, and obtain FDA approval for, a supplemental NDA before implementing a "major" manufacturing change. Other changes may be implemented either after an SNDA has been filed (i.e., a changes-being-effected supplement or a changes being effected in 30 days supplement) or immediately without an SNDA submission (i.e., minor changes to be reported in an NDA annual report). These and related provisions for manufacturing-related SNDAs became effective in November 1999 (see discussion below).

Other aspects of the legislation called for the agency to issue new SNDA standards and guidances for all types of postmarketing changes. To ensure that SNDA reviews received a higher profile, FDAMA called for CDER and other FDA centers to each designate an individual to facilitate efficient SNDA reviews.

When to Submit Supplemental versus Original NDAs

In past years, sponsors often had the option of submitting either full or supplemental NDAs for drug changes that required FDA approval before their formal implementation. Some companies maintained that SNDAs had certain advantages over full submissions, while others held that original NDAs should have been submitted whenever possible.

Under policies instituted as part of the FDA's user-fee program, however, such options no longer exist in most cases. Because different fees apply to certain original and supplemental NDAs, the agency now specifies when each type of application should be used. In a guidance document entitled, *Separate Marketing Applications and Clinical Data for Purposes of Assessing User Fees Under the Prescription Drug User Fee Act of 1992*, the FDA specifies when original and supplemental NDAs are appropriate for changes to approved products:

1. Changes in the composition of an approved product to support a change in the dosage form or route of administration should be submitted in separate original NDAs. Route of administration changes in which the new product remains quanti-

tatively and qualitatively identical to the approved product in composition (e.g., an injectable liquid dosage form intended for use by the intravenous and intraperitoneal routes) can be submitted in SNDAs, however. Also eligible for SNDAs are dosage form changes in which the new product is identical to the approved product in quantitative and qualitative composition (e.g., a sterile liquid in a single dose vial that is intended for use as either an injectable or an inhalation solution).

2. Modifications to an approved product that are based on chemistry, manufacturing, or controls data and bioequivalence or other studies (e.g., safety and immunogenicity) and that change the strength or concentration, change the manufacturing process, equipment or facility, or change the formulation (e.g., different excipients) should be submitted as supplements to an approved application. Ordinarily, such modifications do not warrant a new original application unless they involve a change in the dosage form or route of administration.

3. Requests for approval of a new indication, or a modification of a previously approved indication, should each be submitted individually in a separate supplement to an approved NDA. According to the FDA, "each indication is considered a separate change for which a separate supplement should be submitted. The policy allows FDA to approve each indication when it is ready for approval rather than delaying approval until the last of a group of indications is ready to be approved."

The FDA's user-fee policies have had several other implications for SNDAs. First, sponsors of supplements that require clinical data to support approval must pay user fees for such applications.

On the other hand, the FDA's user-fee program also provides SNDAs with a significantly higher level of review priority. Under PDUFA II, for example, the agency has the following goals for SNDAs submitted in fiscal year 2002 (October 1, 2001–September 30, 2002): to review 90% of priority efficacy supplements within 6 months; to review 90% of standard efficacy supplements within 10 months; and to review 90% of manufacturing supplements for which prior approval is required within 4 months.

Supplemental NDA Submission Requirements

No universal SNDA data submission requirements exist. The nature of the change proposed in an SNDA directly determines the testing and submission requirements applicable to the change. Federal regulations state that "the information required in the supplement is limited to that needed to support the change."

Obviously, changes to a drug's indication, ingredients, or route of administration are likely to require clinical data to prove the product's safety and effectiveness. In contrast, some modifications to a drug's manufacturing or control methods may require only that the change be described and supported by stability and bioequivalence data (Note: No drug produced through a manufacturing change, whether significant or otherwise, may be distributed before the NDA holder validates the change's effects on the product's identity, strength, quality, purity, and potency). Therefore, SNDAs can range from minor filings to documents longer and more complex than some NDAs. All SNDAs, however, must provide an archival copy and a review copy that include an application form, appropriate technical sections, samples, and labeling.

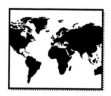

Worldwide Pharmaceutical Regulation Series

The nature of the change proposed in an SNDA also determines when the application must be submitted and whether the sponsor must await FDA approval prior to implementing the change. In its regulations and relevant guidance documents, the FDA has categorized postapproval changes into various classes. Those changes that are most likely to affect the FDA's conclusions about the approved drug's safety and effectiveness require the submission, and FDA approval, of an SNDA before being instituted. Less significant changes do not require FDA approval, but may require either the submission of an SNDA at the time of implementation or a description in the sponsor's annual report.

Postmarketing Manufacturing Changes

Although they have attempted to ease regulatory burdens associated with postapproval manufacturing changes, a variety of legal and regulatory initiatives undertaken in the mid- and late 1990s have done much to complicate any attempt to characterize the regulatory requirements associated with such modifications. At this writing, regulatory requirements facing postmarketing manufacturing changes were dictated primarily by FDAMA provisions, by a November 1999 guidance document that provides agency recommendations on the FDAMA provisions, and by a series of guidances on postapproval manufacturing changes to drugs with certain types of dosage forms (see discussion below on scale-up and postapproval changes (SUPAC) below).

FDAMA and Postmarketing Manufacturing Changes FDAMA's Section 116 first became the basis for SNDA submission requirements facing postapproval manufacturing changes on November 21, 1999, the established effective date for this section of the law. Because the agency was unable to issue final regulations to implement Section 116 by this date, this FDAMA section replaced the existing regulations (C.F.R. 314.70-Supplements and other changes to an approved application), and the agency stated that it would serve as "the sole basis for FDA's regulation of postapproval manufacturing changes for products approved in" NDAs and ANDAs until implementing regulations are published. During this period, the agency established that a November 1999 guidance entitled, *Changes to an Approved* NDA *or* ANDA would represent the agency's position on how it would apply the FDAMA requirements.

By late 2001, the FDA had not yet published the implementing regulations—a final version of a June 1999 proposed rule—and it was unclear how soon they would be released. When the agency does publish implementing regulations, it is also expected to release a revised *Changes to an Approved* NDA *and* ANDA guidance based on the new implementing regulations rather than the FDAMA provisions themselves, on which the current guidance document is based. In January 2001, CDER did release a guidance entitled, *Changes to an Approved* NDA *and* ANDA, *Questions and Answers*, which is based on industry feedback and questions regarding the above-mentioned *Changes to an Approved* NDA *and* ANDA guidance.

The FDA's June 1999 proposed regulation to implement FDAMA's Section 116 was criticized by industry, which recommended that the agency abandon the proposal because it failed to go far enough in fulfilling the intent of FDAMA, which sought to reduce the regulatory burdens associated with postapproval manufacturing changes. Earlier in 1999, industry also recommended that the agency scrap its SUPAC guidance program (see discussion below) in lieu of a decision tree approach that relied on "performance standards rather than command and control regulations."

The November 1999 *Changes to an Approved* NDA *and* ANDA guidance establishes reporting categories (e.g., different types of SNDAs, annual report) for various postapproval changes, most of which are

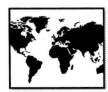

manufacturing-related: components and composition; manufacturing sites; manufacturing process; specifications; packaging; labeling; miscellaneous changes; and multiple related changes.

FDAMA's Section 116 and the November 1999 guidance establish reporting categories that are, in most respects, similar to those defined in earlier SUPAC guidances (see discussion below). Unlike earlier guidances, however, FDAMA provides for two categories of "changes being effected" SNDAs for manufacturing changes. Further, the agency notes that, whenever the November 1999 guidance's reporting categories are inconsistent with those in the SUPAC guidances, the November 1999 guidance supersedes the SUPAC guidances. Because the November 1999 guidance does not provide "extensive recommendations on reporting categories for components and composition changes, however, the agency recommends that sponsors refer to recommendations in previous guidances, particularly the SUPAC guidances. The agency claims that it will be updating the various SUPAC guidances and other documents to make them consistent with the November 1999 guidance on postmarketing changes.

FDAMA and the November 1999 guidance establish four types of changes and reporting categories based on their potential to adversely affect the identity, strength, quality, or potency of a product as they may relate to the drug's safety or effectiveness:

Major Change-Prior Approval Supplement. A change that has a substantial potential to adversely affect a product is considered a major change, and requires the submission, and FDA approval, of a "prior approval supplement" before its distribution using the specified change. A sponsor can request that the FDA expedite the review of a prior approval supplement due to public health reasons (e.g., drug shortage) or extraordinary hardship (e.g., fire). Examples of manufacturing changes that would be considered major changes include modifications that may affect the controlled (or modified) release, metering or other characteristics (e.g., particle size) of the dose delivered to the patient, any fundamental modification in the manufacturing process or technology (e.g., for drug products, changing from a dry to wet granulation or a change from one type of drying process to another), and establishing a new procedure for reprocessing a batch of drug substance or drug product that fails to meet the approved specification.

Moderate Change-Changes Being Effected in 30 Days Supplement. A change that has a moderate potential to adversely affect a product will, unless identified by the FDA as being eligible for a "changes being effected" supplement (see discussion below), require a "changes being effected in 30 days supplemental NDA." This type of moderate change requires the submission of an SNDA at least 30 days before the distribution of the product made using the change. If the agency does not contact the applicant within this 30-day period, the company is free to distribute the product. However, the FDA may contact the sponsor within the 30-day period to inform the company that a prior approval supplement is required for the change or that the supplement is incomplete. The company would then have to delay distribution until a prior approval supplement is submitted and approved (i.e., if one is required) or, if the supplement is deemed incomplete, delay distribution until the supplement is amended with the missing information. After its review, the agency may also order that the manufacturer cease distribution if the FDA disapproves the supplemental application. Examples of changes in specifications that would require a changes being effected in 30 days supplement include the establishment of a new regulatory analytical procedure and a change in the regulatory analytical

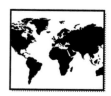

procedure that does not provide the same or increased assurance of the identity, strength, quality, purity, or potency of the material being tested when compared to the regulatory analytical procedure described in the approved application. CDER clarified its processes for handling such supplements in a January 2001 guidance entitled, *Changes to an Approved NDA or NDA, Questions and Answers.*

Moderate Change-Changes Being Effected Supplement. If the agency identifies a change that has a moderate potential to adversely affect a product as a change that can be implemented upon an SNDA's submission, the sponsor can implement the change after the agency receives the supplement supporting the change. This type of supplement is called a "changes being effected" supplement. If the agency disapproves a change under a changes being effected supplement, it can then order the firm to cease distribution of the drugs made using the disapproved change. Examples of moderate labeling changes that can be submitted in a changes being effected supplement include the addition of an adverse event due to information reported to the applicant or agency, the addition of a precaution arising out of a postmarketing study, or the clarification of the administration statement to ensure proper administration of the product.

Minor Change-Annual Report. A change that has a minimal potential to adversely affect a drug product does not require an SNDA. Rather, the applicant need only describe minor changes in its subsequent annual report to the approved NDA. Examples of manufacturing changes that would be considered minor changes include minor modifications in an existing imprint for a dosage form (e.g., changing from a numeric to an alphanumeric code) and a change in the order of addition of ingredients for solution dosage forms or solutions used in unit operations (e.g., granulation solutions).

In discussing these reporting categories, the agency notes that sponsors can use what are called comparability protocols to reduce the reporting category for specific changes. Proposed comparability protocols, which describe the tests, validation studies, and acceptable limits to be achieved in demonstrating the absence of an adverse effect caused by a manufacturing-related change, can be submitted either in an original NDA or as a prior approval SNDA. The agency is developing a guidance document on comparability protocols.

Neither FDAMA nor the November 1999 guidance addresses either SNDA submission requirements or agency review targets for such applications. SNDA submission requirements are addressed more fully in existing agency guidances, the SUPAC guidances in particular (see discussion below), the FDA notes, while review goals are specified in the agency's PDUFA II commitments and in the agency's May 1998 guidance entitled, *Standards for the Prompt Review of Efficacy Supplements, Including Priority Efficacy Supplements.*

SUPAC and SNDAs for Manufacturing Changes Before FDAMA's Section 116 regulations took effect in November 1999, a series of guidances on scale-up and postapproval changes—called SUPAC guidances—had been the key regulatory documents spelling out requirements associated with postapproval manufacturing changes for several types of products (i.e., other than the regulations for such changes). From November 1995 through 1999, CDER published SUPAC guidances applicable to several different types of drug dosage forms.

Although the FDAMA provisions now represent the basis for reporting requirements for all postapproval manufacturing changes, the SUPAC guidances remain relevant in several respects. As noted

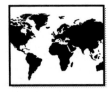

above, they will continue to provide the most detailed guidance on reporting categories for postapproval changes in drug components and composition. And, unlike the November 1999 "changes" guidance, the various SUPAC guidances provide recommendations on the data and information that must be developed and submitted to support various postmarketing manufacturing changes.

Agency officials claim that they will continue to update the existing SUPAC guidances and develop and publish new SUPAC documents. Those currently under development include guidances on postmarketing packaging changes and analytical methods changes, which will address issues that cut across products in all dosage forms.

The FDA's first SUPAC guidance, a 1995 guidance document entitled, *Immediate Release Solid Oral Dosage Forms; Scale-Up and Post Approval Changes (SUPAC-IR): Chemistry, Manufacturing and Controls; In Vitro Dissolution Testing; In Vivo Bioequivalence Documentation*, revised the SNDA requirements applicable to postapproval manufacturing changes for relevant drug products. The November 1995 document was only the first in a series of SUPAC guidances for drugs in a variety of dosage forms. CDER has since released SUPAC guidances for modified release solid oral dosage forms (October 1997) and nonsterile semisolid dosage forms (June 1997), and a January 1999 guidance that addresses immediate release and modified release solid oral dosage form equipment changes. In addition, CDER has released an April 1998 SUPAC guidance for postapproval changes to analytical testing laboratories (PAC-ATLS). In late 1998, CDER released a pair of draft SUPAC guidances: a November 1998 draft guidance on chemistry, manufacturing and controls documentation needed in submissions to support postapproval changes in the manufacturing or specifications of intermediates used in the synthesis of bulk drug ingredients (BACPAC I), and a December 1998 draft manufacturing equipment addendum to the June 1997 nonsterile semisolid dosage form SUPAC guidance.

The published SUPAC-IR guidance—and the subsequent SUPAC guidances—classified postapproval manufacturing changes into as many as three levels—Levels 1, 2, and 3—and established postmarketing reporting requirements for changes within each of these levels (i.e., SNDA, annual report). The agency has defined these levels broadly for each type of change. The following levels apply to SUPAC-IR component, composition, and process changes, for example:

> *Level 1*: changes that are unlikely to have any detectable impact on formulation, quality, or performance.
>
> *Level 2*: changes that could have a significant impact on formulation, quality, or performance.
>
> *Level 3*: changes that are likely to have a significant impact on formulation, quality, or performance.

It is worth noting that some types of changes, such as manufacturing changes, have only two levels in the SUPAC guidances.

For each type of postapproval manufacturing change addressed by the SUPAC-IR document—components and composition changes, manufacturing site changes, scale up/scale down of manufacture, and manufacturing process/equipment changes—the level of the change and the testing and reporting requirements (e.g., SNDA, annual report) associated with the change are established. Generally, the less significant SUPAC-IR changes—most Level 1 changes, for example—require only a description in an annual report. The more important changes—most Level 3 changes, for instance—call for the submission and FDA approval of an SNDA prior to implementation (i.e., a "prior approval" supplement). Many Level 2 changes can be implemented simultaneously with an applicant's submission of a "changes being effected" supplement.

As noted above, however, the reporting categories in the SUPAC guidances are superseded whenever the November 1999 guidance's reporting categories are inconsistent with those in the SUPAC guidances. CDER officials plan to revise the SUPAC guidances to harmonize them with the November 1999 guidance.

Expedited Review for NDA Chemistry Supplements Under agency regulations, NDA holders have traditionally had that right to request that the agency expedite its review of any supplemental NDA requiring prior approval "if a delay in making the change described within it would impose an extraordinary hardship on the applicant." In a June 1999 CDER policy manual, CDER provided guidance on the submission and review of expedited review requests for NDA chemistry supplements.

Expedited review for chemistry SNDAs may be granted when an application is relevant to a public health need (e.g., drug availability), extraordinary hardship on the applicant (e.g., catastrophic event such as a fire) or unforeseeable events (e.g., the abrupt discontinuation of active ingredient supply), or agency need (e.g., government drug purchase program). According to the agency's policy manual entitled, *Requests for Expedited Review of NDA Chemistry Supplements*, expedited review will be considered "only when there is sufficient documentation to support a need for review in less than four months." The document also notes that "granting of an expedited review does not change the information that should be submitted in the supplement to support the change." In such cases, the applicant must mark its supplement and mailing cover with the following statement: "Supplement-Expedited Review Requested."

"Bundled" CMC Supplements In early 2000, CDER established a "bundling coordinator" to coordinate the center's processes for handling so-called "bundled supplements," which are groups or clusters of NDA or ANDA supplements for chemistry, manufacturing, and controls changes that affect more than one original submission and that will be reviewed in multiple review divisions. The center laid out its plans for processing bundled supplements in a January 2000 MaPP entitled, *Review of the Same Supplemental Change to More than One NDA or ANDA in More than One Review Division* (MaPP 5015.6).

After an applicant notifies CDER that it plans to submit a supplement for a change that will affect applications in multiple review teams, divisions, or offices, the bundling coordinator and Office of New Drug Chemistry (ONDC) managers will determine if the change can be submitted in a bundled supplement. If the center decides to accept a bundled submission, it will identify a "lead ONDC chemistry team" for the review based on the team that has the most supplements (within that set, the oldest NDA will be designated the "lead NDA"). After the team assigns a chemistry team leader, a lead reviewer will be assigned. The bundling coordinator will distribute a memo to all chemistry team leaders, project managers, and document room staffers who will be involved in the reviews of the various supplements, and will track the progress of the reviews of the bundled supplements. While the various supplement review teams will work together through the lead reviewer, each team is responsible for issuing its own action letter.

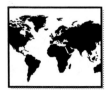

Pending Changes for CMC Supplemental NDAs In addition to the pending FDAMA implementing regulations and other changes highlighted above, other initiatives stand to affect submission requirements for postmarketing manufacturing changes. In late 2000, CDER officials unveiled a proposed "risk-based CMC review" initiative under which the center planned to reduce CMC submission requirements for "low risk" drug products. Under the proposal, CDER would first assess approved products to identify those for which reduced post-marketing filing requirements (i.e., supplements for manufacturing changes, streamlined annual reports) would be highly unlikely to result in product quality problems. Ultimately under this "risk-based" initiative, CDER is planning to reduce manufacturing-related reporting requirements for NDAs and other submissions as well.

Labeling Changes

Although the FDA's *Changes to an Approved* NDA *or* ANDA guidance focuses principally upon postmarketing manufacturing changes, it also addresses postapproval changes in other areas, such as labeling changes. Labeling changes cover a wide array of modifications, ranging from changes in a container label's layout to the addition of new indications.

All significant, or "major," postmarketing drug labeling changes must be approved by the FDA before implementation. Although some labeling changes of lesser importance can be made prior to approval (see discussion below), changes such as the addition of new indications, changes in dosage strengths, changes in dosage form, and changes in recommended dosage schedules require the submission, and FDA approval, of an SNDA before implementation.

In January 2000, CDER Director Janet Woodcock, M.D., claimed that the center would reduce, to one to two weeks, the review of NDA labeling supplements as a quid pro quo for companies willing to submit such applications electronically, although she also noted that the center would consider requiring electronic submissions. This would permit the agency to assemble, and place on the FDA's website, an electronic repository of current drug labeling, Woodcock stated. According to CDER officials, some companies are making e-submissions for drug labeling and labeling changes, although they have not yet provided statistics indicating how frequently such filings are being made.

The *Changes to an Approved* NDA *or* ANDA guidance specifies three different reporting categories for labeling changes:

Major Labeling Changes. As noted, all major changes require the submission and approval of an SNDA before being implemented. The guidance specifies that any change in the labeling, except those designated as a moderate or minor change by regulation or guidance, be submitted as a preapproval supplement. Major changes include labeling changes based on postmarketing study results, the addition of pharmacoeconomic claims based on clinical studies, the addition of superiority claims over another product, and the expansion or contraction of the target patient population based on data. Although the addition of new indications (see discussion below), dosage strengths, and dosage forms, among other labeling changes, are not specifically listed in the guidance, it is assumed that such changes will always require a prior approval SNDA because they are not specifically listed as moderate or minor changes.

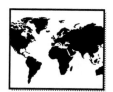

Moderate Labeling Changes. The November 1999 guidance provides examples only of moderate labeling changes for which a changes being effected supplement must be submitted (i.e., there are no references to moderate changes for which a changes being effected in 30 days SNDA must be filed). Moderate changes for which changes being effected supplements are required include: (1) the addition or strengthening of a contraindication, warning, precaution, or adverse reaction; (2) the addition or strengthening of a statement regarding drug abuse, dependence, psychological effect, or overdosage; (3) the addition or strengthening of an instruction regarding dosage and administration intended to further promote the safe use of the product; or (4) the deletion of false, misleading, or unsupported indications for use or claims for effectiveness.

Minor Labeling Changes. Labeling modifications that involve editorial or similar minor changes, or changes in the information concerning the description of the drug product or information on how the drug is supplied (i.e., not involving a change in dosage strength or dosage form) do not require the submission of an SNDA and need only be described in an annual report to the NDA.

Pursuing New Indications for Approved Drugs Despite the level of regulatory activity regarding supplemental applications for postmarketing manufacturing supplements, SNDAs for new indications are more visible and important than most other types of supplements. Because these "efficacy supplements," as they are called, often propose therapeutically significant new uses for approved drugs, they are given a higher regulatory priority than other SNDAs. Under the user-fee program, for example, the FDA's review goals for priority efficacy supplements are identical to those for original NDAs.

Furthermore, FDAMA required the agency to publish standards for the prompt review of "supplemental applications submitted for approved articles," something that the statute's legislative history suggests means efficacy supplements. The agency decided to use the previously established user-fee review goals to fulfill this FDAMA requirement. FDAMA also called for the agency to issue a guidance to specify efficacy supplements that were eligible for priority review, a requirement that the agency met by releasing an industry guidance entitled, *Standards for the Prompt Review of Efficacy Supplements, Including Priority Efficacy Supplements* (May 1998). In this guidance, the agency establishes that SNDAs will be subject to the same priority review criteria to which NDAs are subject—an SNDA will receive priority designation if the product "would be a significant improvement, compared to marketed products, including non-drug products/therapies in the treatment, diagnosis, or prevention of a disease."

Actually, FDAMA was only the latest of several developments that have affected regulatory requirements for SNDAs in the 1990s. In the mid-1990s, the FDA's requirements for efficacy supplements had come under fire during the regulatory reform movement. Following months of efforts to find ways to encourage companies to develop and submit SNDAs for new uses of approved drugs, the FDA unveiled its New Use Initiative in March 1997. This initiative was designed to give "industry clear guidance on whether the agency can determine that a drug is effective for a new use without requiring data from two new clinical trials. In some cases, for example, a drug's effectiveness can be extrapolated from existing efficacy data; it can be shown by evidence from a new single trial supported by already existing related clinical data; or it can be documented by adequate evidence from a single multi-center study."

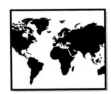

The New Use Initiative comprises two guidelines—*Providing Clinical Evidence of Effectiveness for Human Drug and Biological Products* (May 1998) and FDA *Approval of New Cancer Treatment Uses for Marketed Drug and Biological Drugs* (December 1998). These guidelines provide what might be the FDA's most detailed discussion to date on the agency's efficacy standards for new and supplemental indications (for a further discussion of these guidelines, see Chapter 5). The December 1998 guidance provides the most direct, if brief, discussion of data requirements for supplemental indications:

"To add new use information to the labeling of a marketed product, a holder of an approved marketing application must submit a supplemental marketing application that provides data establishing the safety and effectiveness of the product for the proposed new indication... The application should include all relevant data available from pertinent clinical studies, including negative or ambiguous results as well as positive findings. Data can come from pharmaceutical company-sponsored clinical trials intended to test the safety and effectiveness of a new use of a product, or from a number of alternative sources... To support approval, the data submitted should be sufficient in quality and quantity to establish the safety and effectiveness of the product with a high level of confidence, as required by law and scientific expectations."

In an October 2001 guidance entitled, *Cancer Drug and Biological Products—Clinical Data in Marketing Applications*, however, the FDA suggests that industry may be collecting more data in cancer trials than are necessary for the approval of original or supplemental NDAs for cancer therapies. "Representatives of...noncommercial sponsors [such as cancer cooperative groups] have told FDA that commercial sponsors often encourage collection of more data than the investigators would normally collect," says the guidance. "In fact, many of these data may not be called for in a marketing application for cancer therapy. It is possible that industry representatives are using data submission standards for marketing applications for less serious diseases or assuming standards that could be modified in many situations."

Another FDA action affecting efficacy supplements was the agency's revision of its standards for the "pediatric use" section of drug labeling. In a December 1994 final rule, the agency stated that NDA holders could support the inclusion of pediatric use information in drug labeling without data from controlled clinical trials in children. Under the regulation, the agency established that it would approve a drug for pediatric use "based on adequate and well-controlled studies in adults, with other information supporting pediatric use." The FDA has since supplemented the regulation with *Guidance for Industry: Content and Format for Pediatric Use Supplements*. Further, the FDA Modernization Act of 1997 contains provisions that award additional marketing exclusivity to companies that submit pediatric studies for drugs for which such information is valuable (for a detailed discussion of FDA requirements and incentives regarding pediatric studies, see Chapter 16).

Approval Times for Efficacy Supplements Since the mid-1990s, CDER's approval times for NDA efficacy supplements have been improving. In 2000, the center improved its median review time for such applications for the fifth consecutive year, to 10 months, while approving 134 efficacy supplements, the most in the past several years. In 1995, its median approval time for efficacy supplements was 16 months.

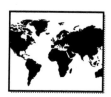

CHAPTER 13

The FDA's Orphan Drug Development Program

Although orphan drugs represent only a minor percentage of the medicines prescribed in the United States, these products have gained an exceptionally high profile in recent decades. Early in the 1980s, for example, orphan drugs became not only the subject of major legislation, but the focus of an FDA office devoted solely to their development as well.

Regulatory, legal, and commercial controversies surrounding better-known orphan drugs, such as Genentech's human growth hormone and Amgen's erythropoietin, have done much to bring widespread attention to orphan products and industry efforts to develop and market these medicines. In part representing the government's response to these controversies, FDA regulations implementing the key elements of the orphan drug laws were released in December 1992.

Despite various legislative and judicial challenges, the FDA's orphan drug development program has stood largely intact over its 18-year history. The program was one of relatively few of the agency's drug approval-related activities that was not earmarked for reform under several FDA reform bills debated in the mid-1990s.[1] In addition, the U.S. orphan drugs program has been the model for similar programs in both Europe and Japan.[2]

The special problems and issues facing orphan product development are well documented. Orphan products are unique because they are potentially useful drugs, biologics, and antibiotics that have limited commercial value. There are several reasons why they may lack profit potential—for example, a product may be used to treat a disease with a small patient population, it may be used only in minute doses, or it may have an unfavorable patent status.

In the past, few companies were willing to invest in an experimental drug whose potential sales did not justify, or whose actual sales might not even recover, these expenditures. Individuals suffering from such rare conditions as Turner's Syndrome, central precocious puberty, acute graft v. host disease (GVHD), and cystinosis were caught between the medical reality that few others shared their plight and the economic reality that a drug's development can cost more than $200 million.

Thanks to orphan drug legislation and the FDA's own efforts to shepherd these products through the development process, however, the 1980s and 1990s brought no dearth of firms willing to invest in

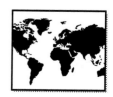

Worldwide Pharmaceutical Regulation Series

orphan products. According to FDA statistics, the agency had granted approximately 1,200 orphan designations and had approved 218 orphan drugs and biologics as of year-end 2000.

The FDA and Orphan Drugs: A Brief History

During the late 1970s, government leaders became increasingly concerned that the therapeutic abilities of many drugs went unexplored while millions of patients with one of an estimated 5,000 rare or orphan diseases went untreated. A 1979 report by the FDA-organized Interagency Task Force on Significant Drugs of Limited Commercial Value stated that, "whenever a drug has been identified as potentially life-saving or otherwise of unique major benefit to some patient, it is the obligation of society, as represented by government, to seek to make that drug available to that patient." The formal government response to the problem came several years later in the form of the Orphan Drug Act of 1983, a law that provides incentives for manufacturers to develop and market orphan products, including drugs, antibiotics and biologics.

Responsibility for administering the law was given to the FDA's Office of Orphan Product Development (OPD), which was founded in 1982. Today, the 19-person office continues to encourage orphan drug development by awarding financial incentives available under the law to sponsors of qualifying products, coordinating the efforts of investigators and drug companies, acting as a mediator between orphan sponsors and the FDA's drug and biologic review divisions, administering a grant program, and performing other promotional and educational activities.

The Importance of Orphan Drug Designation

The incentives offered under the Orphan Drug Act are seen as the keys to the development of future orphan products. The law provides major financial and marketing incentives to companies and investigators willing to research and develop qualified products. But before outlining the orphan product incentives themselves, it is worthwhile discussing orphan drug designation, a status that drugs must attain to become eligible for the most valuable incentives.

Tax advantages and marketing exclusivity are perhaps the two most important incentives that the U.S. Congress made available to orphan product sponsors through the Orphan Drug Act of 1983. Since Congress did not want these incentives to be awarded indiscriminately, it wrote into law that only products meeting specific criteria would be eligible for the two principal benefits.

Today, there are at least five basic eligibility criteria for orphan drug designation. To be eligible, a product:

- Must be a drug, biologic, or antibiotic. Medical devices, medical foods, and other products do not qualify for designation.

- Must have a sponsor that is testing or is planning to test the product for use in a "rare disease or condition." According to the Orphan Drug Act, a rare disease or condition is one that: "A) affects less than 200,000 persons in the United States, or B) affects more than 200,000 persons in the United States but for which there is no reasonable expectation that the costs of developing and making available in the United States a drug for such disease or condition will be recovered from sales in the United States

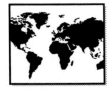

for such drug." The under-200,000 provision applies not only to diseases or conditions with a total patient prevalence of less than 200,000, but to subpopulations of more common diseases as well. The FDA insists that sponsors of orphan products for such indications be able to test the product in, and clearly label the product for, use in the relevant subpopulation. For prophylactic products such as vaccines and blood products, the figure of 200,000 applies to the number of patients receiving the product per year.

- Must not have been previously approved under a new drug application (NDA) or product license application/biological license application (BLA) for the disease or condition for which the sponsor is seeking orphan status. In other words, eligible products include both new chemical entities (NCE) —substances never before approved as medicines in the United States—and products that have been approved for any indication other than the indication for which the sponsor is seeking orphan designation. When granted by the FDA, designation applies only to the subject product for use in the specific rare disease or condition.

- Must be shown to have an adequate pharmacologic rationale for use in the orphan indication. This requirement is not one that the FDA enforces rigidly. Dr. Marion Finkel, former director of the FDA's Office of Orphan Products Development, stated in a 1984 speech that "a plausible hypothesis backed by some experimental evidence would be sufficient for orphan drug designation."

- Must not be the subject of a submitted marketing application prior to the filing of an orphan status request. This requirement was added in mid-1988 through the Orphan Drug Amendment Act of 1987. The amendment was an attempt by Congress to reserve marketing exclusivity and tax incentives for those firms whose initial intentions were to develop orphan drugs, and to withhold the incentives from companies that pursue designation simply as an afterthought to optimize the profitability of their products.

Obtaining Orphan Drug Designation Congress gave the FDA the authority to determine which drugs meet the criteria outlined above. To have its product designated, a firm must submit to the FDA an application called a Request for Designation of a Drug as an Orphan Drug.

The FDA's 1992 orphan drug regulations specify nine basic submission requirements for designation requests. According to these regulations, a sponsor must submit two copies of a completed, dated, and signed designation request that contains the following:

- A statement that the sponsor requests orphan-drug designation for a rare disease or condition, which must be identified with specificity.

- The name and address of the sponsor; the name and address of the sponsor's primary contact person and/or resident agent, including the person's title, address, and telephone number; the drug's generic and trade name (if any); and the name and address of the source of the drug if it is not manufactured by the sponsor.

- A description of the rare disease or condition for which the drug is being or will be investigated, the proposed indication or indications for the drug, and the reasons why such therapy is needed.

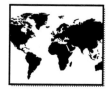

- A description of the drug, and a discussion of the scientific rationale for the use of the drug for the rare disease or condition, including all data from nonclinical laboratory studies, clinical investigations, and other relevant data that are available to the sponsor, whether positive, negative, or inconclusive. Copies of pertinent unpublished and published papers are also required.

- When the sponsor of a drug that is otherwise the same as an already-approved orphan drug seeks orphan-drug designation for the same rare disease or condition, an explanation of why the proposed variation may be "clinically superior" to the first drug (see discussion below).

- When a drug is under development only for a subset of persons with a particular disease or condition, a demonstration that this patient subset is medically plausible.

- A summary of the regulatory status and marketing history of the drug in the United States and in foreign countries (e.g., IND and marketing application status and dispositions; the specific uses under investigation in each country; the indication(s) for which the drug is approved in foreign countries; and any "adverse regulatory actions" that have been taken against the drug in any country).

- Documentation, with appended authoritative references, to demonstrate: (1) that the disease or condition for which the drug is intended affects fewer than 200,000 people in the United States or, if the drug is a vaccine, diagnostic drug, or preventive drug, that the persons to whom the drug will be administered in the United States are fewer than 200,000 per year as specified in federal regulations, or (2) for a drug intended for diseases or conditions affecting 200,000 or more people, or for a vaccine, diagnostic drug, or preventive drug to be administered to 200,000 or more persons per year in the United States, that there is no reasonable expectation that costs of research and development of the drug for the indication can be recovered by sales of the drug in the United States (e.g., cost data, a statement and justification of future development costs the sponsor expects to incur, and an estimate of, and justification for, the expected revenues from drug sales during its first seven years of marketing).

- A statement as to whether the sponsor submitting the request is the "real party in interest" in the development and the intended or actual production and sales of the product.

Drug sponsors may request orphan drug designation any time prior to the submission of a marketing application for the product. Once a request for designation is submitted, the FDA's OPD attempts to issue a decision within 60 days. In most cases, the office handles the review itself, although it may refer certain technical or scientific questions to one of the agency's drug or biological product review divisions. Within 14 months of a drug's designation, and annually thereafter, the sponsor must submit to OPD a brief progress report that includes a short account of the progress of drug development, the investigational plan for the coming year, and any changes that may affect the product's orphan-drug status.

When OPD denies these designation requests, the reasons range from poorly prepared designation request documents to the selection of invalid subpopulations. Before sponsors submit designation requests, OPD officials recommend that companies educate themselves about designation request

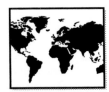

submission requirements, and have a defined rationale for the use of a drug for a selected indication, a reasonable strategy for the product's development, and a highly specific indication and patient population that can be studied and for which the drug can be labeled if ultimately approved.

The practical advantages of orphan drug designation essentially are limited to tax incentives and marketing exclusivity. Although some believe that designation makes FDA drug reviewers more aware of a specific orphan drug, there are probably no real advantages during the drug approval process (see discussion below). FDA staffers claim that many sponsors are surprised to learn that orphan drug designation itself affords no competitive advantages. For example, a drug's designation does not stop another firm from requesting or obtaining a designation for the same drug and indication. Also, the seven-year marketing exclusivity is awarded to the first designated orphan drug to obtain marketing approval, not designation.

There seem to be few, if any, disadvantages to obtaining orphan drug designation. Having to prepare a designation request and having general information published about the drug upon designation are, in many cases, small inconveniences when compared to the benefits designation offers.

Still, some drug firms do not pursue designation when developing a product that would qualify as an orphan drug. In some cases, these firms do not seek orphan designation because they view it as their corporate responsibility as health-care companies to develop these products. Others speculate that companies, knowing that orphan drugs may prove useful in additional, more profitable ways, do not want the possible public relations burden of profiting from a drug developed using public monies.

A Look at Orphan Drug Incentives

Currently, the Orphan Drug Act and the FDA offer orphan drug sponsors four primary incentives: marketing exclusivity, tax credits, protocol assistance, and grants and contracts. More recently, under the Food and Drug Administration Modernization Act of 1997, NDAs for orphan drugs were statutorily exempted from user fees unless "non-orphan" indications are sought in the application.

Marketing Exclusivity Marketing exclusivity may be the single most important incentive to orphan drug sponsors. Under the law, the first sponsor to obtain marketing approval for a designated orphan drug is awarded a seven-year period of marketing exclusivity for the product. During this period, no other sponsor can obtain FDA approval for the drug for the orphan indication. The agency can, however, approve identical versions of the drug for other indications.

The rewards of marketing exclusivity are linked directly to FDA approval. Although orphan designation makes a drug eligible for exclusivity, that exclusivity is not awarded until a product's NDA is approved. Therefore, several identical products could be designated for the same orphan indication, but only the first company to receive approval will obtain marketing exclusivity rights.

Marketing exclusivity has at least two main advantages over traditional patent protection. First, designation and product approval are virtually the only eligibility requirements for exclusivity. The product need not be new or unobvious, or meet any of the criteria used in determining a drug's patent eligibility. Because of this, natural substances and other products that are unable to receive any form of patent protection are eligible for marketing exclusivity.

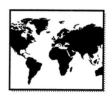

The second significant advantage marketing exclusivity has over patent protection is that its life begins on the date of approval. Although a patent award grants a 20-year monopoly, a drug's patent life begins on the date the patent is awarded, and several years of that life are generally lost during the drug testing and evaluation process. Since exclusivity is awarded upon approval, its seven-year life is not eroded during product development.

While marketing exclusivity may be the most important orphan drug incentive, it is also the most complex. In the past, some critics have argued that the FDA's inability or unwillingness to deny marketing approval to drugs that are similar in structure to drugs that have already been awarded marketing exclusivity has unfairly denied orphan product innovators the protection afforded to them under the Orphan Drug Act.

In fact, the FDA's criteria for determining when two orphan drugs designated for the same indication are considered identical have been tested at least four times, the last of which was ongoing as of this writing. During the late 1980s, the FDA faced a pair of widely publicized cases involving two human growth hormone products and two erythropoietin products. The issue, in both cases, involved the FDA's then-unpublished criteria for differentiating between medical compounds, particularly biologics and biotechnology products, for the purposes of marketing exclusivity.

Then, in December 1992, the FDA's orphan drug regulations first established the conditions under which the agency would consider two drugs to be the same and, therefore, take action to block the approval of the second designated product:

> "(i) If it is a drug composed of small molecules, a drug that contains the same active moiety as a previously approved drug and is intended for the same use as the previously approved drug, even if the particular ester or salt (including a salt with hydrogen or coordination bonds) or other noncovalent derivative such as a complex, chelate or clathrate has not been previously approved, except that if the subsequent drug can be shown to be clinically superior to the first drug, it will not be considered to be the same drug.
>
> (ii) If it is a drug composed of large molecules (macromolecules), a drug that contains the same principal molecular structural features (but not necessarily all of the same structural features) and is intended for the same use as a previously approved drug, except that, if the subsequent drug can be shown to be clinically superior, it will not be considered the same drug. This criterion will be applied as follows to different kinds of macromolecules:
>
> > (A) Two protein drugs would be considered the same if the only differences in structure between them were due to post-translational events, or infidelity of translation or transcription, or were minor differences in amino acid sequence; other potentially important differences, such as different glycosylation patterns or different tertiary structures, would not cause the drugs to be considered different unless the differences were shown to be clinically superior.
> >
> > (B) Two polysaccharide drugs would be considered the same if they had identical saccharide repeating units, even if the number of units were to vary and even if there were postpolymerization modifications, unless the subsequent drug could be shown to be clinically superior.

(C) Two polynucleotide drugs consisting of two or more distinct nucleotides would be considered the same if they had an identical sequence of purine and pyrimidine bases (or their derivatives) bound to an identical sugar backbone (ribose, deoxyribose, or modifications of these sugars), unless the subsequent drug were shown to be clinically superior.

(D) Closely related, complex partly definable drugs with similar therapeutic intent, such as two live viral vaccines for the same indication, would be considered the same unless the subsequent drug were shown to be clinically superior."

These regulations established the concept of clinical superiority, and made it the criterion upon which the agency could base its approval of a second designated drug that is otherwise identical to, and is marketed for the same indication as, a previously approved designated orphan drug. To be considered clinically superior, a drug must offer a "significant therapeutic advantage" over the existing product. According to FDA regulations, this advantage can be based upon evidence of greater effectiveness, improved product safety in a significant segment of the target population, or, in exceptional cases, "a major contribution to patient care."

The FDA's application of these provisions was challenged in early 1996, when Berlex Laboratories filed suit to block the agency's approval of Biogen's Avonex (interferon beta), a competitor to Berlex' Betaseron (interferon beta), which was already marketed as a treatment for relapsing/remitting multiple sclerosis. Based on what is viewed as a safety advantage—fewer injection site reactions—the agency approved Avonex, stating that "a small demonstrated improvement in efficacy or diminution in adverse reactions may be sufficient to allow a finding of clinical superiority." In late 1996, the U.S. District Court dismissed the Berlex suit.

A more recent challenge to the FDA's "sameness" provisions came in mid-1999, when Baker Norton, a generic drug company, challenged the agency's regulations for determining when two products are the same. The company sued the agency because it was seeking to market a generic version of Bristol-Myers Squibb's Taxol (paclitaxel), even though Taxol has orphan exclusivity for Karposi's sarcoma. Specifically, the company asked the court to establish that the orphan drug regulation's definition of the term "drug" is inconsistent with the provisions of the Orphan Drug Act. In arguments made before the court in May 1999, Baker Norton contended "that FDA's reliance on active moieties to distinguish one small molecule drug from another is not permissible under the statute." The company also argued that the concept of "clinical superiority," through which the agency can determine that two identical drugs are different, has no basis in the Orphan Drug Act. Baker Norton argued that the plain meaning of "drug" is the "drug product," rather than simply the active moiety. In other words, the company wanted to force the agency to consider factors other than the active moiety, including differences in formulation and labeling, in determining when two drugs are different. Ultimately, however, the Baker Norton arguments failed, as the court ruled in favor of the FDA and its interpretation of the Orphan Drug Act's provisions.

At this writing, Serono was attempting to use the FDA's clinical superiority provisions to gain marketing approval for Rebif, its interferon beta-1a product for relapsing-remitting multiple sclerosis. To accomplish this, Serono would have to break Biogen's orphan exclusivity for Avonex, something the company hoped to due by establishing Rebif's clinical superiority through a comparative head-to-head efficacy trial against Avonex. After submitting the results of this trial during 2001, Serono was hoping to gain FDA approval for Rebif by mid-2002.

Tax Credits Sponsors of designated orphan drugs are eligible for a 50 percent tax credit for funds spent on clinical development. Therefore, a firm can subtract directly from its annual tax bill one-half of the money spent on the clinical testing of an orphan drug.

However, there are several important limitations to the tax credit incentive:

- Sponsors can receive credits only for clinical testing conducted within the United States. The one principal exception to this is a situation in which the sponsor must go outside the United States to find the patients necessary to conduct the trial.

- The credits can be used only for clinical testing actually paid for and conducted by the sponsor. For example, a sponsor could not receive credits for another company's testing that is referenced in the sponsor's drug application.

- The credits are available only for products that are formally designated by the FDA.

- The credit can be applied only to testing conducted for the orphan indication for which a drug is designated.

- Tax credits do not apply to nonclinical testing. OPD staffers claim that this can be a problem, since basic animal toxicity and carcinogenicity testing alone can cost well over a million dollars.

Through the enactment of the Small Business Job Protection Act of 1996, Congress addressed what was, at least for many biotechnology and other fledgling companies, perhaps the most notable limitation to the Orphan Drug Act's tax incentives: Originally, tax credits were only beneficial to companies that were profitable. Under previous law, orphan product tax credits could be applied against taxes on profits, but could not be used to increase a company's losses or be carried forward into a year in which the company would post profits.

Tax code revisions made under the Small Business Job Protection Act permit companies to carry forward tax credits into a year in which they can be applied against profits. The law's provisions allow credits to be carried forward for 15 years, something that can impart immediate value on small, startup firms interested in partnering or other business arrangements (i.e., because a firm can pass along the tax credit to a larger firm that can use it immediately).

Because the orphan drug tax credit provisions traditionally had to be reauthorized periodically by Congress, there was considerable uncertainty in this area. Recently, however, Congress passed legislation making the tax credit provisions permanent.

Protocol Assistance Protocol assistance is an incentive for which orphan designation is unnecessary. If a sponsor can show the FDA that a drug will ultimately be used for a rare disease or condition, the agency provides written recommendations on the nonclinical and clinical studies needed for the product's approval. With CDER and sponsors working so closely on most drug development programs today, however, the value of this incentive is likely minimal.

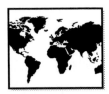

To obtain protocol assistance, a sponsor must submit a formal request providing information on the drug, including its intended use, available test data, regulatory and marketing status, and proposed testing plans. The FDA's 1992 orphan drug regulations specify 16 content requirements for such requests. OPD staffers warn that, unless sponsors ask specific questions in these requests, firms are likely to receive extremely vague recommendations. Protocol recommendations are made by product review divisions within CDER.

FDA Grants and Contracts The Orphan Drug Act authorizes the U.S. Congress to appropriate funds for grants and contracts to physicians, companies, and others who are developing orphan drugs. In recent fiscal years, the Office of Orphan Product Development was granted $11 to $11.5 million for such purposes.

More common than contracts, grants are awarded to university-based investigators and some smaller companies, particularly biotechnology firms, for the clinical testing of orphan drugs. Contract funds, on the other hand, are available to investigators and companies that agree to conduct testing for a drug or in a therapeutic area of particular interest to the FDA.

Orphan Drug Designation and Approval Statistics, 1990–2000

	1990	1991	1992	1993	1994	1995	1996	1997	1998	1999	2000
Orphan Designation Applications Received*	131	84	77	72	81	73	78	72	123	94	88
Orphan Designations Made*	89	80	56	65	58	56	60	55	67	79	68
Average NDA Approval Time (months) (all NDAs)	35.4	28.6	32.6	33.1	25.3	19.2+	17.8+	17.6	12.8	13.5	15.0
Average Orphan NDA Approval Time (months)	24.4	20.2	17.6	12.8	25.1	14.3+	19.2+	17.5+	13.4+	12.0+	6.3+
# of Orphan Drug Approvals	12	12	13*	13*	11*	11*	23*	19*	20*	20*	14*
# of Active Orphan Designations	–	–	–	–	–	–	–	708*	752*	807*	858*
Cumulative # of Orphan Product Approvals	–	–	–	–	–	–	–	167*	185*	197*	218*

* drugs and biologics
+ New Molecular Entities only

Source: FDA

The FDA Approval Process: Advantages for Orphan Drugs?

Generally, orphan products receive no preferential treatment in terms of testing and submission requirements, and face the same safety and effectiveness criteria and review processes as undesignated products. FDA staffers do claim, however, that the agency will modify the drug testing and approval process for orphan products when appropriate. In the past, issues such as the availability of patients with orphan conditions and the lack of competitive therapies have forced the agency to consider alternative testing requirements and review criteria.

NDAs submitted for orphan products are reviewed within one of the FDA's drug review divisions. There, reviewers evaluate products strictly on the basis of safety, efficacy, and risk-benefit analyses.

Worldwide Pharmaceutical Regulation Series

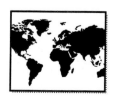

Although the product's status as an orphan drug may appear to be of little or no benefit, OPD staffers do work to make agency reviewers more sensitive to the special issues that orphan products present.

One advantage that many orphan drugs have over other products is that they often—although not always—receive priority reviews. This is related not to the fact that the products are designated orphan drugs, but that they are frequently the only treatments available for certain conditions. Because of this, the FDA generally classifies them as high-priority drugs, and expedites their review. The FDA has denied at least one petition requesting that all orphan drugs automatically receive the FDA's highest review priority, however.

Historically, approval times for orphan drugs have compared favorably with those of conventional drugs, according to FDA statistics (see exhibit below). In 2000, the agency approved NDAs for orphan drug NMEs in an average of 6.6 months, compared to 18.5 months for all other NME NDAs. In most years, however, the review-time difference has not been as dramatic.

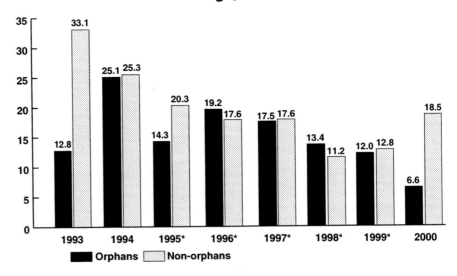

Mean Orphan Drug Approval Times vs. Approval Times of Other Drugs, 1993–2000

* 1995, 1996, 1997, 1998, 1999 and 2000 analyses include only New Molecular Entity (NME) drugs

What is the OPD's role in the review of an orphan drug? The office actively monitors the progress of orphan reviews, but has no formal authority in product approvals or real influence in the decisions of FDA reviewers. OPD staffers do attend FDA-sponsor meetings, however, and act as mediators to help resolve special regulatory problems presented by orphan drugs.

References

1. Shulman, S.R. and Manocchia, M. (Tufts Center for the Study of Drug Development), The U.S. Orphan Drug Program: 1983-1995.
2. Ibid.

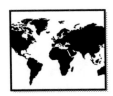

CHAPTER 14

CDER's Bioresearch Monitoring Program

Given that its regulatory decisions are based directly on research data, CDER has a vested interest in the accuracy and validity of clinical and nonclinical study results submitted in NDAs and other applications. Under CDER's Bioresearch Monitoring Program (BIMO), agency investigators conduct on-site inspections of laboratories, clinics, and offices where scientific data are developed and stored to ensure the quality of the data submitted in such filings.

Specifically, CDER inspects clinical investigators, drug firms, IRBs, and nonclinical laboratories to ensure: (1) that data submitted in product applications are accurate and valid; and (2) that the rights and welfare of human subjects are protected in clinical studies. During these inspections, FDA investigators evaluate how well sponsors, monitors, contract research organizations, IRBs, and clinical and nonclinical investigational site staff have fulfilled their various responsibilities and commitments under GCP, study protocols, and other standards and regulatory requirements.

In the late 1990s, a series of disclosures shook CDER's confidence in the data collected by clinical investigators and in the pharmaceutical industry's ability to detect investigator noncompliance—and even fraud—through their routine monitoring practices. Primary among these was the case of Southern California Research Institute President and Principal Investigator Robert Fiddes, M.D., who was sentenced in 1998 to 15 months in prison and was fined $800,000 for falsifying and fabricating clinical trial data used in NDAs for multiple drug products and for prescribing prohibited medications to manipulate clinical data. During 1998 and 1999, this case prompted a series of congressional inquiries into CDER's actions in the Fiddes case, FDA efforts to detect research fraud and the extent of fraud-related problems in clinical research, the agency's authorities to conduct oversight of and to discipline clinical investigators, and the general practices that clinical investigators employ to recruit patients for trials.

Although CDER since has released data indicating that the incidence of research fraud is small (i.e., less than 5%), the disclosures in the Fiddes case, and the congressional attention and widespread press coverage that they prompted, helped to set in motion several agency initiatives and responses that are having fundamental effects on CDER's BIMO program. In addition, CDER has looked in recent years to evaluate how it should modernize its BIMO program in response to emerging realities in the clinical research process, among them the commercialization of clinical research, the increasing use of computers to collect clinical data, the flood of new clinical investigators participating in trials, and the increasing use of pivotal trial data from foreign trial sites.

Sporadic, but high profile, reports of compliance problems in clinical trials have kept the public and political pressure on the U.S. government to respond. In June 2001, for example, the agency cited Johns Hopkins Asthma and Allergy Clinic for its failure to submit an IND for a clinical investigation involving the administration of hexamethonium bromide by inhalation to three human subjects, and for failing to report an unanticipated adverse event to its IRB. A healthy 24-year-old volunteer died of acute distress syndrome after developing a cough following hexamethonium inhalation.

In response to these and other developments, CDER has taken several steps under, or relevant to, the center's BIMO program:

- As the federal government mobilized to respond to the above-mentioned disclosures and perceptions regarding an undermined public confidence in the clinical research process, the NIH and FDA both reorganized to form offices to spearhead initiatives in the human research subject protection area. In March 2001, the FDA formed the Office for Human Research Trials (OHRT) within the Office of the FDA Commissioner to coordinate the agency's human subject protection policies and activities, and to direct the agency's international harmonization, outreach and GCP regulation initiatives. In late 2001, the FDA renamed OHRT the Office for Good Clinical Practice in an effort to highlight the distinct roles of the FDA office from those of the Department of Health and Human Services' Office for Human Subject Protections. The formation of OGCP has taken a toll on the management of CDER's Division of Scientific Investigations (DSI), which has lost both David Lepay, M.D., Ph.D., and Stan Woollen, the former DSI director and deputy director, respectively. In late 2001, CDER named DSI Acting Director Joanne Rhoads, M.D., who was on a 90-day detail from her post as medical team leader within the Division of Antiviral Drug Products, as the permanent director of DSI.

- Acknowledging that "a major gap" exists between its current clinical research inspectional capability and the monitoring level necessary to assure the protection of volunteers in clinical research, the FDA moved to "significantly increase the number inspections, focusing on high-risk situations and responding rapidly to potential problems," the agency stated in its annual performance plan for FY2001. In the FDA's view, "high-risk" trials include those conducted by "sponsor-investigators" who have a proprietary interests in the product under study and studies enrolling vulnerable populations (e.g., mentally impaired, pediatric). Further, FDA officials spoke about closing "loopholes" in current regulations, including one that allows sponsors to avoid reporting investigator misconduct by keeping an investigator "on their books" and not formally terminating the investigator from the study. The agency plans to close this loophole in its regulations, which require sponsors to report investigator misconduct only when an investigator is terminated, by requiring reporting whenever there are serious compliance problems or misconduct, including data falsification, fraud, and human subject protection abuses.

- CDER's BIMO, whenever extremely problematic investigator noncompliance is discovered, is continuing its attempts to link such physicians back to specific drug sponsors to assess where such noncompliance should have been detected through the companies' routine monitoring practices. In early 1998, CDER completed an analysis of six particularly problematic clinical investigators, one of whom was conducting studies for 43 sponsors under 91 different INDs. Center officials said that there was "a pool of sponsors" that several of these investigators shared.

- In 1999, physicians from CDER's Division of Scientific Investigations (DSI) first began to participate in protocol design meetings, IND reviews, end-of-Phase 2 meetings, and related activities in an effort consider clinical monitoring issues early in the development process and to build quality into the development process up front. Through their participation in end-of-Phase 2 meetings with sponsors, DSI physicians are reviewing and commenting on sponsors' planned monitoring and quality assurance programs for Phase 3 trials. The prospective involvement of DSI staff, who fulfilled a purely compliance role previous to this initiative, was thought to be a first within the drug center. In part to reflect this emerging role, DSI was moved from CDER's Office of Compliance to the center's Office of Medical Policy in mid-1999.

- To ensure that complaints of investigator misconduct are addressed in a timely fashion, DSI has developed and implemented a set of new policies and procedures for handling reports of possible investigator misconduct. This action is said to be a response to criticism that many months passed between the initial complaint to CDER and the center's initial action in the Fiddes case. In turn, DSI has seen an increase in reports of possible investigator misconduct. Of 13 complaints made by sponsors in FY1999, 7 involved the possible falsification of clinical data. DSI officials are hoping that increasing numbers of sponsors become more proactive in reporting possible misconduct on a voluntary basis. Complaints of possible misconduct from all sources, including sponsors, the public, and others, surged from 9 in FY1998 to 101 in FY1999. During 2001, FDA officials reiterated their commitment to promoting patient reporting of clinical trial problems by establishing and creating awareness of "channels" for such reports to the FDA, the investigator, and the investigator's institution.

- To communicate its expectations for remote data entry systems and other computerized systems employed in the clinical development process, CDER released a May 1999 industry guidance entitled, *Computerized Systems Used in Clinical Trials*. The guidance, which center officials acknowledge is vague due to the rapid evolution of computer systems and clinical settings, "addresses how data quality might be satisfied where computerized systems are being used to create, modify, maintain, archive, or transmit clinical data."

- Under a regulation that took effect in 1999, CDER is requiring NDA sponsors to submit information concerning the financial interests of, and compensation paid to, investigators who conduct key clinical studies (see Chapter 7). This regulation is the result of emerging concerns regarding the effects of investigator financial interests on the validity of research data. When NDA reviewers determine that such interests or compensation "raise a serious question about the integrity of the data," CDER could order DSI to conduct an audit of the data collected by the clinical investigator in question.

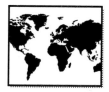

CDER's Bioresearch Monitoring Program

Chapter 14

- In May 2000, the FDA and Department of Health and Human Services (HHS) unveiled a "plan of action" in response to what FDA Commissioner Jane Henney, M.D., called "the failure of some researchers at prestigious institutions...to follow the most basic elements of what it takes to properly conduct clinical studies." The action plan came in response to investigator noncompliance (i.e., failure to report adverse experiences) in highly publicized gene therapy trials. As part of this plan, which seeks to heighten government oversight of clinical research and to reinforce to research institutions their responsibility to oversee their clinical researchers and IRBs, HHS was to pursue legislation authorizing the FDA to levy civil monetary penalties of up to $250,000 per clinical investigator and $1 million per research institution for violations of informed consent and "other important research practices." As of late 2001, HHS and members of Congress were still considering this legislative proposal. In addition, the FDA/HHS action plan comprised several other moves focusing largely on upgraded training and guidance for clinical investigators (see Chapter 6). Although the FDA claimed to be in the process of upgrading its informed consent-related and IRB-related guidance documents, it was facing increasing criticism for not having acted on many of these initiatives, particularly in the informed consent area, by mid-2001. At the same time, a pair of HHS reports concluded: (1) that the growing demands that multi-center trials are placing on IRBs are making it increasingly difficult for such boards to fulfill their duties: and (2) that the FDA should, through its site inspections, look more closely at strategies used to recruit study subjects (e.g., enrollment incentives). In part a response to the first of these HHS reports, a June 2000 House bill entitled, "Human Research Subjects Protection Act" (HR 4605), which ultimately failed, sought to establish standards for IRBs and IRB membership and to discourage IRB "shopping" by requiring clinical investigators to disclose prior IRB study protocol rejections.

- Continuing its several-year focus on industry monitoring practices, FDA officials in early 2001 encouraged sponsors to broaden their monitoring efforts to include assessments of the trial-related activities of clinical research staff at various clinical sites being inspected. Traditionally, industry monitoring inspections have focused largely on the activities of clinical investigators. In late 1997, BIMO officials first announced that they would be looking more closely at industry's monitoring practices, which was part of a larger effort to further educate themselves on evolving monitoring practices and how they may need to be upgraded. Beginning in January 1998, all CDER inspectional assignment packages contained new instructions for FDA field inspectors to examine specific aspects of sponsor monitoring during inspections of clinical investigators. The center used the inspectional results to help establish a "baseline" of industry's monitoring activities in the late 1990s. Although this initial data-gathering effort has been completed, CDER's increased focus on monitoring practices is now showing itself in compliance-related actions: After issuing a combined 15 clinical investigator warning letters (i.e., a formal notification of noncompliance) in 1998 and 1999, the drug center issued 13 in the first nine months of 2000.

- In 2000, the HHS and FDA contracted with the Institute of Medicine (IoM) to form an independent panel to examine, and make recommendations for improving, the human subject protection systems in clinical trials. Since beginning its work in December 2000, the panel has issued its first report, which focuses on IRBs and

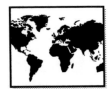

which recommends an accreditation system for such boards. In the second and final phase of its work, the panel is examining other areas, including informed consent and the work of IRBs and clinical investigators. Its second report, which is expected to include broader recommendations on improving human subject protections in clinical research, is due in September 2002.

- An increasing focus on international clinical trials also may have implications for CDER's BIMO program. A September 2001 HHS report entitled, *The Globalization of Clinical Trials: A Growing Challenge in Protecting Human Subjects* discussed the implications of the ever-increasing number of foreign clinical investigators providing data to be used in NDAs—the number of foreign investigators conducting studies under INDs has grown 16-fold from 1990 to 1999, the report claims. Due to concerns regarding the adequacy of foreign IRBs, and the fact that the FDA's lack of information on foreign IRBs makes it difficult to assure the same level of human subject protections in foreign trials as domestic studies, the HHS report made several recommendations, including that the FDA: (1) work with foreign regulators to obtain more information regarding foreign IRBs; (2) help newly formed foreign IRBs "build capacity" to conduct effective human subject reviews; (3) encourage sponsors to obtain attestations from foreign investigators stating that they will adhere to ethically sound research principles (as is required under IND regulations); (4) encourage more rigorous sponsor monitoring of foreign trials; (5) develop a database to track the growth and location of foreign research; and (6) work with HHS to encourage all IRBs to participate in a voluntary accreditation system.

While clinical investigators are the focus of most CDER bioresearch inspections, there are several reasons why the results of such inspections are of great importance to clinical trial sponsors. First, drug sponsors are ultimately responsible for the conduct of clinical studies, and FDA inspections are designed, today more than ever, to determine how well sponsors perform in that role. Secondly, these inspections, should they uncover serious problems, can result in the agency's rejection of data essential to a drug's approval. As mentioned above, a sponsor also may now face inspectional and compliance implications whenever it is found to have worked with noncompliant clinical investigators.

Like virtually all other CDER drug review and compliance efforts, the Bioresearch Monitoring Program has been affected by the agency's prescription drug user fee program. Since the center faces mandated deadlines for NDA reviews, preapproval bioresearch monitoring inspections must be conducted within short time frames so that inspection results may be evaluated promptly. The compressed inspectional time frames have presented new challenges for FDA field investigators. This pressure is likely increasing given FDAMA provisions establishing that review division actions cannot be delayed due to the unavailability of information from, or action by, field inspectors, unless the review division determines that a delay is necessary to assure a drug's safety or effectiveness.

In addition, CDER reviewers and clinical investigations staff have been forced to carefully scrutinize the need for various inspectional assignments given resource limitations. Therefore, although inspectional activity may have risen in recent years because the agency was approving more NDAs, the number of studies and sites inspected per application may be lower today than in the past. CDER's DSI continues to be asked to focus its inspectional resources on those studies that are truly pivotal to a drug's approval.

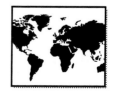

A Brief History of the Bioresearch Monitoring Program

The origin of the FDA's authority to inspect research data and related records lies in the Food, Drug and Cosmetic (FD&C) Act. The law states that every person required to maintain records must, upon the FDA's request, allow access to clinical data for review and copying. FDA regulations and Form FDA-1572 *Statement of Investigator*, which clinical investigators sign before undertaking the study of an investigational drug, state that "…the investigator will make such records available for inspection and copying."

Because of physicians' importance in the development and collection of clinical safety and efficacy data, inspections of investigators represent the core of CDER's Bioresearch Monitoring Program. FDA inspections of clinical investigators began in 1962, although only three inspections were conducted by 1965. The agency expanded its efforts in the years following, and established a four-person office to organize and conduct inspections. Since government authorities outside the FDA believed that only physicians should inspect other physicians, however, inspectional activities were limited (i.e., only seven or eight inspections were conducted annually).

By 1972, the U.S. government had gained a new respect for the importance and abilities of FDA inspectors. As a result, the FDA initiated a survey of 162 commercially sponsored clinical investigators, 70 noncommercial clinical investigators, and 15 manufacturers. The results of this multi-year study, and increased FDA staff and budget, led to the founding of the agency's Bioresearch Monitoring Program in June 1977.

Although this chapter focuses on clinical investigator and sponsor/monitor compliance activities, today's Bioresearch Monitoring Program consists of five separate compliance inspection programs, each designed to evaluate the activities of a key entity in the conduct of a scientific study:

- Clinical Investigator Compliance Program;
- Sponsor/Monitor Compliance Program;
- Institutional Review Board (IRB) Compliance Program;
- Nonclinical Laboratory Compliance Program (for information on the inspection of nonclinical laboratories, see Chapter 2); and
- In Vivo Bioequivalence Compliance Program.

These inspectional programs are managed by three branches within CDER's Division of Scientific Investigations (DSI): Good Clinical Practices Branch I, Good Clinical Practices Branch II, and the GLP and Bioequivalence Investigations Branch. DSI's former Human Subject Protection Team, which dealt with IRB issues, has been absorbed into the division's two GCP branches.

Due in part to rising government concerns about the abilities of IRBs to fulfill their responsibilities in the growing and increasingly complicated clinical research market, the FDA has stepped up its inspections of the estimated 1,600 IRBs. From 1997 to 1999, for example, the number of IRB inspections surged 34 percent (see exhibit below). Still, notes the agency, only 4% to 5% of all IRB inspections require formal regulatory action.

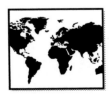

CDER Investigator, Foreign Investigator, IRB, and Sponsor/Monitor/CRO Compliance Inspectional Activity, 1995-2000

(# of inspection of each type)

	1995	1996	1997	1998	1999	2000
U.S. Clinical Investigators	312	393	297	246	293	296
Foreign Clinical Investigators	28	40	42	64	61	49
Institutional Review Boards	170	158	143	184	191	155
Sponsors, Monitors, CROs	4	7	1	4	10	28

Source: CDER

The Clinical Investigator Compliance Program

As stated previously, inspections of clinical investigators represent the core of CDER's Bioresearch Monitoring Program. CDER has three separate investigator inspection programs:

- Study Oriented Inspection Program;
- Investigator Oriented Inspection Program; and
- Bioequivalency/Bioavailability Inspection Program.

Study Oriented Inspection Program Formerly called the Data Audit Program, the Study Oriented Inspection Program is a routine surveillance effort that involves the inspection of 300 to 400 clinical investigators per year. During these inspections, which are conducted during an NDA's review, an FDA field inspector looks at the conduct of the study and performs a data audit. In evaluating the investigator's conduct of a clinical study, the inspector considers several factors, including the following:

- what the investigator, each of his/her staffers, and others did during the study;
- the degree of delegation of authority;
- when and where specific aspects of the study were performed;
- how and where data were recorded;
- how the drug substance was stored and accounted for;
- the monitor's interaction with the physician;
- evidence that proper informed consent was obtained from subjects; and
- evidence that IRB approval was obtained for studies performed.

In the typical audit, data submitted in an NDA are compared with the on-site records that should support their validity. On-site records to which an FDA inspector must be given access include a physician's office records, hospital records, and various laboratory reports. Records obtained prior to the initiation, and following the completion, of the study may be reviewed and copied.

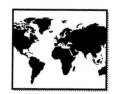

As noted above, CDER leveraged its investigator inspections in the late 1990s to gain insights on how well sponsors monitored investigations. Although this initial data-gathering effort is now complete, DSI officials maintain that the sponsor's performance in monitoring a trial continues to be evaluated on some levels.

Because of the inspectional program's nature, CDER's DSI does not publicize its criteria for selecting studies and sites for routine inspections. Obviously, however, a particular study's importance to the approval decision will have a direct bearing on its likelihood of being inspected.

The division also uses a sampling method for determining the number of sites within a particular study to be inspected, although the number is often influenced by other factors, including a protocol's complexity. CDER drug reviewers and DSI staff will also consider the number of patients at a site (i.e., sites with the most patients), the number of adverse experiences reported (i.e., sites with far fewer or greater reports), and the number of dropouts at a site. Although CDER had been developing an internal policies and procedures manual to describe the study and site selection and assignment process, that project has been on hold since mid-1999.

When CDER has targeted key clinical studies and sites for inspection, agency staffers send a field inspector an "assignment package," which includes copies of a representative case report form (CRF), case report form tabulations, the protocol, and other pertinent information. The assignment package will indicate the number of subject records to be inspected at the site. If the field inspector discovers potential problems, he or she can then inspect other site records.

Due to the nature of physicians' work and schedules, study oriented inspections are made by appointment. Therefore, investigators are alerted as to which study is to be audited, and are given the opportunity to locate, collect, and organize all relevant records.

Because sponsors increasingly are relying on foreign data in their drug applications, CDER is now conducting significantly more inspections of foreign clinical investigators per year. In FY1999, for example, CDER conducted 64 inspections of foreign clinical trial sites, almost triple the number conducted just four years earlier. Overall, foreign inspections represented 21 percent of all CDER investigator inspections in FY1999, up from just 7% in FY1995.

"Investigator Oriented" Inspection Program The "investigator oriented" site inspection is, in most respects, similar to the study oriented, or routine, inspection. Investigator oriented inspections are not routine, however, and may be initiated for one or more of several reasons:

- the investigator is suspected of impropriety;
- the investigator is responsible for a large volume of work, particularly if that work involves different medical disciplines;
- the investigator has done work outside his or her specialty;
- the investigator reports drug effectiveness that appears to be too optimistic when compared to the reports of other physicians studying the same drug;
- the investigator reports no toxicity or few adverse reactions when other physicians report numerous reactions of a certain type;

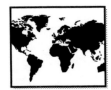

Cumulative Results of CDER Study-Oriented (Surveillance)[1] Inspections of Clinical Investigators (6/1/77–1/1/2001)

6139 surveillance inspections have been issued since 6/1/77*
5992 have been received to date. Of these:

Cancellations	344
Washouts	125
Reviewed	5504
Under Review	19

Classifications (New classification structure as of 1/1/94)	No.	% of 5504
Number of investigators in full compliance; no deficiencies noted (NAI)	1491	27
Number of investigators with objectionable practices which do not represent major departures from regulations (VAI)	3693	67
Number of inspections where objectionable conditions or practices represent significant departures from regulations (OAI)**	320	6

Most Common Deficiencies*

Inadequate patient consent form	2328	42
Failure to adhere to protocol	1743	32
Inadequate and inaccurate records	1421	26
Inadequate drug accountability	1008	18

Other Deficiencies

Failure to keep IRB informed of changes, progress	324	6
Inappropriate follow-up of adverse reactions	274	5
Unapproved concomitant therapy	115	2
Problems with records availability	113	2
Failure to obtain IRB approval if necessary	116	2
Failure to list additional investigators on Form 1572	81	2
Failure to obtain patient consent****	69	1
Inappropriate payment to volunteers	28	-
Submission of false data	24	-
Inappropriate delegation of authority	14	-
Commercialization of drug	10	-
Use of drug before obtaining IND status	4	-
Subjects receiving simultaneous investigational drugs	5	-

[1]Note: Previous category of "surveillance" inspections is changed to "study-oriented." But the new category is not exactly parallel to the old.

*Included are 68 Biologics inspections conducted between 10/1/85 and 1/1/88.

**Includes warning letters as of 1/1/94.

***One inspection may contain no deficiencies or several deficiencies. Therefore the total of percentages will not equal 100.

****FY 77-80 summaries' category "problems with patient consent" has been included under "inadequate patient consent form."

Source: FDA

- the investigator seems to have too many patients with a given disease for the locale or the setting in which he or she practices;
- the investigator reports laboratory results that are consistent beyond the usual biologic variation or that are inconsistent with results submitted by other investigators;
- representatives of the sponsor have reported to the FDA that they are having difficulty obtaining case reports from the investigator, or that they have found the investigator to be deficient in some other manner;
- a routine audit revealed problems too serious to be handled by correspondence; or
- the FDA receives letters or phone calls claiming violations of subject's rights, variations in protocol, or some other violation or noncompliance.

As noted above, an investigator may also be selected for inspection as the result of questions raised regarding the effects of the investigator's financial interests or compensation on clinical data. Under new regulations that went into effect in early 1999, NDA applicants are required to submit information regarding the financial interests of, and compensation paid to, clinical investigators who developed the data submitted in the application. Although DSI physicians will not review such disclosures in NDAs routinely, DSI will receive inspection requests whenever these financial disclosures raise questions regarding the validity of clinical data in the minds of review division medical officers, who will be responsible for evaluating these disclosures.

In mid-2000, CDER gave the first indications of how such financial disclosures were affecting NDA reviews and investigator inspections. When an NDA sponsor discloses financial ties with a clinical investigator, CDER reviewers will specifically look at the number of subjects the investigator recruited and if he or she had any reporting outliers in terms of adverse experiences, according to center officials. If such analyses turn up questionable findings, the reviewer will initiate data audits with DSI, which might ask that the data be analyzed further, request additional studies to confirm the study's results, or reject the study as a pivotal trial in the NDA. Of 129 marketing applications submitted between February 2, 1999, and April 30, 2000, 33 provided financial disclosure information on at least one investigator (i.e., rather than a certification that no financial arrangement was involved or a claim that the disclosure requirements were not relevant to the study). At that time, the agency had not rejected any study as a pivotal study because of a disclosed financial arrangement with a sponsor.

Investigator oriented inspections are usually conducted by a DSI reviewer and a field investigator. Although the procedures used parallel those of routine inspections, the inspection team probably reviews more data. For instance, the inspection team will probably evaluate more case reports—sometimes for the entire study—and may audit studies of more than one drug. Patient interviews may be conducted when there are questions as to whether a subject participated in a study, whether the subject had the condition being studied, or whether informed consent was obtained. In addition, investigator oriented inspections are more likely to focus on the particular aspect of a study in question (e.g., delegation of authority) rather than attempting to review all aspects of a study.

Many investigator oriented inspections also differ from study oriented inspections in that they are unannounced inspections. In cases in which the agency suspects an investigator of study fraud, manipulation of records, or other misconduct, DSI will not contact the investigator prior to the inspection.

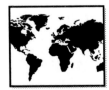

Cumulative Results of CDER Investigator-Oriented (For Cause)[1] Inspections (6/1/77–1/1/2001)

598 for cause inspections have been issued since 6/1/77*
561 have been received to date. Of these:

Cancellations	5
Washouts	9
Reviewed	511
Under Review	26

Classifications (New classification structure as of 1/1/94)	No.	% of 511
Number of investigators in full compliance; no deficiencies noted (NAI)	117	23
Number of investigators with objectionable practices which do not represent major departures from regulations (VAI)	210	41
Number of investigators where objectionable conditions or practices represent significant departures from regulations (OAI)**	184	36

Most Common Deficiencies***	No.	% of 489****
Failure to adhere to protocol	267	55
Inadequate and inaccurate records	261	53
Inadequate patient consent form	207	42
Inadequate drug accountability	138	28

Other Deficiencies		
Failure to keep IRB informed of changes, progress	61	12
Unapproved concomitant therapy	48	10
Submission of false data	50	10
Problems with records availability	38	8
Inappropriate follow-up of adverse reactions	35	7
Inappropriate delegation of authority	21	4
Failure to list additional investigators on Form 1572	13	3
Failure to obtain IRB approval if necessary	12	3
Subjects receiving simultaneous investigational drugs	11	2
Failure to obtain patient consent*****	8	2
Use of drug before obtaining IND status	6	1
Commercialization of drug	3	1
Inappropriate payment to volunteers	0	-

[1] Note: Previous category of "for cause" inspections is changed to "investigator-oriented." But the new category is not exactly parallel to the old.

* Included are 68 Biologics inspections conducted between 10/1/85–1/1/88.

** Includes warning letters as of 1/1/94.

*** One inspection may contain no deficiencies or several deficiencies. Therefore the total of percentages will not equal 100.

**** There are 22 missing or incomplete files for which no deficiencies could be abstracted.

***** FY 77-80 summary contained a category "problems with patient consent" which has been included under "inadequate patient consent form."

Source: FDA

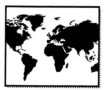

Despite the well-publicized cases of investigator misconduct in recent years, agency statistics indicate that few CDER site inspections are uncovering major regulatory violations. In FY1999, about 1% of investigator inspections in the United States were found to have objectionable conditions or practices representing significant departures from federal regulations. Roughly 45% of U.S. sites were found to be in full compliance, while 50% of the sites were able to address minor violations through voluntary actions.

Despite the more frequent use of trial sites in countries that have never before conducted trials for use in U.S. submissions (sites in some countries, such as Canada and England, have long been used), foreign site compliance has generally improved in recent years, CDER compliance data suggest. In FY1998, for example, 43% of foreign sites were found to be in full compliance, more than triple the rate for the FY1995/FY1994 period. Surprisingly given that foreign sites are generally less familiar with U.S. standards, the prevalence of foreign sites with significant noncompliance was slightly less than at U.S. sites during FY1998.

For all clinical sites, the most common categories of deficiencies in FY1999 included protocol violations (27% of sites), records (20%), adverse experience reporting (15%), drug accountability (9%), and informed consent (8%).

Bioequivalency/Bioavailability Inspection Program Bioequivalency/bioavailability inspections involve the inspection of both a clinical and an analytical facility. According to FDA staffers, these inspections are more important for the verification of biopharmaceutic data submitted for generic drugs than for new drugs. An FDA field inspector and an FDA laboratory scientist qualified in the evaluation of analytical techniques conduct this audit.

During the inspection of a biopharmaceutic facility, where a drug is administered to, and blood samples are then taken from, human volunteers, the inspection team will verify that IRB approval was given for the study and that all regulatory requirements were met. The inspector might review such records and factors as drug accountability records, prescreening laboratory data, the presence of medical supervision, the handling of biological samples, and the assessment of situations in which the health and safety of the subjects are placed at risk.

In the analytical audit, the inspection team reviews standard operating procedures for the technology utilized, the status of the samples to be analyzed, qualifications of the personnel performing the analyses, raw documentation of the reported results, and the presence of quality control techniques such as the use of standard curves.

Post-Inspectional FDA Actions

At the conclusion of all three types of inspections, the FDA inspector conducts what is called an "exit interview" with the clinical investigator. During this exchange, the two individuals discuss the inspector's findings, which will be reported to the FDA in the form of an Establishment Inspection Report (EIR).

In some cases, the inspector may leave the investigator with a written statement of his/her observations on Form FDA-483, the *Inspectional Observation Form*. This statement identifies the relevant deviations from regulations, which may include protocol deviations, IRB noncompliance, or inadequate informed con-

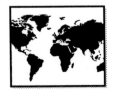

New Drug Approval in the United States

sent. The inspection results are discussed in detail with the clinical investigator, whose responses are recorded as part of the EIR. CDER provides a detailed discussion of the Clinical Investigator Compliance Program in its *Compliance Program Guidance Manual for Clinical Investigators* (7348.811).

When the agency determines that an investigator has repeatedly or deliberately failed to comply with regulatory standards or has submitted false information to the study's sponsor, it may disqualify that investigator from receiving investigational drugs, and thereby prevent the physician from participating in future clinical trials. After regulatory violations are discovered, some investigators may agree to certain restrictions (e.g., participate in only a limited number of studies as a principal investigator at once, be personally involved in specified aspects of a study) in their activities regarding future studies. In rare instances in past years, the agency has agreed not to impose sanctions on certain violative investigators because the investigators have given assurances for their performance in future studies (e.g., will use specific SOPs, will participate in single dose studies only).

From 1964 through 1999, CDER had disqualified 99 clinical investigators, prosecuted or convicted 20, and imposed restrictions on or obtained assurances from another 26. In 1999, the drug center disqualified 2 clinical investigators and issued 8 warning letters. In 1998 and 1999, CDER issued a total of 15 warning letters to clinical investigators after having issued only 22 from 1993 through 1997. Just 9 months into 2000, however, CDER had already issued 13 investigator warning letters. CDER's Disqualified/Restricted/Assurances List for Clinical Investigators is available on the center's website.

The Sponsor/Monitor Compliance Program

Historically, CDER's Sponsor/Monitor Compliance Program has not been one of the center's most active monitoring programs. In the past, FDA officials claimed that this has been due to several factors, including relatively broad regulations on sponsor requirements and CDER's greater concerns about investigator activities and compliance. Agency officials also maintained that, in comparing an NDA's data tabulations with site records during investigator inspections, CDER is also indirectly inspecting the sponsor's records.

Not surprisingly given the increased focus on monitoring practices, however, CDER revised its approach to sponsor/monitor inspections in late 1999. CDER's DSI was not only planning to conduct more sponsor/monitor inspections going forward, but also to evolve such inspections from the "information-gathering investigations" (i.e., quick and focused reviews directed at specific records, such as randomization reports) to more traditional compliance inspections, which are more comprehensive.

DSI's increased activity became obvious in 2000. The division conducted 28 sponsor/monitor/CRO inspections in 2000, after having conducted only 26 in the previous 5 years combined.

"For cause" sponsor/monitor inspections, which have been less common in the past, are performed when there are indications that a sponsor is not fulfilling its responsibilities. Due to CDER's upgraded clinical trials complaint process, DSI officials point out that such inspections have been on the rise.

CDER initiates sponsor inspections to determine: (1) if a sponsor, a sponsor's employee, or a contract research organization (CRO) is monitoring a clinical investigation adequately; and (2) if the sponsor

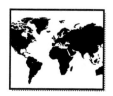

is fulfilling each of its requirements as outlined in existing federal regulations. The clinical sponsor and its research-related activities are the primary focus of inspections conducted under this program. It is worth mentioning, however, that the activities of two other entities, because they may assume some of the sponsor's responsibilities during a clinical study, may also be investigated by the FDA:

- Clinical Monitors. Monitors are those individuals selected by either a sponsor or contract research organization to oversee the progress of the clinical investigation. The monitor may be an employee of the sponsor, a contract research organization, or a consultant.

- Contract Research Organization (CRO). CROs are organizations or corporations that enter into contractual agreements with sponsors to perform one or more of the sponsor's duties in the clinical research process. Sponsors may delegate several of their responsibilities to a CRO, including the design of a protocol, the monitoring of clinical studies, the selection of investigators and study monitors, the evaluation of reports, and the preparation of materials to be submitted to the FDA.

Initially under its reinvigorated sponsor/monitor inspectional program, DSI was to pursue sponsor/monitor inspectional assignments only for new molecular entities (NME), and planned to tie them to clinical investigator assignments. In other words, whenever DSI is called on to conduct a clinical site inspection regarding a pending NDA for an NME, it will also conduct a sponsor/monitor inspection.

As noted above, today's sponsor/monitor inspections are also be more traditional compliance inspections. This means that the inspections are comprehensive investigations of the sponsor/monitor's practices, and that such inspections sometimes trigger formal regulatory communications, such as notices of adverse findings and warning letters. CDER issued only one warning letter to a sponsor in 1999.

The Inspection of Drug Sponsors Sponsor inspections take place at the company's headquarters, and generally involve the evaluation of records from recently conducted or active studies. According to the FDA's *Compliance Program Guidance Manual for Sponsors, Contract Research Organizations, and Monitors* (7348.810), the field inspector evaluates at least six elements of a clinical study: (1) the selection of, and directions to, a monitor; (2) test article accountability; (3) assurance of IRB approval; (4) the adequacy of facilities; (5) continuing evaluation of data; and (6) records retention.

Monitor Selection and Directions. In this aspect of the inspection, the FDA investigator determines if the clinical monitor is adequately qualified, and whether the sponsor has given the monitor sufficient direction. Specifically, the inspector must determine:

- whether at least one individual has been charged with monitoring the progress of the investigation (if there are two or more monitors, the inspector must determine how the responsibilities are divided);

- what training, education, and experience qualify the monitor to oversee the progress of the clinical investigation;

- whether written procedures have been established for the monitoring of the clinical investigation; and

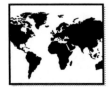

- whether the sponsor has assured that the monitor has met his or her obligations.

Test Article Accountability. The inspector must evaluate whether the sponsor maintained adequate drug accounting procedures before, during, and, if applicable, after a clinical investigation. The inspector is instructed to make six separate determinations:

- whether the sponsor maintained accounting procedures for the test article, including records showing: (1) the shipment dates, quantity, serial, batch lot or other identification number of units sent; (2) the receipt dates and the quantity of returned articles; and (3) the names of investigators;
- whether the records are sufficient to allow a comparison of the total amount of the drug shipped against the amounts used and returned by the investigator;
- whether all unused or reusable supplies of the test article were returned to the sponsor when either (1) the investigator discontinued or finished participating in the clinical investigation, or (2) the investigation was terminated;
- if all unused or reusable supplies of the test article were not returned to the sponsor, a determination of the alternate disposition of the test article and a description of how the sponsor determined the manner in which the investigator accounted for unused or reusable supplies of the test article dispensed to a subject and not returned to the investigator;
- whether the alternate disposition was adequate to ensure that humans or food-producing animals were not exposed to experimental risk; and
- whether records were maintained for alternate disposition of the test article.

Assurance of IRB Approval. For a clinical investigation subject to IRB approval, the FDA inspector must determine whether the sponsor maintains documentation showing that the clinical investigator obtained IRB approval before any human subjects were allowed to participate in the investigation.

Ascertaining the Adequacy of Facilities. The FDA inspector must determine whether the monitor assessed the adequacy of all facilities used by the study investigator (e.g., office, clinic, hospital).

Continuing Evaluation of Data. The inspector must examine records to evaluate the clinical sponsor's efficiency in reviewing data submitted by the investigator and in responding to reports of adverse reactions. In this aspect of the inspection, the investigator must make six determinations:

- whether the sponsor reviews all new case reports and other data received from the investigator regarding the safety of the test article within ten working days after receipt;
- whether all case reports and other data received from the investigator are periodically evaluated for effectiveness as portions of the study are completed (included in this determination are the practices of the monitor);
- what actions are taken in response to incomplete case report forms;
- whether there is a system for tabulating the frequency and character of adverse reactions;

- whether existing evidence indicates that the sponsor's present data receipt system is operating satisfactorily; and
- whether any deaths occurred among study subjects, and what actions were taken to determine whether the deaths were related to the use of the test article.

Record Retention. Finally, the inspector must determine the sponsor's compliance with whichever of the following two record retention requirements is applicable: (1) records must be retained for a period of two years after a drug's marketing application is approved; or (2) records must be retained for a period of two years following the date on which the sponsor discontinues the shipment and delivery of the drug for investigational use and so notifies the FDA.

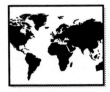

Chapter 15

Accelerated Drug Approval/Expanded Access Programs

Over the past two decades, various medical crises and political pressures have spurred the FDA to develop and implement several programs under which patients could gain access to desperately needed new drugs earlier than would otherwise be permitted under the conventional drug development and approval process. In creating such programs, the FDA has acknowledged that the traditional drug development process is a compromise in many respects, and that the system can be particularly costly to those in dire need of new therapeutic alternatives. After all, it is during this process that potentially valuable drugs may be withheld from patients who may need them while clinical testing and the NDA review move forward.

It is important to point out, however, that this process also protects such patients from unproven experimental drugs that may hurt them or that may keep them from using alternative and perhaps more appropriate therapies. And while critics have charged that some aspects of the drug approval process are unethical and even cruel, the FDA continues to hold that the randomized, placebo-controlled clinical trial remains the single best and most efficient vehicle for determining whether new drugs are safe and effective.

Under efforts that were sometimes called "compassionate drug use" or "emergency drug use," companies developing experimental therapies were permitted to provide the drugs to physicians not involved in the formal clinical trials in an attempt to help desperately ill patients. During the 1980s and early 1990s, however, the AIDS crisis thrust the FDA into a crucible of victim desperation and public and political pressure. Ultimately, the medical realities and politics of AIDS spurred the FDA to develop and implement several plans under which promising new therapies could reach desperately ill patients more quickly. From 1987 through 1992, the FDA developed and implemented four programs that were designed to expedite patients' access to emerging therapies, either by allowing patients access to unapproved therapies or by accelerating the drug development and approval process: the treatment IND, a mechanism that provides patients with access to promising, but as-yet unapproved drugs for serious and life-threatening diseases; parallel track, a plan that provides patients suffering from AIDS or AIDS-related diseases with early access to experimental-stage

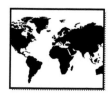

Accelerated Drug Approval/ Expanded Access Programs

Chapter 15

therapies; an accelerated drug development program for drugs designed to treat life-threatening and seriously debilitating diseases; and an accelerated drug approval program for therapies designed to treat serious or life-threatening illnesses.

For at least two reasons, the desperation and public pressure that prompted government action began to abate at least somewhat beginning in the early 1990s. First, victims of AIDS and AIDS-related conditions had a growing number of approved therapeutic options to treat their conditions. Secondly, increasing numbers of experts began to question the wisdom of providing early and expanded access to therapies whose risks and benefits have not been characterized in traditional drug development processes. Since the early 1990s, for instance, some have questioned the relevance of the surrogate endpoints on which the approval of the first AIDS therapies were based.

Further, some agency advisors pointed to several patient deaths during a Phase 2 trial involving the hepatitis B treatment fialuridine (FIAU) as both a warning about the dangers of expanded access plans and a confirmation of the value of traditional drug development schemes. Although FIAU was not used in an expanded access program, members of the FDA's Antiviral Drugs Advisory Committee pointed out that, if the drug had shown early activity against AIDS, it might have been used in such a scheme. Five trial-related deaths might have become dozens or even hundreds under an expanded access program, they speculated during a 1993 meeting. One member of the committee, which reviews AIDS treatments as well, suggested that the pendulum had begun to swing away from early drug access and expedited development plans and back toward conventional drug development programs.

During the mid-1990s, the very patient advocacy groups that had most aggressively sought earlier access to unproven therapies seemed to seek what a traditional drug development process could offer: Better labeling and a more thorough assessment of a drug's safety and effectiveness. At FDA advisory committee meetings and in communications with agency officials, it was the AIDS community itself that had begun to question the use of surrogate markers, which could speed drug development but which would require validation following a therapy's approval.

In the late 1990s, other factors seemed to undermine the appeal of these programs. For example, with CDER approving new drugs in an average of 12 months or less (less than half the time required in the early 1990s), and AIDS treatments in an average of less than 6 months, some companies may no longer consider participation in these programs necessary to ensure rapid approvals and rapid patient access to new therapies.

Despite this, the FDA's four initial expanded access and accelerated development/approval programs stand largely as they did when introduced, although they are now, in most cases, less active than they once were. Further, a pair of programs designed to expedite drug approvals have taken their places alongside the programs mentioned above.

On March 29, 1996, the FDA unveiled a formal program designed to expedite the development and approval of new cancer treatments. In response to mounting criticism over the imbalance of resources targeted to AIDS drug reviews versus those targeted to other life-threatening illnesses, the FDA established what it called the Oncology Initiative. This program brought several reforms that some analysts estimated would reduce cancer drug development times by at least a year and cut average oncology drug review times from 12.4 to 6 months (see discussion below).

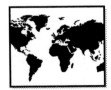

The most recent evolution in the FDA's various expanded access/accelerated development programs came in the form of a new program authorized under the FDA Modernization Act of 1997 (FDAMA). Through this law, Congress added a new program designed to expedite the development and approval of new drugs for unmet medical needs associated with serious or life-threatening conditions. Under the "fast track" program, which incorporates and, therefore, mirrors the accelerated approval program and similar programs in many respects, Congress introduced certain new provisions, including the submission of "rolling"—or incomplete—NDAs for agency review (see discussion below).

Congress also used FDAMA to codify, in the Food, Drug and Cosmetic Act, some of the FDA's existing expanded access programs for which federal regulations already provided:

Access to Experimental Drugs in Emergency Situations. FDAMA added to the FD&C Act a new section specifically allowing the FDA to authorize the shipment of investigational drugs designed to diagnose, monitor, or treat a serious disorder or condition in so-called "emergency situations." This element of the law essentially codifies existing FDA regulations, which permit the agency to authorize the shipment of a drug for a specified emergency use in advance of an IND submission (see Chapter 3). In recent FDA discussions of experimental drug access programs, the agency also mentions "special exemptions," or "compassionate exemptions," which can be used when a particular patient cannot meet the eligibility criteria of a certain study protocol. If a sponsor and investigator agree to treat a patient under a special exemption, a request that includes the rationale for the request and a brief patient history must be submitted to the agency.

"Individual Patient Access" to Investigational Drugs. FDAMA also adds to the FD&C Act provisions that permit a patient, through a licensed physician, to request from a manufacturer or distributor access to an investigational drug intended to diagnose, monitor, or treat a serious disease or condition. A manufacturer or distributor may provide such a drug to a physician under the following circumstances: (1) the physician determines that the patient has no comparable or satisfactory alternative therapy and that the probable risk from the investigational drug does not surpass the probable risk from the disease or condition; (2) the FDA determines that there is sufficient evidence of the drug's safety and effectiveness to support its use in this situation; (3) the FDA determines that permitting the use of the drug in this instance will not interfere with the initiation, conduct, or completion of the clinical investigations designed to support marketing approval; and (4) the drug's sponsor or clinical investigator submits a clinical protocol consistent with the regulations associated with treatment use in a single patient or a small group of patients (see discussion on treatment INDs below). The FDAMA provisions regarding "individual patient access" essentially codified existing FDA regulations, which already provided for such access.

Treatment INDs. FDAMA essentially codified in law the FDA's existing treatment IND regulations (see discussion below). Upon the submission of what FDAMA terms an "expanded access protocol," which is equivalent to a treatment IND or treatment protocol, by a sponsor or clinical investigator, the FDA will permit an investigational drug to be made available for widespread patient access under a treatment IND, provided that specific conditions are met, including that the drug is for the diagnosis or treatment of a serious or life-threatening disease or condition. FDAMA also authorizes the agency to inform national, state, and local medical associations, health organizations, and other appropriate groups about the availability of investigational drugs under expanded access protocols.

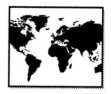

Worldwide Pharmaceutical Regulation Series

Accelerated Drug Approval/ Expanded Access Programs

Chapter 15

In late 2001, CDER was developing a proposed regulation on compassionate drug use that will outline the agency's criteria for a variety of drug access options under which patients not enrolled under formal clinical trials can gain access to experimental therapies. At June 2001 congressional hearings prompted by the increased attention that FDA policies regarding patient access to experimental therapies have received due in part to the promise of developmental-stage cancer treatments, FDA officials emphasized that they "actively support" wider access to drugs prior to approval. The new regulation, they claimed, would give the agency its first formal policy on compassionate drug use, even though such use has been permitted for many years.

The following discussions highlight the six principal expanded access/accelerated approval programs mentioned above.

The Treatment IND

Although the FDA had been pressured to reform clinical testing methodologies in the past, the unique issues posed by AIDS highlighted the drawbacks of the drug development process perhaps as never before. As Burroughs Wellcome's AZT, or Retrovir, emerged as the first therapy to show promise in treating AIDS, victims of the disease not fortunate enough to be enrolled in clinical trials refused to die silently in the name of science. While the intense public debate that followed was often bitter, it was not unproductive. After early clinical studies of AZT showed promising results, the FDA quickly approved what it called a treatment IND, under which more than 4,000 patients were allowed access to AZT while the drug underwent final FDA review.

The realities of AIDS first brought formal changes to FDA regulations on May 22, 1987, when the agency published a final rule allowing the treatment use and sale of investigational drugs intended to treat desperately ill patients. Specifically, the regulations were "intended to facilitate the availability of promising new drugs as early in the drug development process as possible…to patients with serious and life-threatening diseases for which no comparable or satisfactory alternative drug or other therapies exist."

In many respects, the treatment IND was a compromise that attempted to satisfy those who believed that the desperately ill should have unlimited access to an emerging therapy, and those who believed that a developmental-stage drug should be withheld from patients outside the clinical trial setting until such testing is completed and is judged to have demonstrated the drug's safety and effectiveness. Under a treatment IND, desperately ill patients gain access to a promising drug while the all-important clinical development and FDA review of a drug continue.

Although it was the AIDS crisis that eventually brought the FDA to formalize the treatment IND as it is now known, agency officials point out that the treatment IND has its roots in the 1960s and 1970s. At that time, applications commonly referred to as "compassionate INDs" were used to make unapproved antiarrhythmics, calcium channel blockers, and beta blockers accessible to patients intolerant to other therapies. In the early 1980s, FDA regulations formally recognized the treatment IND, allowing its use in cases in which: (1) there was sufficient evidence of safety and effectiveness; (2) the potential benefits outweighed the risks; and (3) the medical condition under study was a serious disease with no satisfactory therapies.

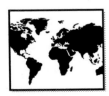

The 1987 regulations took a relatively loose concept and, for the first time, defined the treatment IND's purpose, established more specific criteria for FDA approval, and described how and when the treatment IND could be used. The regulations specify the point in a product's development at which treatment use may begin, a key factor since preapproval accessibility was the primary goal of the treatment IND.

To qualify for treatment use under the FDA's treatment IND regulations, a drug must meet four principal criteria. According to federal regulations, "FDA shall permit an investigational drug to be used for a treatment use under a treatment protocol or treatment IND if: (i) The drug is intended to treat a serious or immediately life-threatening disease; (ii) There is no comparable or satisfactory alternative drug or other therapy available to treat that stage of the disease in the intended patient population; (iii) The drug is under investigation in a controlled clinical trial under an IND in effect for the trial, or all clinical trials have been completed; and (iv) The sponsor of the controlled trial is actively pursuing approval of the investigational drug with due diligence." In FDAMA's codification of the FDA's treatment IND regulations, the law reiterates the four criteria above and specifies one additional criterion: For drugs being tested in a controlled clinical trial, the availability of an investigational drug under a treatment use must not interfere with the enrollment of patients in the ongoing investigation.

The second criterion noted above deserves a brief discussion, primarily because the entire treatment IND concept is designed for desperately ill individuals with no therapeutic alternatives. Responding to concern about its interpretation of the "no comparable or satisfactory alternative drug or other therapy available" requirement for treatment IND eligibility, the FDA has clarified that this standard is met "when there are patients who are not adequately treated by available therapies, even if the particular disease does respond in some cases to available therapy. This criterion would be met, for example, if the intended population is for patients who have failed on an existing therapy (i.e., the existing therapy did not provide its intended therapeutic benefit or did not fully treat the condition); for patients who could not tolerate the existing therapy (i.e., it caused unacceptable adverse effects); or for patients who had other complicating diseases that made the existing therapy unacceptable (e.g., concomitant disease making available therapy contraindicated) for the patient population."

In reality, FDA regulations provide for two different treatment IND vehicles—one for drugs designed to treat immediately life-threatening illnesses, and the other for drugs intended to treat serious diseases. The timing of, and FDA criteria for granting, treatment INDs for the two types of indications differ considerably.

Treatment Use for Immediately Life-Threatening Conditions Under the May 1987 regulations, the FDA defined "immediately life-threatening disease" as a stage of a disease in which there is a reasonable likelihood that death will occur within a matter of months or in which premature death is likely without early treatment. The agency claimed that it would apply a common sense definition so that death within more than a year would not normally be considered immediately life-threatening, but that death within several days or even several weeks would fall under the definition.

For illustrative purposes, the FDA identified in the regulations nine diseases that would "normally" be considered immediately life-threatening: advanced cases of AIDS, advanced congestive heart failure

(New York Heart Association Class IV), recurrent sustained ventricular tachycardia or ventricular fibrillation, herpes simplex encephalitis, most advanced metastatic refractory cancers, far advanced emphysema, severe combined immunodeficiency syndrome, bacterial endocarditis, and subarachnoid hemorrhage (see listing below of treatment INDs approved).

Provided that a drug meets the four principal criteria outlined above, the FDA may only deny a treatment IND "if the available scientific evidence, taken as a whole, fails to provide a reasonable basis for concluding that the drug: (A) May be effective for its intended use in its intended patient population; or (B) Would not expose the patients to whom the drug is to be administered to an unreasonable and significant additional risk of illness or injury." The rather vague efficacy standard was discussed just briefly in the regulation's preamble, which stated that, "...the level of evidence needed is well short of that needed for a new drug approval—and may be less than what would be needed to support treatment use in diseases that are serious but not immediately life-threatening."

One of the more hotly debated aspects of the treatment IND regulations was the timing of treatment programs for drugs used against immediately life-threatening conditions. Some regarded the FDA's criteria as too liberal, and claimed that these criteria allow general accessibility before a drug development program can be expected to provide sufficient evidence of safety and/or effectiveness. The FDA, however, held to the provisions of its early proposals, and allows drugs for immediately life-threatening conditions to be "made available for treatment use...earlier than Phase 3, but ordinarily not earlier than Phase 2."

The FDA emphasizes, however, that available scientific evidence, rather than simply the phase of development, is more important to its decision-making process: "FDA expects that data from controlled clinical trials will ordinarily be available at the time a treatment IND is requested. However, FDA is committed to reviewing and considering all available evidence, including results of domestic and foreign clinical trials, animal data, and, where pertinent, in vitro data. FDA will also consider clinical experience from outside a controlled trial, where the circumstances surrounding an experience provide sufficient indication of scientific value."

Treatment Use for Serious Conditions The FDA's criteria for granting treatment INDs for serious conditions were considerably less controversial than those for immediately life-threatening illnesses. Interestingly, however, the FDA provided no specific definition of "serious" in either the treatment IND proposal or final rule. The agency did give examples of serious conditions: Alzheimer's disease, advanced multiple sclerosis, advanced Parkinson's disease, transient ischemic attacks, progressive ankylosing spondylitis, active advanced lupus erythematosus, certain forms of epilepsy, nonacidotic or hyperosmolar diabetes, and paroxysmal supraventricular tachycardia.

To qualify for treatment use, drugs intended to treat serious illnesses must meet a tougher, if more vague, safety and effectiveness standard than that described above for life-threatening conditions. The FDA "may deny a request for treatment use...if there is insufficient evidence of safety and effectiveness to support such use."

Considering this requirement, it is not surprising that treatment INDs for serious illnesses are more likely to be granted later in the clinical development process than are therapies for immediately life-

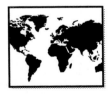

threatening conditions: "In the case of serious diseases, a drug ordinarily may be made available for treatment use...during Phase 3 investigations or after all clinical trials have been completed; however, in appropriate circumstances, a drug may be made available for treatment use during Phase 2."

Obtaining FDA Permission for Treatment Use Both drug sponsors and practicing physicians may pursue FDA approval for a treatment use. The sponsor of a drug's IND may do so through a treatment protocol, while "licensed practitioners" must submit a treatment IND.

According to FDA regulations, a sponsor-submitted treatment protocol must provide:

- the intended use of the drug;
- an explanation of the rationale for use of the drug, including, as appropriate, either a list of what available regimens ordinarily should be tried before using the investigational drug, or an explanation of why the use of the investigational drug is preferable to the use of available marketed treatments;
- a brief description of the criteria for patient selection;
- the method of administration and the dosages of the drug; and
- a description of clinical procedures, laboratory tests, or other measures designed to monitor the effects of the drug and to minimize risk.

Additionally, a treatment protocol must "be supported" by an informational brochure for each treating physician, technical information relevant to the safety and effectiveness of the drug for the intended treatment purpose, and a commitment by the sponsor to ensure the compliance of all participating investigators with informed consent requirements.

Like a traditional IND submission, a treatment protocol becomes active 30 days after the FDA receives the protocol, or on earlier notification by the FDA that the treatment use may begin. Of course, treatment protocols are also subject to clinical holds any time after submission.

If a practicing physician wants to obtain for treatment use a drug whose sponsor will not establish a treatment protocol for this purpose, the practitioner must submit his or her own treatment IND. Such applications must contain:

- a cover sheet (Form FDA 1571);
- information on the drug's chemistry, manufacturing, and controls, and prior clinical and nonclinical experience with the drug (when not provided by the sponsor either directly or through the incorporation-by-reference of information in the existing IND);
- a statement of the steps taken by the practitioner to obtain the drug from the sponsor under a treatment protocol;
- a treatment protocol containing all the information required for such a submission (see discussion above);
- a statement of the practitioner's qualifications to use the investigational drug for the intended treatment use;

Accelerated Drug Approval/Expanded Access Programs

Chapter 15

- the practitioner's statement of familiarity with information on the drug's safety and effectiveness derived from previous clinical and nonclinical experience with the drug; and
- the practitioner's commitment to report to the FDA safety information in accordance with current regulations.

The licensed practitioner who submits a treatment IND is the "sponsor-investigator" for such an IND, and is responsible for meeting all applicable sponsor and investigator responsibilities. Like standard INDs and treatment protocols, treatment INDs may be initiated 30 days after submission or upon earlier notification by the FDA.

The Sale of Investigational Drugs The FDA's treatment IND regulations also contain provisions that allow sponsors to sell investigational drugs under some conditions. Drug sponsors may not "commercialize an investigational drug by charging a price larger than that necessary to recover costs of manufacture, research, development, and handling of the investigational drug," however.

According to federal regulations, a sponsor may charge for an investigational drug under a treatment protocol or treatment IND, provided that: "(i) There is adequate enrollment in the ongoing clinical investigations under the authorized IND; (ii) charging does not constitute commercial marketing of a new drug for which a marketing application has not been approved; (iii) the drug is not being commercially promoted or advertised; and (iv) the sponsor of the drug is actively pursuing marketing approval with due diligence."

At least 30 days prior to selling an investigational drug, a sponsor must notify the FDA in writing and, with this notification, include a certified statement that the requested price is not greater than the amount necessary to recover costs associated with the drug's manufacture, research, development, and handling. If the FDA does not contact the sponsor within the 30-day review period, the sponsor is free to begin selling the drug.

A sponsor may also sell a drug in any clinical trial, provided the sponsor can gain the FDA's prior approval. To obtain this approval, the sponsor must provide an adequate explanation of why sale of the drug is necessary to either begin or continue a trial.

Unfortunately, the final regulations give few details on how a company can show that the sale of a drug is necessary or how this necessity should be determined. The regulation's preamble states that "charging for investigational drugs during a clinical trial would normally not be allowed... FDA believes that cost recovery is justified in clinical trials only when necessary to further the study and development of a promising drug that might otherwise be lost to the medical armamentarium. The agency believes that this situation is most likely to arise in the context of new products derived through biotechnology which are produced by small, medium and large firms alike."

The FDA has approved the sale of several investigational products under the treatment IND program. A 1995 Tufts Center for the Study of Drug Development study found that 9 of the first 33 drugs granted treatment IND status were also approved for sale during development, including Serono's Serostim, Teva/Lemmon's Copolymer-1, Gynex' Oxandrin, Warner-Lambert's Cognex, Genzyme's

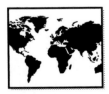

Ceredase, Lyphomed/Fujisawa's Nupent, Somerset's Eldepryl, and Massachusetts Department of Public Health's Cytomegalovirus immunoglobulin.

Although 39 treatment INDs, including 11 for HIV/AIDS and 13 for cancer, have been granted, the submission and approval of treatment INDs have diminished somewhat since 1991 (see listing below). From 1991 through September 1999, the agency granted just 21 treatment INDs. The reasons, many believe, are related partly to continuing industry ambivalence toward the IND program, perhaps because of issues related to the potential costs, complexities and liabilities associated with expanded access. And while the agency still recommends treatment INDs to some sponsors, it is also obvious that the FDA has never been as aggressive in recruiting treatment INDs as it once was under Frank Young, M.D., who was the FDA commissioner when the program was introduced and who left the agency in 1989.

It is worth noting that another expanded access program, called the Group C program, is considered to be a subset of the larger treatment IND program. Established under an agreement between the FDA and National Cancer Institute (NCI), the Group C treatment IND provides a mechanism for distributing investigational cancer agents to oncologists outside a controlled clinical trial. Group C drugs, which are typically in Phase 3 trials and have shown evidence of relative and reproducible efficacy in a specific tumor type, are distributed only by the NCI under an NCI protocol.

Designated Treatment INDs: June 1987-September 1999
(drugs and biologics)

Generic (Trade Name)	Sponsor	Indication	Designation Date
Cytomegalovirus immunoglobulin[b,o]	Mass. Dept. of Public Health	Prevention of cytomegalo-virus infections in certain renal transplant patients	10/19/87
Ifosfamide[c,e,o] (Ifex)	NCI/BMS	Testicular cancer (in conjunction w/mesna)	12/24/87
Mesna[c,o] (Mesnex)	NCI/Asta	Hemorrhagic cystitis (in conjunction w/ifosfamide)	12/24/87
Trimetrexate[e,o] (Neutrexin)	NIAID/Warner-Lambert (licensed to U.S. Bioscience)	PCP	2/12/88
Clomipramine (Anafranil)	Ciba Geigy	Severe OCD	6/3/88
Selegiline[o] (Eldepryl)	Somerset	Parkinson's	6/16/88
Pentostatin[c,e,o] (Nipent)	NCI/Warner-Lambert	Hairy cell leukemia	7/28/88
Teniposide[c,o] (Vumon)	NCI/BMS	Refractory acute lymphoblastic leukemia	10/7/88
Gancyclovir[e] (Cytovene)	NIAID/Syntex	Cytomegalovirus retinitis	11/28/88
Aerosolized Pentamadine Isethionate[e,o] (Nebupent)	Lyphomed/Fujisawa	PCP (AIDS) [new formulation]	2/3/89
Levamisole HCL[c] (Ergamisol)	NCI/Janssen	Colon cancer (in conjunction w/ 5-flurouracil)	5/4/89

—continued—

Accelerated Drug Approval/ Expanded Access Programs

Chapter 15

Generic (Trade Name)	Sponsor	Indication	Designation Date
Erythropoietin[b,o] (Eprex)	Ortho	AIDS-associated anemia [new indication]	6/27/89
Colfosceril Palmitate[e,o] (Exosurf neonatal)	Burr. Wellcome	Neonatal respiratory distress syndrome	7/26/89
Didanosine/ddI[a] (Videx)	NIAID/BMS	AZT-intolerant AIDS-related Complex	9/28/89
Beractant[b,e,o] (Survanta)	Abbott	Neonatal respiratory distress syndrome	9/29/89
Zidovudine/AZT[a] (Retrovir syrup)	Burr. Wellcome	AIDS in children [new indication]	10/26/89
Alglucerase[b,e,o] (Ceredase)	NINDS/Genzyme	Gaucher's disease	11/7/89
Fludarabine Phosphate[c,e,o] (Fludara)	NCI/Triton Biosciences*	Chronic lymphocytic leukemia	11/24/89
Baclofen Intrathecal[d,o] (Lioresal)	Medtronic	Spasticity in oral baclofen-intolerant MS/SCI patients [new formulation]	3/7/90
Sargramostim/ GM-CSF[b,o] (Leukine)	Immunex	Neutropenia due to bone marrow transplant	9/24/90
Zalcitabine/ddC[a,o] (Hivid)	Hoffmann La Roche	AZT-intolerant ARC/AIDS patients	5/30/91
Perfosfamide/4-HC[o] (Pergamid)	Scios-Nova	Ex vivo treatment of bone marrow	6/14/91
Oxandrolone[o] (Oxandrin)	Gynex**	Boys with constitutional delay of puberty [new indication]	10/17/91
Atovaquone[e,o] (Mepron)	Burr. Wellcome	PCP	11/8/91
Tacrine (Cognex)	Warner-Lambert	Alzheimer's disease	12/02/91
Rifabutin[e,o] (Mycobutin)	Adria	Prophylaxis of myco-bacterium avium complex	3/6/92
Cladribine/2-CDA[c,o] (Leustatin)	Ortho	Hairy cell leukemia	3/6/92
Paclitaxel[c] (Taxol)	BMS	Ovarian cancer	7/15/92
Oxandrolone[o] (Oxandrin)	Gynex**	Girls with Turner's Syndrome [new indication]	10/21/92
Copolymer-1[o] (Copaxone)	Teva Marion Partners	Multiple sclerosis	1/5/93
Metformin (Glucophage)	Lipha	Non-insulin dependent diabetes mellitus	9/10/93
Vinorelbine (Navelbine)	Burr. Wellcome	Non-small cell lung cancer	4/14/94
Human Growth Hormone[b,e,o] (Serostim)	Serono	AIDS-associated wasting/weight loss	12/20/94
Gemcitalbine HCl (Gemzar)	Lilly	Locally advanced or metastatic pancreatic cancer	1/27/95
Atorvastatin (Lipitor)	Warner-Lambert	Homozygous familial hypercholesterolemia or severe refractory hypercholesterolemia	2/9/95

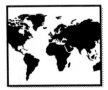

Generic (Trade Name)	Sponsor	Indication	Designation Date
Riluzole[o] (Rilutek)	RPR	Amyotrophic lateral sclerosis (ALS)	6/20/95
Cell Therapy[b,o] Autologous Peripheral Blood Lymphocytes	Cellcor	Treatment of metastatic (Stage IV) renal cell carcinoma	9/15/95
Cidofovir[b] (Vistide)	Gilead	Relapsing cytomegalovirus retinitis	9/1/95
Carmustine Wafer[o] (Gliadel)	Guilford/RPR	Recurrent malignant glioma-intracranial therapy	10/27/95
Insulin-like Growth Factor IGF[o] (Myotrophin)	Cephalon/Chiron	Protein-based therapeutic treatment of amyotrophic lateral sclerosis	6/24/96
Nelfinavir mesylate (Viracept)	Agouron	Protease inhibitor for use by patients for whom other treatments have failed	9/12/96
Progestereone Vaginal Gel (Crinone)	Columbia Research Labs	In vitro fertilization	2/7/97
Xyrem (sodium oxybate)	Orphan Medical	Narcolepsy	12/16/98

a=accelerated approval; b=biological; c=group C cancer drug; d=device; e=Subpart E designation; o=orphan drug designation. * Berlex acquired Triton Biosciences in 1990; ** Gynex merged with Bio-Technology General in 1993.

Source: Shulman, SR, Tufts Center for the Study of Drug Development, June 1997; FDA

The FDA's Accelerated Drug Development Program (Subpart E)

By mid-1988, the FDA had successfully implemented several initiatives designed to make drugs more accessible through both preapproval availability plans and speedier reviews. At that time, the treatment IND regulations were in effect, and seven experimental therapies had been available to patients with AIDS, cancer, Parkinson's disease, and other life-threatening conditions. In addition, the agency had established a new level of review priority for all AIDS products, and had created a new drug review division to focus on evaluating these therapies. The FDA credited such initiatives with the rapid availability and review of AZT, which the agency approved only 107 days after the submission of Burroughs Wellcome's NDA.

In August 1988, then-Vice President George Bush, in his capacity as the chairman of the Presidential Task Force on Regulatory Relief, asked the FDA to build on these "successes" by developing procedures for expediting the marketing of new therapies intended to treat AIDS and other life-threatening illnesses. In the two months that followed, FDA officials met with representatives from other government agencies, AIDS groups, and consumer, health, and academic organizations to obtain input on developing this program.

The FDA released such a plan on October 21, 1988: its *Interim Rules on Procedures for Drugs Intended to Treat Life-Threatening and Severely Debilitating Illnesses*, or Subpart E procedures. The interim rule, which the FDA claims is based on its experience with AZT, is described by the agency as an attempt "to speed the availability of new therapies to desperately ill patients, while preserving appropriate guarantees for safety and effectiveness. These procedures are intended to facilitate the development, evaluation, and marketing of such products, especially where no satisfactory therapies exist. These procedures reflect the recognition that physicians and patients are generally willing to accept greater risks or side effects from products that treat life-threatening and severely debilitating illnesses than

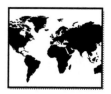

they would accept from products that treat less serious illnesses. These procedures also reflect the recognition that the benefits of the drug need to be evaluated in light of the severity of the disease being treated. The procedures apply to products intended to treat acquired immunodeficiency syndrome (AIDS), some cancers, and other life-threatening and severely debilitating illnesses."

Like the treatment IND, the FDA's accelerated development plan was announced with considerable fanfare and, in turn, was met by some degree of skepticism. Even officials within the FDA review units responsible for the approval of AIDS and cancer therapies claimed that the plan's primary elements—close sponsor consultation and an accelerated clinical testing scheme—were already common practice.

But because it provides for a drug's approval before its sale, the accelerated development program has three key advantages over the treatment IND, according to the FDA: (1) no limitations are put on the pricing or profitability of FDA-approved drugs; (2) consumers who buy FDA-approved drugs are eligible for third-party reimbursement, for which patients under treatment INDs cannot qualify; and (3) FDA approval confers some liability protection to manufacturers.

Essentially, there are four key components to the FDA's expedited development plan: (1) early and increased FDA and sponsor consultation aimed at formulating agreements on the design of preclinical and clinical studies needed for marketing approval; (2) the "compression" of Phase 3 clinical trials into Phase 2 testing; (3) the FDA's adoption of a modified medical risk-benefit analysis when assessing the safety and effectiveness of qualifying drugs; and (4) the use of Phase 4 postmarketing studies to obtain additional information about drug risks, benefits, and optimal use.

Eligibility for Accelerated Development Eligibility was perhaps the most fascinating aspect of the interim regulation when it was first released. Recognizing the great opportunities that expedited approval could offer, the drug industry quickly turned to the agency for guidance on which products might qualify for the plan.

In general terms, the expedited development program applies to new drugs, antibiotics, and biologics under study for treating life-threatening or severely debilitating diseases. As is true for every other regulation, the scope of this interim rule is subject to FDA interpretation, which the agency bases on two primary definitions:

- *Life-Threatening Conditions.* For the purposes of the plan, "life-threatening" illnesses include: "(1) Diseases or conditions where the likelihood of death is high unless the course of the disease is interrupted; and (2) Diseases or conditions with potentially fatal outcomes, where the end point of clinical trial analysis is survival." Any disease whose progression is likely to lead to death, particularly in a short period (e.g. six months to one year), would also fall under this definition, as would any "condition on which a study is to be carried out to determine whether the treatment has a beneficial effect on survival (e.g., increased survival after a stroke or heart attack)."

- *Severely Debilitating Conditions.* The FDA has defined "severely debilitating" illnesses as "diseases or conditions that cause major irreversible morbidity," such as severe function deficits in multiple sclerosis, Alzheimer's disease, or progressive ankylosing spondylitis, and blindness due to cytomegalovirus infection in AIDS patients."

The agency cautioned that accelerated development would be relevant only for studies that "will examine the treatment's capacity to prevent or reverse what would otherwise be irreversible damage such as putting ankylosing spondylitis into remission and stopping joint damage and deformity, or preventing blindness."

Despite these definitions, eligibility remained a widely discussed issue in the months following the interim rule's publication. To help educate industry as well as its own staff, the FDA completed a retrospective review of approximately 200 new molecular entities (NME) approved during the 1980s to determine which of these would have been eligible under the new rules. The agency also reviewed its existing inventory of approximately 10,000 drug INDs, and reportedly contacted the sponsors of qualifying drugs.

The Cornerstone of Accelerated Development: Early FDA-Sponsor Consultation Despite serious questions about whether the agency should involve itself in the research process, FDA officials have maintained that early consultation is the single most critical element of this program. The FDA believes that the insights it has gained in reviewing both acceptable and unacceptable drug applications could prove invaluable to sponsors, and that close consultation will allow the agency to share its expertise in the planning and design of both preclinical and clinical development programs.

According to the FDA's interim rule, FDA-sponsor consultations would take two forms:

- Pre-Investigational New Drug Application (IND) Meetings. Prior to an IND submission, the sponsor may request a meeting "to review and reach agreement on the design of animal studies needed to initiate human testing. The meeting may also provide an opportunity for discussing the scope and design of Phase 1 testing, and the best approach for presentation and formatting of data in the IND."

- End-of-Phase 1 Meetings. In the FDA's ideal accelerated drug development program, Phase 3 clinical trials are "compressed" into Phase 2 studies, which then provide the data on which the drug is to be approved. Therefore, after Phase 1 data are available, the sponsor may again request a meeting to "review and reach agreement on the design of Phase 2 controlled clinical trials, with the goal that such testing will be adequate to provide sufficient data on the drug's safety and effectiveness to support a decision on its approvability for marketing."

Restructuring Clinical Trials In attempting to use data derived from Phase 2 trials as the basis for the final approval of a new drug, the FDA brought about, in theory at least, a reasonably significant departure from the traditional drug development and approval path. Interestingly, however, the FDA drug review divisions responsible for evaluating AIDS and cancer therapies claimed to have approved desperately needed new drugs based upon Phase 2 clinical data well before the plan's introduction.

Under the accelerated development scheme, Phase 3 trials are "compressed" into Phase 2 studies, with Phase 1 trials taking on the significance of conventional Phase 2 studies. According to the interim rule, "to increase the likelihood that phase 2 testing can provide sufficient results, sponsors could need to plan phase 2 studies that are somewhat larger and more extensive than is currently the norm, including a mode for replication of key findings. Moreover, to avoid missing an effect by using too little drug, or to avoid studying a dose that proves toxic, it may be necessary to study several doses in

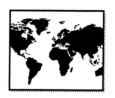

the first formal trials, an approach that may require a larger study but can plainly save time, thereby enabling physicians to treat patients with life-threatening illnesses more rapidly. However, it should be appreciated that if a drug has only minor or inconsistent therapeutic benefits, its positive effects may be missed in this stage of clinical testing, even if the drug ultimately proves to be beneficial following more extensive phase 3 trials."

On the issue of the quantity of data needed for approval, the FDA has stated that, in most cases, two pivotal Phase 2 studies will be necessary: "...the agency cautions that persuasively dramatic results are rare and that two entirely independent studies will generally be required." The approvals of the first AIDS drugs under the accelerated program, however, indicated that the FDA was willing to base the approval of desperately needed drugs on a single pivotal study.

Other Provisions of the Interim Rule The FDA's interim rule contained key provisions in several other areas, including the following:

- Treatment IND. The accelerated development plan was not meant to eliminate the need for treatment INDs. In fact, when the preliminary analyses of Phase 2 results appear promising, the FDA may ask the sponsor to submit a treatment IND, under which the test drug could be made available while the sponsor prepares, and the FDA reviews, the NDA.

- FDA Risk-Benefit Analysis. According to the interim rule, the "FDA will consider the seriousness of the disease being treated in balancing risks and benefits... Clearly, for a life-threatening illness, a relatively high level of known risks and some uncertainty about potential risk from the drug can be acceptable in exchange for the improved survival provided by effective drug treatment for a condition that, if left untreated, would result in death. Similarly, for the same life-threatening illnesses, evidence of effectiveness must be weighed against risks of the drug and the knowledge that death would result in the absence of treatment."

- Phase 4 Testing. Although FDA officials state that approvals granted under the accelerated plan are in no way conditional on sponsor willingness to conduct postmarketing testing, the agency says that it "...may seek agreement from the sponsor to conduct certain postmarketing (phase 4) studies to delineate additional information about the drug's risks, benefits, and optimal use. These studies could include, but would not be limited to, studying different doses or schedules of administration than were used in phase 2 studies, use of the drug in other patient populations or other stages of the disease, or use of the drug over a longer period of time."

The limited data that are available suggest that the Subpart E program may have become less relevant given the availability of other options for industry. According to research by the Tufts Center for the Study of Drug Development, the FDA had approved 48 drugs under the Subpart E regulations from October 1988 through December 1999. However, the research also indicates that only 2 of these 48 drugs were approved from 1997 through 1999. The program appeared to have reached its peak of approval activity in 1991, when the FDA approved 12 drugs under the Subpart E program.

By most accounts, the Subpart E program has become less relevant given the agency's successes under the prescription drug user fee program and given the availability of the fast track program and

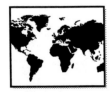

related provisions under FDAMA. In addition, the agency now routinely works with sponsors of all drugs so early in the development process that the accelerated development program's focus on early sponsor-FDA interaction is probably no longer viewed as a worthwhile incentive to participate.

Accelerated Drug Approval Program (Subpart H)

With its 1988 accelerated drug development program in place, the FDA wanted to take "additional steps...to facilitate the approval of significant new drugs...to treat serious or life-threatening diseases." The agency did so under a final regulation (Subpart H) published in December 1992.

Today, the Subpart H program remains perhaps the most active and relevant of the accelerated development and early/expanded access programs that the FDA introduced in the late 1980s and early 1990s. In part reflecting this fact, the Food and Drug Administration Modernization Act codified, in law, the key concepts of the accelerated drug approval program by creating the fast track program (see discussion below).

Unlike the FDA's accelerated development program, which focused largely on expediting the drug testing process, the Subpart H regulations focused on accelerating the agency's review and approval of promising therapies. The regulations attempted to do so by modifying the criteria on which the agency can base marketing approval for desperately needed new drugs, and by giving the agency greater authority regarding the study and use of the drugs following approval.

Specifically, the accelerated approval program allows the agency to base marketing approval on a drug's effect on a surrogate endpoint or on a clinical endpoint other than survival or irreversible morbidity. According to the regulation, "FDA may grant marketing approval for a new drug product on the basis of adequate and well-controlled clinical trials establishing that the drug product has an effect on a surrogate endpoint that is reasonably likely, based on epidemiologic, therapeutic, pathophysiologic, or other evidence, to predict clinical benefit or on the basis of an effect on a clinical endpoint other than survival or irreversible morbidity. Approval under this section will be subject to the requirement that the applicant study the drug further, to verify and describe its clinical benefit, where there is uncertainty as to the relation of the surrogate endpoint to clinical benefit, or of the observed clinical benefit to ultimate outcome. Postmarketing studies would usually be studies already underway. When required to be conducted, such studies must also be adequate and well controlled."

In its April 1992 regulatory proposal for the accelerated approval plan, the FDA discussed the benefits of not requiring companies to study the effects of desperately needed new drugs on primary endpoints (i.e., mortality or morbidity). "Approval of a drug on the basis of a well-documented effect on a surrogate endpoint can allow a drug to be marketed earlier, sometimes much earlier, than it could if a demonstrated clinical benefit were required... Approval could be granted where there is some uncertainty as to the relation of that endpoint to clinical benefit, with the requirement that the sponsor conduct or complete studies after approval to establish and define the drug's clinical benefit."

Ironically, it was controversy over the use of surrogate endpoints that led FDA officials to begin considering possible improvements in the accelerated approval program in the mid-1990s.[1] At FDA advisory committee meetings and in communications to the agency, it was the AIDS community itself that had begun to question the wisdom of basing approval on largely unvalidated surrogate endpoints.

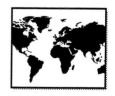

Despite such concerns, the FDA's accelerated approval program has been perhaps the most active of the agency's expedited development and review initiatives in recent years. According to CDER data, 35 NDAs for 32 drugs were approved under its Subpart H program from its inception through September 2001 (see listing below). It is interesting to note that more than a third of these NDAs gained approval in 1998, 1999, and 2000. After four Subpart H approvals in 2000, CDER approved only one drug under the program in 2001 (i.e., through September 2001).

Given that the majority of the Subpart H approvals were for AIDS or AIDS-related conditions, it is not surprising that many of these approvals received some of CDER's fastest reviews ever. More than two-thirds of the Subpart H drugs were approved in less than 10 months, for example.

Eligibility for Accelerated Approval Under the FDA's regulations, the accelerated approval program "applies to certain new drug and antibiotic products that have been studied for their safety and effectiveness in treating serious and life-threatening illnesses and that provide meaningful therapeutic benefit to patients over existing treatments (e.g., the ability to treat patients unresponsive to, or intolerant of, available therapy, or improved patient response over available therapy)."

Although the agency stated in its April 1992 proposal that it would apply the terms "serious" and "life-threatening" as it had in its treatment IND program and other programs, the FDA did discuss their application once again in the context of the accelerated approval plan. "The seriousness of a disease is a matter of judgement, but generally is based on its impact on such factors as survival, day-to-day functioning, or the likelihood that the disease, if left untreated, will progress from a less severe condition to a more serious one. Thus, acquired immunodeficiency syndrome (HIV) infection, Alzheimer's dementia, angina pectoris, heart failure, cancer, and many other diseases are clearly serious in their full manifestations. Further, many chronic illnesses that are generally well managed by available therapy can have serious outcomes. For example, inflammatory bowel disease, asthma, rheumatoid arthritis, diabetes mellitus, systemic lupus erythematosus, depression, psychoses, and many other diseases can be serious for certain populations or in some or all of their phases."

The Parallel Track Program

In mid-1989, National Institute of Allergy and Infectious Diseases (NIAID) Director Anthony Fauci, M.D., publicly proposed a new experimental drug accessibility plan called "parallel track." As proposed, the plan would allow the availability of experimental AIDS therapies earlier than ever in clinical development.

The federal government officially unveiled the parallel track program in April 1992 as a plan "intended to make promising new investigational drugs for AIDS and other HIV-related diseases more widely available as early as possible in the drug development process." The approach called for AIDS drugs to be made available after the completion of Phase 1 studies to subjects who are unable to enroll in the controlled trials or are unable to benefit from current therapies. Although similar to the treatment IND concept, parallel track is a more liberal mechanism in that it can provide for expanded drug access when the evidence of a drug's effectiveness cannot meet the threshold necessary to qualify for a treatment IND.

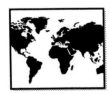

NDAs Approved Under CDER's Accelerated Approval Program (Subpart H), 1992-September 2001

Drug	Indication	Approval Time (months)
Hivid	Combination w/ zidovudine in advanced HIV	7.6
Biaxin (suspension)	Disseminated mycobacterial infections	13.7
Zerit	Advanced HIV in adults	5.9
Zinecard	Reduce incidence/severity of cardiomyopathy assoc. w/ doxorubicin administration in certain breast cancer patients	9.7*
Casodex	Combination w/ LHRH analogue for treating advanced prostate cancer	12.7
Epivir	HIV infection	4.4
Doxil	AIDS-related Kaposi's sarcoma in unresponsive patients	14.3
Invirase	Advanced HIV in combination w/ nucleoside analogues	3.2
Norvir (2 NDAs)	HIV infection as monotherapy or in combination w/ nucleoside analogues	2.3
Crixivan	HIV infection in adults	1.4
Taxotere	Patients with locally advanced or metastatic breast cancer who have relapsed or progressed during anthracycline-based therapy	21.6
Camptosar	Refractory colorectal cancer	5.6
Viramune	Combination w/ nucleoside analogues for HIV-1-infected adults experiencing clinical or immunologic deterioration	3.9
Serostim	AIDS wasting assoc. w/ catabolism loss or cachexia	11.4
ProAmatine	Symptomatic orthostatic hypotension	11.4**
Viracept (2 NDAs)	HIV infection	2.6
Rescriptor	Treatment of HIV infection in combination w/ antiretroviral agents	8.7
Xeloda	Treatment of patients w/ metastatic breast cancer who are resistant to both paclitaxel and an anthracycline-containing chemotherapy regimen or resistant to paclitaxel and for whom further anthracycline therapy may be contraindicated	6
Sulfamylon	Adjunctive topical antimicrobial agent to control bacterial infection of excised burn wounds	14.2***
Priftin	Pulmonary tuberculosis	6
Thalidomide	Cutaneous manifestations of erythema nodosum leprosum	18.8
Sustiva	Use in combination w/ other antiretroviral agents for HIV-1	3.2
Actiq	Breakthrough cancer pain	23.7
Ziagen	Treatment of HIV-1 in combination w/ other antiretroviral agents	5.8
DepoCyt	Intrathecal treatment of lymphomatous meningitis	5.9
Temodar	Adults w/ refractory anaplastic astrocytoma	5.9
Synercid	Vancomycin resistant Enterococcus faecium	7.8****
Mylotarg	Treatment for patients 60 or older with CD33 positive acute myeloid leukemia in first relapse	6.6
Kaletra (2 NDAs)	Treatment of HIV in combination w/ other antiretroviral agents	3.5
Mifeprex	Termination of pregnancy through 49 days of pregnancy	18.0†
Trizivir	Alone or in combination w/ other antiretroviral agents in treating HIV	10.9
Gleevec	Treatment of chronic myeloid leukemia	2.4

* Review time based on date of submission of significant new clinical data. ** Review time based on date of submission of significant new clinical data. *** Review time based on date of submission of significant new clinical data supporting a new indication. **** Total approval time adjusted because of negative plant inspection. †Time adjusted due to manufacturing issues, submission of final study report late in review.

Source: CDER

Accelerated Drug Approval/ Expanded Access Programs

Chapter 15

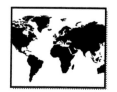

There are other, if more subtle, differences between the two experimental access programs. While the treatment IND requires approval at the commissioner's office level, parallel track is technically a protocol amendment, which needs the approval of review division directors. Also, sponsors can submit their parallel track proposals for review by the AIDS Research Advisory Committee of the National Institute of Allergy and Infectious Diseases in addition to the FDA.

In October 1992, Bristol-Myers Squibb's AIDS drug Zerit (stavudine) became the first drug made available under parallel track. The company established the parallel track arm during Phase 2/3 trials, and at a time when the controlled trials were enrolling rapidly. Just six weeks into the parallel track program, the company's controlled trials were fully enrolled, while the parallel access arm had enrolled several hundred patients. Ultimately, more than 13,000 patients received the drug under the parallel track program. Two earlier expanded drug access programs—for Hoffmann-La Roche's Hivid (zalcitabine or ddC) and Bristol-Myers Squibb's Videx (didanosine or ddI)—were said to be the models for the parallel track program.

Since this time, however, the parallel track program has failed to attract willing industry participants. Although some companies have discussed parallel track programs with the FDA, Zerit remains the only drug made available in the program's history.

While it is generally acknowledged that AIDS patients have many more therapeutic options than they did in the early 1990s, FDA officials are uncertain why the program has not been more active. Like the treatment IND program and any other expanded access plan, however, parallel track access can be extremely expensive. Some point out that other drug access mechanisms, such as large, open-label safety studies, are easier for industry to implement. In addition, since parallel track drugs would be made available even earlier in drug development than they would under other expanded access mechanisms, it is likely that many sponsors and AIDS patients have been reluctant to participate in this program.

The Oncology Initiative

One of CDER's newer accelerated drug development and approval programs is its Oncology Initiative. Unveiled in March 1996, the Oncology Initiative was, at least in part, a response to public criticism and congressional inquiries regarding why there was such an imbalance of agency resources dedicated to the review of therapies for AIDS compared to the review of drugs for illnesses that kill far more Americans each year, including cancer and heart disease. Responding to such inquiries, then-FDA Commissioner David Kessler, M.D., agreed to evaluate the perceived inequalities in resource allocations and to evaluate methods of expediting cancer drug reviews.

Over the past several years, the focus on the Oncology Initiative as a distinct program or initiative has faded to some degree. During this time, however, the Division of Oncologic Drug Products has assimilated the Oncology Initiative's goals and provisions into standard divisional practices and policies.

Introduced as "a uniform policy" rather than as a regulation, CDER's Oncology Initiative (formally called "Reinventing the Regulation of Cancer Drugs") was designed to reduce cancer drug development times by at least a year and to cut FDA oncology drug review times from an average of 12.4

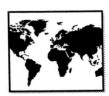

months to 6 months. The initiative itself comprised four separate elements, each of which the FDA claimed to have the authority to implement immediately:

- Accelerated Approval for Cancer Drugs. "To speed the availability of cancer drugs, FDA may now rely on partial response (such as measurable but incomplete shrinkage of a tumor) to a therapy, in addition to the current criteria such as a patient's survival and improved quality of life," the agency stated in the policy document. "While the predictive value of partial responses may still be a matter of discussion and study for all types of cancer patients, FDA has concluded that for patients with refractory malignant disease or for those who have no adequate alternative, clear evidence of anti-tumor activity is a reasonable basis for approving the drug. In these cases, studies confirming a clinical benefit may appropriately be completed after approval. By basing accelerated approval on surrogate markers such as tumor shrinkage for patients who have no satisfactory alternative therapy, and by allowing more definitive data on survival or other criteria to be developed after marketing approval, FDA believes that many cancer therapies will reach patients sooner." Under the policy, the agency will also apply the accelerated approval provisions to certain products intended to remove a serious or life-threatening toxicity associated with a particular cancer treatment.

    In effect, this aspect of the Oncology Initiative simply extended the accelerated approval process (Subpart H) to cancer drugs. While the FDA pointed out that the accelerated approval program has been applicable to promising drugs for cancer patients who do not benefit from or cannot tolerate available therapy, the agency stressed that, in the past, "this approval mechanism has not been frequently utilized, largely because general agreement on reasonable surrogate endpoints has been lacking." Post-approval studies would be required for most drugs approved on the basis of tumor shrinkage and for all products that remove treatment-associated toxicities.

- Expanded Access for Drugs Approved in Other Countries. Under this aspect of the Oncology Initiative, the FDA was to contact the U.S. sponsor and encourage the company to pursue an expanded access protocol "whenever a cancer therapy for patients who are not curable or well-treated by currently available therapies is approved by a recognized foreign regulatory authority." To qualify, a drug must be in a controlled clinical trial in the United States and be approved by "an identified regulatory agency in a foreign country." Although the FDA did not specifically identify any "recognized" regulatory authorities, it did state that the authorities must have "review practices, review standards, and access to specialized expertise in the evaluation of agents for use in cancer treatment that are sufficient to allow FDA to conclude that a marketing approval action by that authority is likely to provide an adequate basis for proper consideration of an expanded access protocol for U.S. patients."

    In considering such expanded access protocols, the agency will accept an English-language version of the data submitted to the foreign regulatory authority. The expanded access protocols should be directed at the "same general type of patient condition and similar dosage and schedule" as approved by the foreign regulatory authority.

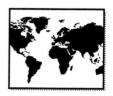

Accelerated Drug Approval/ Expanded Access Programs

Chapter 15

In following up on the expanded access component of the Oncology Initiative, the FDA's Office of International Affairs originally wrote to regulatory authorities in 25 "major" countries to request a list of all cancer or cancer-related therapies approved in each country during the previous 10 years. According to the agency, "no further action is indicated for a number of these drugs, which are not needed for patients in the U.S. due to the availability of other similar or superior drugs." As of 1999, the other drugs that were approved in these countries were either approved in the United States or were actively being reviewed for approval in this country.

- Cancer Patient Representation at FDA Advisory Committee Meetings. The FDA agreed to expand the "consumer member" concept in the context of its advisory committees, each of which typically includes a consumer member. "Because cancer is not one disease but many, FDA will now include a person who has experienced the specific cancer on each cancer-therapy advisory committee... FDA will now ensure that an individual who has personal experience with the specific cancer being studied be included as an ad hoc member of each cancer therapy committee."

- Clarification of the FDA's Policy for Studies of Marketed Cancer Products. To reduce the number of unnecessary INDs submitted by clinical investigators, the agency clarified its policy on INDs for studies of marketed drugs and announced that it would now refuse to accept INDs for exempt studies of marketed drugs. The agency states that it will not accept an IND for a study of a lawfully marketed drug if: (1) the study is not intended to support approval of a new indication or a significant change in product labeling or advertising; (2) the study does not involve a route of administration or dosage level or use in a patient population or other factor that significantly increases the risks (or decreases the acceptability of the risks) associated with the use of the product; and (3) the study meets the requirements for IRB approval and informed consent and does not commercialize the investigational product. The agency also clarified that it will not view a drug company's act of providing a marketed drug free of charge for an investigator-initiated study as constituting a promotional activity.

Since the Oncology Initiative's introduction, the Division of Oncology Drug Products has granted accelerated approvals to several cancer drugs, including Taxotere (docetaxel), Camptosar (irinotecan), Celebrex (new indication), Temidor, Depocit, Zeloda, and Doxil (new indication).

Fast Track Initiative

The so-called "fast track" initiative is not only the newest of CDER's accelerated drug development/approval programs, it is also the only one that was implemented directly by statute. Under the FDA Modernization Act of 1997, Congress established the fast track process to facilitate the development, and expedite the review, of products that demonstrate the potential to address unmet medical needs in the treatment of serious or life-threatening conditions.

Through its fast track provisions, FDAMA authorizes CDER to:

- Approve a new drug that qualifies for fast track status "upon a determination that the product has an effect on a clinical endpoint or on a surrogate endpoint that is

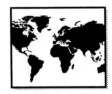

reasonably likely to predict clinical benefit." The agency has pointed out that this element of FDAMA in effect codifies in law the Subpart H program, which permits the agency to approve a new drug product on the basis of the product's effect "on a surrogate endpoint that is reasonably likely, based on epidemiologic, therapeutic, pathophysiologic, or other evidence, to predict clinical benefit or on the basis of an effect on a clinical endpoint other than survival or irreversible morbidity." Similar to approvals under the Subpart H program, drugs approved under the fast track program may require appropriate postapproval studies to validate the surrogate endpoint or otherwise confirm the effect on the clinical endpoint.

- Accept for review portions of a marketing application prior to the receipt of the complete application. Sponsors of designated fast track products can request, by submitting clinical data indicating that the product may be effective, that the agency accept for formal review completed portions of an NDA before the other sections of the application are submitted. If the agency permits this submission—sometimes called a rolling submission—the sponsor is required to provide a schedule for submitting the information necessary to make the NDA submission complete.

Although industry encouraged Congress to include the fast track program in FDAMA, it was unclear to many what real advantages the program offered aside from those that were already available under other programs. The agency itself concedes that, with the exception of the "rolling NDA" provisions, other elements of the fast track program have been available under regulations authorizing the other accelerated development/approval programs. In many ways, FDA officials note, the fast track program is an amalgamation of the provisions of these various other programs.

Still, industry had sought 138 fast track designations as of October 2001, and companies appeared to be fairly aggressive in seeking such designations. While many industry officials did not see the benefits offered under the fast track program as intrinsically valuable, they had begun to view a fast track designation as a valuable "staging mechanism" for what they increasingly saw as the real gateway to rapid drug approval—priority review status. With priority NMEs being approved, on average, 15.3 months faster than their standard counterparts (i.e., for 2000-approved drugs), companies are attempting to get whatever edge they can in obtaining the prized priority status for their products. Although priority review status is not necessarily automatic once a firm obtains a fast track designation, industry officials note that such a designation does seem to help a company set the expectation at the agency that the drug will be a significant new therapy—an expectation that the company can use to its advantage. CDER's September 1998 guidance entitled, *Fast Track Drug Development Programs—Designation, Development, and Application Review* specifically notes that "a fast track product would ordinarily meet [the agency's] criteria for priority review." And, since a fast track designation can be sought and obtained so early in the development process (as early as the IND filing), a firm can leverage that designation throughout the process to obtain meetings and to set the stage for seeking priority review status for an NDA.

Qualifying for Fast Track Status To become eligible for the benefits offered under the fast track program, a drug sponsor must first apply for, and obtain, a fast track designation for its drug product. In its September 1998 fast track guidance, the agency establishes the specific eligibility criteria that sponsors, drugs, and product development programs must meet to qualify for designation.

Accelerated Drug Approval/Expanded Access Programs

Chapter 15

In outlining the fast track eligibility criteria, which industry has applauded as being fairly liberal, the agency emphasizes that a fast track classification applies not to a product alone, but to a combination of the product and specific indication for which it is being studied. "The indication, for the purposes of [the fast track guidance], includes both the condition for which the drug is intended (e.g., heart failure) and the anticipated or established benefits of use (e.g., improved exercise tolerance, decreased hospitalization, increased survival)," the agency states. "It is therefore the development program for a specific drug for a specific indication that will receive fast track designation. Such a program is referred to...as a fast track drug development program."

Although the fast track program applies to drugs that are designed to treat, diagnose, or prevent serious or life-threatening conditions and that demonstrate the potential to address unmet medical needs, the agency chooses not to distinguish between serious or life-threatening conditions in its guidance. Rather, the agency points out that all life-threatening conditions, as defined under the accelerated drug development (Subpart E) program (see discussion above), automatically qualify as serious conditions, which the guidance document focuses on defining.

To qualify for a fast track development program, a drug must "not only be used in patients with a serious condition, it must be intended to treat a serious aspect" (i.e., either a serious manifestation or serious symptom) of the condition, the agency emphasizes. "Products intended to ameliorate or prevent a side effect of therapy of a condition would be considered to treat a serious condition if the side effect is serious (e.g., serious infections in patients receiving immunosuppressive therapy).

The agency notes that a preventive product will be considered to treat a serious condition if it is being evaluated for its ability to prevent a serious manifestation of the condition, or if it is being studied for its ability to prevent the condition and it is scientifically reasonable to assume that prevention of the condition would prevent its serious consequences.

"A product that is intended, and is being studied for its ability, to treat a condition while avoiding the side effects of currently accepted treatments of the condition may be considered to treat a serious condition if such side effects are serious (e.g., a less myelosuppressive treatment for a tumor or an anti-inflammatory drug that does not cause gastrointestinal bleeding)," the guidance states. "The potential for a new drug to avoid the serious sequelae of existing drugs would qualify that drug development program for fast track designation only in limited circumstances. Many therapies, even those intended to treat non-serious conditions, are associated with rare, serious, adverse reactions, and new therapies, despite initial hopes, often are associated with their own set of serious reactions. Nonetheless, some adverse reactions are significant public health problems, and the development of therapies that do not cause such serious reactions would merit close attention."

In addition to being intended for a serious or life-threatening condition, a drug must also meet a second critical criterion—it must demonstrate the potential to address an unmet medical need—to qualify for fast track status. While an unmet medical need is obvious when no therapy exists for a qualifying condition, it is not as apparent when alternative therapies exist. In such cases, the agency's guidance indicates that programs for new agents would qualify if they evaluate any of the following:

- improved effect(s) on serious outcomes of the condition that are affected by alternate therapies;

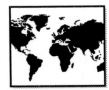

- effect(s) on serious outcomes of the condition not known to be affected by the alternatives;
- the ability to provide benefit(s) in patients who are unable to tolerate or are unresponsive to alternative agents;
- the ability to provide benefits similar to those of alternatives while avoiding serious toxicity present in existing therapies, or avoiding less serious toxicity that is common and causes discontinuation of treatment of a serious disease; or
- the ability to provide benefit(s) similar to those of alternatives but with improvement in some factor, such as compliance or convenience, that is shown to lead to an improved effect on serious outcomes.

Seeking a Fast Track Designation As noted, a firm must apply for and obtain a formal fast track designation before its drug becomes eligible for the program's benefits. According to the FDA's September 1998 guidance, designation requests can be made as early as the IND submission stage, but generally should not be made later than the pre-NDA meeting. The request must be submitted either with the IND or as an IND amendment.

About the content of the designation request, the agency states that the sponsor should "identify the serious condition and the unmet medical needs, provide a plausible basis for the assertion that the drug has the potential to address such unmet medical needs, and include in the development plan (at a level of detail appropriate to the stage of development) trials designed to evaluate this potential." Although the agency claims that the submission "should not be voluminous," it should contain the discussion and supporting documentation necessary to allow a reviewer to assess whether the criteria for fast track designation are met without having to refer to information located elsewhere.

The nature and quantity of data submitted in a designation request will depend on several factors, including whether the drug is designed to treat a fatal or non-fatal condition (i.e., less discussion/data if for a fatal condition), the availability of alternative therapies (i.e., less discussion/data if no alternatives available), and the stage of a drug's development (i.e., only animal and pharmacology data may be available). The evidentiary standard for obtaining a fast track designation was modest by design so that firms would be able to seek designation as early as the IND submission (i.e., because many of the benefits of designation are more valuable early in the development process).

The FDA will respond to a designation request within 60 calendar days of receiving the request. If the agency determines that the sponsor and drug/development program have met the criteria for fast track designation, it will forward a "designation letter" to inform the sponsor that designation has been granted and that the sponsor must design and perform studies that can show whether the product fulfills unmet medical needs, and to emphasize that the develoment program must continue to meet the fast track designation criteria. Alternatively, the agency may issue a "non-designation letter" informing the sponsor that the request was incomplete or that the development program failed to meet the criteria for fast track designation. Sponsors can re-apply for designation after receiving non-designation letters.

Accelerated Drug Approval/ Expanded Access Programs

Chapter 15

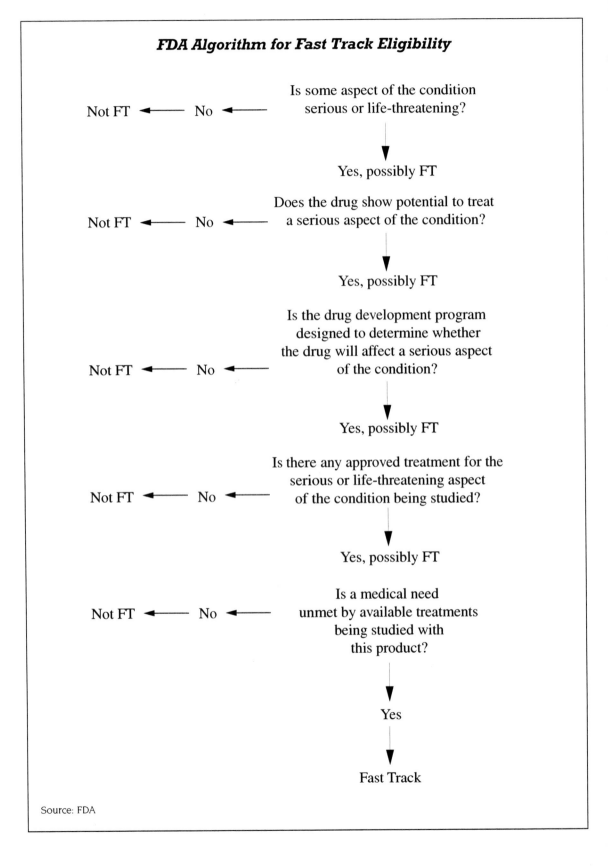

FDA Algorithm for Fast Track Eligibility

Source: FDA

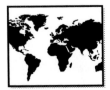

New Drug Approval in the United States

FDA performance data released in late 2001 showed that CDER had taken action on 78.3% of fast track designations within the 60-day goal. At the time, CDER had taken action on the requests in a median time of 53.5 days.

Fast Track and the Rolling NDA As noted above, the right to submit rolling NDAs is really the only new element of the fast track program that was not already available under previous accelerated drug development and approval regulations. The theory behind the rolling NDA, which some CDER review divisions have accepted in the past, is that the review process may be expedited if the agency can begin its review of parts of an NDA while the final elements of the application are being completed. Although the rolling NDA is addressed under FDAMA's fast track provisions, CDER officials have maintained that FDAMA permits the rolling NDA's use under existing programs, including the priority review and accelerated approval programs.

It is important to note that FDAMA establishes only that the FDA "may consider" a sponsor's request that the agency accept and begin the review of portions of a marketing application before the complete NDA is submitted. According to the fast track guidance, "after the sponsor submits to the IND a preliminary evaluation of data from the clinical trials, the Agency may consider accepting portions of the application if (i) the clinical trials that would form the basis for the Agency's determination of the safety and effectiveness of the product and that would support drug labeling are nearing completion or have been completed, (ii) the Agency agrees that the product continues to meet the criteria for fast track designation, and (iii) the Agency agrees that preliminary evaluation of the clinical data supports a determination that the product may be effective." Typically, the sponsor's request to submit a rolling NDA should be included in the company's information package submitted in advance of the pre-NDA meeting (i.e., so that the firm and review division can discuss relevant issues during the meeting).

Applicants seeking to submit a rolling NDA must first provide a schedule for the submission of portions of the NDA and obtain the agency's agreement to accept portions of the application as well as its agreement to the submission schedule. About the standards that partial NDA submissions must meet, the agency states that, "it is expected that a section submitted for review will be in a form adequate to have been included in a complete...NDA submission. Drafts should not be included in a submission... Occasionally, the Agency may, in its discretion, accept less than a complete section (e.g., a CMC section lacking final consistency lot data and long-term stability data; an acute toxicology section lacking chronic toxicology data or final study reports for some or all of the principal controlled trials without integrated summaries) if it determines that such a subsection would constitute a reviewable unit and would be useful in making the review process more efficient overall." The agency also emphasizes that its acceptance of a rolling NDA does not necessarily guarantee that its review will begin prior to the complete dossier's submission, and that review assignments are based on several factors, including staffing and workload.

A sponsor must submit the full user fee associated with an NDA when it submits the initial portion of the application for review. In addition, the review clock applicable to the NDA (i.e., likely the six-month timeframe for priority products) will not begin until the complete application is submitted, the agency notes.

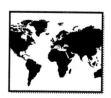

The agency establishes in its September 1999 guidance that applicants with fast track drug programs can seek traditional approval based on data demonstrating an effect on clinically meaningful endpoints or well-established surrogate endpoints, or under the existing accelerated approval regulations based on evidence of a drug's effect on a less than well-established surrogate endpoint. Generally, approval based on clinical endpoints other than survival or irreversible morbidity would be granted under traditional procedures rather than under the accelerated approval process. Approval based on clinical endpoints other than survival or irreversible morbidity would "be considered under the accelerated approval regulations only when it is essential to determine effects on survival and irreversible morbidity in order to confirm the favorable risk/benefit judgement that led to approval," the agency notes in quoting the accelerated approval regulations.

Assessing the Activity of the Fast Track Program Although it seemed that industry was somewhat slow to embrace the fast track program, perhaps due to ill-defined benefits and the lack of a formal guidance document initially, there has been considerable effort to seek designations in the program's first four years. According to CDER statistics, drug companies had submitted 138 fast track designation requests as of October 2001.

Based on the 124 designation requests acted on as of October 2001, industry is enjoying a roughly 71% success rate in obtaining fast track designations for their drugs.

Not surprisingly given the intent of the fast track program, industry's designation request activity centers on a handful of divisions. In fact, just over half of all designation requests have been submitted to either the Division of Antiviral Drug Products or the Division of Oncologic Drug Products. Seventy percent of fast track designation requests have been submitted to just four divisions. In June 2000, CDER released a partial list of the indications for which fast track designations had been granted, including coronary syndrome, CVA, ALS, malignancies, acute pancreatitis, platelet adhesion, HIV, SLE, ARDS, and acromegaly.

Given that CDER has approved only a handful of drugs with fast track designations to date, it is premature to assess the degree to which such designations are affecting review times. As of September 30, 2001, CDER had approved eight drugs with fast track designations: Ziagen (approved December 18, 1999 for HIV); Agenerase (approved April 15, 1999 for HIV); Taxotere (efficacy supplement approved December 23, 1999 for locally advanced metastatic non-small cell lung cancer); Sustiva (approved September 17, 1998 for HIV); Kaletra (approved September 15, 2000 for HIV); Trisenox (approved September 25, 2000 for acute promyelocytic leukemia); Cancidas (approved January 26, 2001 for aspergillus infections); and Gleevec (approved May 10, 2001 for chronic myeloid leukemia).

References

1. Shulman, S.R. and Brown, J.S. (Tufts Center for the Study of Drug Development), The Food and Drug Administration's Early Access and Fast-Track Approval Initiatives: How Have They Worked? *Food and Drug Law Journal*, 1995, pp. 503-531.
2. Ibid.
3. Hewitt, P. (Tufts Center for the Study of Drug Development). Data from Tufts Center for the Study of Drug Development Marketed Drugs and Expedited/Accelerated Datasets, March 1997.

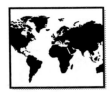

CHAPTER 16

The Pediatric Studies Initiative

by Christopher-Paul Milne
Assistant Director
Tufts Center for the Study of Drug Development

After nearly a century of being neither seen nor heard, pediatric drug studies have become the rallying point during the last decade for a crusade spearheaded by pediatricians, child health advocates, and public health officials. The culmination of these efforts, which sought to make the development of pediatric use information a standard component of the pharmaceutical research process, was the launch of the pediatrics studies "initiative" in the late 1990s. This precedent-setting combination of reinvigorated regulations and statutory incentives truly embodies the meaning of the word "initiative"—a fresh start or new departure—as clinical investigations of formerly overlooked pediatric indications will now be incorporated routinely into drug development programs. The pediatric studies initiative's controversial carrot-and-stick approach was necessitated by the complicated circumstances of studying drugs in children.

Amid all the complexity and controversy, however, two realities have shaped the initiative. First, drugs—even those commonly used in pediatric patients—lack labeling on such pediatric uses. Various studies have determined that 70% to 80% of marketed drugs are not labeled for pediatric use, and that the situation is even worse for neonates. The off-label use of drugs without adequate pediatric dosing information can present significant problems, including an increased risk of adverse drug reactions, ineffective treatment due to underdosing, suboptimal utilization of therapeutic advances for pediatric patients, and the increased use of extemporaneous formulations that may be poorly or inconsistently bioavailable.

The second reality is that there are significant disincentives facing companies that might otherwise conduct pediatric studies for drugs developed primarily for adult use. These include a limited return on investment, potential product liability and medical malpractice issues, the complexities of enrolling pediatric patients, and difficulties with drug administration and patient compliance.

Thus, the goal of the initiative was to maintain the economic viability of drug development while promoting better medicines for patients of all ages. Ultimately, the government determined that there were two ways to reach this goal—economic incentive and regulatory mandate.

Worldwide Pharmaceutical Regulation Series

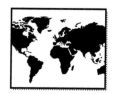

Historical Development

Although most of the early legislation regulating drugs and biologics in the United States was influenced by poisoning tragedies largely involving children, neither the Public Health Service Act nor the Food, Drug, & Cosmetic Act (FD&C Act) were particularly concerned with children. In fact, the 1962 amendments to the FD&C Act actually made children "therapeutic orphans" (a term coined by Dr. Harry Shirkey) by establishing that, if a drug is not tested in children, then the label should discourage its use in such patients.

A few years later, an article in a pediatrics journal noted that 78% of all medications listed in the 1973 Physician's Desk Reference (PDR) either included a disclaimer or lacked adequate dosing information for pediatric patients. In recognition of this problem, the American Academy of Pediatrics (AAP) Committee on Drugs issued guidelines on the evaluation of drugs for pediatric use in 1974. Three years later, the organization released guidelines to encourage ethical conduct in studies evaluating drugs in pediatric populations. The FDA responded in 1979 by publishing regulations requiring sponsors to conduct pediatric clinical trials before including pediatric information on the label.

In 1990, a resurgence of concern about the lack of labeling for pediatric use drugs prompted the Institute of Medicine (IOM) to convene a workshop on the topic. The emergence of AIDS as a pediatric disease had resulted in a renewed sense of urgency regarding the need for new drugs in pediatric medicine. At the IOM workshop, speakers highlighted the long delay in the pediatric availability of AZT, and the fact that 70% of the drugs used to treat infants in hospitals lacked pediatric labeling. Although the FDA noted an increase in pediatric studies at the time, that meeting can be viewed as the seminal event for the current pediatric studies initiative.

The early FDA response was to initiate the so-called "Pediatric Page" and "Pediatric Plan," which were intended to encourage industry to focus attention voluntarily on pediatric patients throughout the new drug development process. The real impetus for manufacturers "to think pediatric," however, was the FDA's 1994 pediatric labeling regulation, which required manufacturers to decide if existing data warranted a change to the label for pediatric use and to submit supplemental new drug applications accordingly. The 1994 regulation was considered "voluntary" because it did not impose a general requirement for manufacturers to conduct pediatric studies. The FDA later noted, in fact, that industry's response to the regulation did not substantially address the need for more information. Labeling supplements were submitted for only a small fraction of the prescription drugs and biologicals on the market, and 75% of the supplements that were filed did not significantly improve the pediatric use information.

In response, the FDA began crafting what would become the 1998 pediatric rule, which shape-shifted the regulatory nature of the pediatric initiative from voluntary to mandatory. Chris Jennings, the Clinton Administration's deputy assistant for health policy development, trumpeted the arrival of the proposed rule by declaring that the government had tried it industry's way (i.e., through voluntary programs) and that the approach had failed. In recognition of both the public health needs and the difficulties inherent in conducting pediatric studies, Congress viewed the Clinton Administration's efforts as a clarion call to add pediatric research incentives to ongoing legislative efforts to reform the FDA. Congress grafted an earlier version of pediatric research incentive legislation—The Better

Pharmaceuticals for Children Act—onto the FDA Modernization Act of 1997 (FDAMA). FDAMA's pediatric provision offered an incentive—six months of market exclusivity—to manufacturers that would, in response to an FDA request, conduct pediatric studies of drugs with potential use as medicines for children. To render the statute and pediatric regulations mutually re-enforcing, the provision contained a harmonization clause that allowed studies conducted for the purpose of applying for FDAMA exclusivity to potentially do "double-duty" by also fulfilling FDA regulatory requirements for pediatric studies. Thus, the pediatric initiative assumed its current form of a carrot and stick—a limited and temporary legislative "carrot" under FDAMA framed by the regulatory "stick" of the FDA's 1998 regulation requiring the assessment of pediatric safety and effectiveness.

The Carrot: FDAMA's Pediatric Provision

On November 21, 1997, the FDA Modernization Act became law. The law included the pediatric studies provision, under which a six-month period of market exclusivity would be awarded to a drug sponsor that conducted pediatric studies of drugs that the FDA believes may have health benefits for the pediatric patient population. Only drugs that have indications occurring in children are eligible. Other than that, however, eligible drugs may currently be approved only in adults, or they may be drugs whose only indication is for children. During this so-called "pediatric exclusivity" period, the agency cannot approve another company's abbreviated new drug application (ANDA) that is submitted for the same drug or biological and that relies on the safety and effectiveness data in the original company's full new drug application (NDA).

New drugs and already-marketed drugs are both eligible for this incentive. New drug applications that qualify for pediatric exclusivity include: (1) new drug applications for new chemical entities (i.e., the first approval of a new drug); (2) new drug applications or supplemental new drug applications for a new indication or other change in an already-approved drug; and (3) new drug applications or supplemental new drug applications for a pediatric use of a currently unapproved indication (i.e., in contrast to drugs in the second category, the indication in question is not even approved in adults, but the drug itself is already approved).

Already-marketed drugs are eligible if they appear on a list that FDAMA required the FDA to compile. This list comprises approved drugs for which additional pediatric information may produce health benefits in the pediatric population (the "FDAMA list"). Drugs that are not on the FDAMA list but that have an approved adult indication with potential use in children, and that have some patent or market exclusivity life remaining are also eligible. The original FDAMA list was published in May of 1998 and is updated at least annually as products (currently numbering about 450) are added or removed from the list. Over-the-counter drugs that are the subject of approved NDAs are eligible, as are a small number of CBER-regulated biological products that are subject to section 505 of the FD&C Act. Biological products subject to the Public Health Service Act are not eligible, even if they have orphan exclusivity or patent protection. Antibiotics that were the subject of any marketing application received before November 21, 1997, are not eligible for the pediatric exclusivity program, unless such antibiotics also received orphan drug exclusivity (see Chapter 13).

In addition to the unique eligibility requirements, pediatric exclusivity differs from other forms of exclusivity in several ways. Pediatric exclusivity is not a patent extension per se, but is a period of

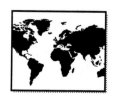

market exclusivity that attaches to the end of the existing patent or exclusivity period listed in the *Orange Book* (a compendium of patent and market exclusivity and other information published by CDER, formally entitled, *Approved Drug Products With Therapeutic Equivalence Evaluations*) instead of running concurrently. It accrues not only to the drug product that was investigated in the pediatric study, but also to any drug product containing the same active moiety (including all dosage forms and indications) for which the sponsor of the pediatric study holds the approved NDA. Finally, the awarding of pediatric exclusivity is not conditional upon the FDA's approval of the labeling information that may (or may not) result from the study reports submitted in support of the pediatric exclusivity application, but may be granted merely upon acceptance of the study reports themselves.

An added incentive "to think pediatric," a sponsor can earn an additional six-month period of pediatric exclusivity if it submits a supplement for a new use (i.e., one not already covered in the approved labeling) in response to a written request. If approved, the supplement qualifies for three-year Hatch-Waxman exclusivity, to which the six-month pediatric exclusivity extension would attach. This would be an additional 3.5 years of exclusivity for the products with the active moiety that was the subject of an earlier pediatric exclusivity award. In the case of a second award, however, the supplement (including the labeling) must be approved before the pediatric exclusivity would have anything to which it could attach. The FDA has pointed out that this approach could also provide a way for sponsors to take advantage of pediatric exclusivity even if they do not have any remaining patent or exclusivity protection remaining. Although the circumstances under which the FDA will grant a second period of pediatric exclusivity are limited, the FDA now lists Lamivudine as having received one.

The *quid pro quo* for receiving the enviable reward of pediatric exclusivity under FDAMA is that the sponsor must submit pediatric studies in response to a specific FDA "written request"—a detailed legal and scientific document from the agency. This process involves five basic steps: (1) an FDA determination as to what types of pediatric studies will be necessary; (2) the sponsor's receipt of an FDA written request for pediatric studies; (3) developing a sponsor/FDA agreement regarding what studies need to be undertaken; (4) the sponsor's efforts to conduct the studies; and (5) the sponsor's submission of the pediatric study reports.

Step 1-Pediatric Studies Pediatric studies are defined in the statute as "at least one clinical investigation (that at the Secretary's discretion may include pharmacokinetic studies) in pediatric age groups in which the drug is anticipated to be used." In practice, safety studies and pharmacokinetic studies are commonly required. Efficacy studies have also been frequently requested, especially when the course of the disease and the drug's effects in pediatric patients are not known to be similar to those in adults.

The agency will determine what studies must be conducted by asking the following question: "What information do health care providers or parents need to use this active moiety appropriately in the pediatric population?" The FDA will first examine what pediatric labeling exists for the drug products, any additional pediatric information submitted for labeling, and pediatric information contained in NDAs for other products with the same active moiety. The agency will evaluate the need for studies in all pediatric subpopulations and for all indications (approved and pending indications, as well as unapproved uses) for which the active moiety is being used in the pediatric population.

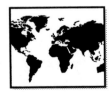

Step 2-The Written Request Unless the FDA issues a written request to a sponsor on its own initiative (22% of written requests issued as of November 2001), the written request process begins with the sponsor submitting a proposed pediatric study request (PPSR) to the appropriate FDA reviewing division. The PPSR should address the following 15 issues at a minimum: study objective; the indications to be studied; types of studies; study design; number of patients; age groups; inclusion/exclusion criteria; clinical endpoints; study evaluation; safety concerns; statistical analysis; potential label changes; report format; timeframes; and dosage form, regimen, route of administration, and formulation information on the drug. Within approximately 120 days (an FDA-suggested timeframe), the agency will decide if the PPSR is acceptable and issue either an inadequacy letter or a written request that asks the sponsor to submit certain studies to determine if the use of a drug could have meaningful health benefits in the pediatric population.

In developing its written request, the agency may use the sponsor's PPSR or other information. A general sample written request template as well as templates for particular categories of drugs are available on the agency's Pediatric Web Page (see Information Sources Checklist below). Since this program is voluntary, a sponsor is not required to respond to a written request.

In general, the FDA will not accept pediatric study reports unless they are submitted in response to a formal agency written request. The written request will cover similar issues to those addressed in the PPSR, including a timeframe (typically no longer than two to three years, although extensions may be requested) for submitting the study and provisions for amending the written request to account for deviations—from the study protocol, for example—before the data are submitted. This last item may be of particular interest to sponsors, since there have already been 124 amendments to the 208 written requests issued as of November 2001.

Step 3 - Reaching Agreement with the FDA After receiving a written request, the sponsor can take one of two approaches. The sponsor can negotiate a written agreement with the FDA on the study's protocol, the study's timeframe, and a plan for addressing other details specified in the written request. Written agreements are usually pursued to clarify remaining ambiguities, but also may be used either to agree on a particular method when several options exist or to confirm the number of patients considered adequate in a study. Once it is concluded, the written agreement may be modified only in writing by mutual agreement, and pediatric protocols submitted under a written agreement must be followed to the letter unless they are amended. In the several years following implementation, such written agreements have been rare and are even discouraged because they appear to impede rather than facilitate implementation.

When they are submitted for FDA comment, pediatric protocols relevant to pediatric exclusivity are considered special protocols and should be answered within 45 days of the FDA's receipt of the request for protocol review. Other than this requirement, there are no specific timeframes, suggested or mandated, within which the written agreements must be concluded.

In an alternative approach, the sponsor would not execute a written agreement. Instead, the sponsor could request a voluntary protocol review and conduct the study according to commonly accepted scientific principles and protocols.

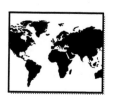

Step 4-Conducting the Studies Studies must be conducted according to the written agreement and/or commonly accepted scientific principles and protocols. In particular, the FDA recommends that the following documents be consulted: FDA regulations 21 CFR 312.23 (describing protocol contents) and 314.126 (describing adequate and well-controlled studies); ICH guidelines E3 (Structure and Content of Clinical Study Reports), E4 (Dose-Response Information to Support Drug Registration), E6 (Good Clinical Practices: Consolidated Guideline), E8 (General Considerations for Clinical Trials), and E11 (Clinical Investigation of Medicinal Products in the Paediatric Population (Draft); and FDA guidances regarding the format and content of pediatric use supplements and the clinical and statistical sections of the NDA (see Information Sources Checklist below). The types of studies that the FDA will accept include new studies conducted by the sponsor or new studies performed by third parties. Studies conducted prior to the written request are acceptable, unless they provide no additional useful information. Data already submitted to an NDA may not be used, although data submitted to an IND are acceptable. The FDA states that, although such studies may be new or previously conducted studies, studies conducted prior to the issuance of the written request generally will not be accepted unless they would potentially support a labeling change. Reviews of the published literature, in particular, are not considered "pediatric studies" by the FDA.

Step 5-Submitting the Study Reports Lastly, the study reports must be submitted according to the FDA's filing requirements (i.e., accompanied by an NDA, supplement, or NDA amendment). Although the NDA or supplement need not be approved for the pediatric studies to qualify for pediatric exclusivity, the completed study reports must be filed before the product's existing patent or exclusivity protection expires. As specified in FDAMA, the FDA will notify a sponsor within 60 days (with a written agreement) or 90 days (without a written agreement) of its decision as to whether pediatric exclusivity will be granted or denied. Acceptance of the study reports is determined by the Pediatric Exclusivity Board with little opportunity for the sponsor to intercede on its own behalf if a dispute

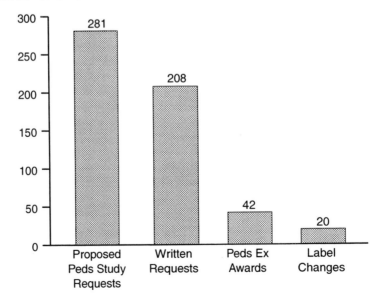

Status of the Pediatric Studies Iniative as of Q4 2001

- Proposed Peds Study Requests: 281
- Written Requests: 208
- Peds Ex Awards: 42
- Label Changes: 20

regarding both the nature of the process and the time frame for the decision arises. The recent implementation history indicates that the FDA has required strict compliance with the terms of a written request in addition to the conduct of studies consistent with the specifications of any written agreements or commonly accepted scientific principles.

If all goes well, six months of pediatric exclusivity will be added to all patents and exclusivity periods listed in the *Orange Book* for all the sponsor's products that have the same active moiety as the one studied. If the studies were conducted for an unapproved indication, then the additional period of exclusivity will accrue upon approval.

The Stick: The FDA's 1998 Rule for Assessment of Pediatric Safety and Effectiveness

In August 1997, the FDA made a controversial proposal to counteract the widespread practice of using adult drugs in children on an off-label basis. Its proposal called for companies submitting applications for new medicines considered "therapeutically important and/or likely to be used in children" to provide pediatric clinical study data to support pediatric use at the time of, or soon after, marketing approval. Subsequently, the agency published a December 1998 final rule "that created a presumption" that all new drugs and biological products (i.e., every application submitted after the December 2, 2000 compliance date for a new active ingredient, new indication, new dosage form, new dosing regimen, or new route of administration) would be studied in pediatric patients, but that allowed manufacturers to obtain a waiver or deferral from the requirement under certain circumstances.

The 1998 rule, in fact, contains five "bailout" options from the requirement that sponsors submit assessments of pediatric safety and effectiveness with their applications. First, the FDA could conclude that pediatric effectiveness may be extrapolated from adult data supplemented with other information, such as pediatric pharmacokinetic studies (as permitted under the 1994 FDA pediatric labeling regulation).

Second, the submission of pediatric studies may be deferred until after the drug product's approval for use in adults. In the formal language of the rule, the FDA states that such deferrals can be granted, among other reasons, if the drug is set for approval in adults before studies in pediatric patients are complete, or if pediatric studies should be delayed until additional safety and effectiveness data have been collected.

The third and fourth bailout provisions involve waivers and partial waivers. A full waiver may be granted if the drug product has no therapeutic advantage or anticipated use in pediatric patients, if the studies are impossible or impractical, or if the drug product is ineffective or unsafe for the pediatric population. A partial waiver can be granted for similar reasons, but would be related to the drug's use in specific age groups of the pediatric population. Partial waivers are also available when the applicant can demonstrate that reasonable attempts to produce a pediatric formulation for that specific age group have failed. The fifth and last bailout clause comprises an exemption for approved orphan indications of any drug or biological product.

The FDA will be able to track the progress of pediatric studies in a number of ways. Initially, tracking will be accomplished through IND annual reports, in which sponsors are required to include a discussion of pediatric patients enrolled in clinical trials. Advance submissions for end-of-Phase 1 (EOP1), end-of-Phase 2 (EOP2), and/or pre-NDA/BLA meetings will be required to include reports on the progress of the sponsor's investigation of the product's pediatric use. Sponsors may also utilize such submissions to support requests for waivers, deferrals, or pediatric exclusivity (see Reporting Requirements Checklist below). The FDA will also be able to ascertain the status of a pediatric investigation of the drug or biological product by evaluating the integrated summary of existing pediatric research, the pediatric assessment reports, and information contained in waiver and deferral requests (see Reporting Requirements Checklist below).

In addition, sponsors must submit other relevant information in their postmarketing annual reports: (1) a summary briefly stating whether labeling supplements for pediatric use have been submitted and whether new studies in the pediatric population have been initiated; (2) when possible, an estimate of patient exposure to the drug product with specific reference to the pediatric population (although this is not required when no such data exist, the FDA notes the existence of commercial data bases designed to estimate the use of marketed drugs); (3) an analysis of available safety and efficacy data in the pediatric population and changes proposed in the label based on this information (see Reporting Requirements Checklist below); (4) an assessment of data necessary to ensure appropriate labeling for the pediatric population; and (5) a statement as to whether the sponsor has been required to conduct postmarketing pediatric studies and, if so, a report on the status of those studies. According to the FDA, analyses referred to in this section should involve already collected data.

1998 Pediatric Rule Reporting Requirements Checklist

1) Reports on planned pediatric studies in IND (s. 312.23 (a) (10) (iii))
2) Reports for EOP1, EOP2, and pre-NDA/BLA meetings (s. 312.47 (b)(1)(iv),s. 312.47 (b) (2))
3) Summaries of data on pediatric safety and effectiveness in NDA (s. 314.50 (d) (7))
4) Reports assessing the safety and effectiveness of certain drugs and biological products for pediatric use in NDA, BLA, or SNDA (s. 314.55 (a), s. 601.27 (a))
5) Requests seeking deferral of required pediatric studies (s. 314.55 (b), 601.27 (b))
6) Requests seeking waiver of required pediatric studies (s. 314.55 (c), 601.27 (c))
7) Postmarketing reports of analyses of data on pediatric safety and effectiveness (s. 314.81 (b) (2) (vi) (c), s. 601.37 (a) (1))
8) Postmarketing reports on patient exposure to certain marketed drug products (s. 314.81 (b) (2) (i), s. 601.37 (a) (2))
9) Postmarketing reports on labeling changes initiated in response to new pediatric data (s. 314.81 (b) (2) (vi) (c), s. 601.37 (a) (3))
10) Postmarketing reports on the status of required postapproval studies in pediatric patients (s. 314.81 (b) (2) (vii), s. 601.37)

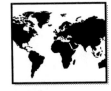

Products already on the market are subject to the 1998 pediatric rule as well, but only under "compelling circumstances." Compelling circumstances are triggered when: (1) a product is used (or is likely to be used) in a "substantial number of pediatric patients;" or (2) the product provides a "meaningful therapeutic benefit" for pediatric use over existing treatments, and inadequate labeling could pose significant risks.

The "substantial number of pediatric patients" threshold is met when there are 50,000 pediatric patients with the disease or condition for which the drug or biological product is indicated. Currently, such assessments are predicated on physician-mention data from the National Disease and Therapeutic Index (a database maintained by IMS America Ltd.), which tracks the use of drugs by measuring the number of times physicians mention drugs during outpatient visits. The FDA has noted, however, that this definition of "substantial number" is not codified, and may be modified at some point after consultation with pediatric experts (see discussion of Pediatric Advisory Subcommittee below).

The term "meaningful therapeutic benefit," which was derived, in part, from CDER's definition of a priority drug, attaches to a drug when it provides an improvement over existing products labeled for pediatric use. The term may be applied, for example, when there is evidence supporting any of the following: (1) increased effectiveness in the treatment, prevention, or diagnosis of disease; (2) elimination or substantial reduction of a treatment—limiting reaction; (3) documented enhancement of patient compliance; or (4) safety and effectiveness in a new subpopulation. In addition, a product can be considered to provide "meaningful therapeutic benefit" if it is in a class of products or has an intended indication for which there is a need for additional therapeutic options, even if it is not necessarily considered a priority drug. This second criterion was developed to cover instances in which a drug might not be the first product in its class labeled for pediatric use, and therefore would not be considered a priority drug. Depending upon the severity of the disease and the adverse reaction profile of existing treatments, however, such a product may still be necessary to ensure that a range of products is available for pediatric patients.

When the FDA decides that the use of a marketed product in children crosses the compelling circumstances threshold, the agency will consult with the manufacturer on the types of pediatric studies needed and the applicable time frame. It will then notify the manufacturer by letter of its tentative conclusion regarding the need for a pediatric study. In the penultimate step, the agency will provide the manufacturer with an opportunity to provide a written response and to participate in a meeting, perhaps even an advisory committee meeting. Ultimately, if after reviewing the manufacturer's response, the FDA determines that there is still a need for a study, it will order the manufacturer (in the form of a letter) to submit a "supplemental application" containing pediatric safety and effectiveness data within a specified time. However, the FDA, either on its own initiative or at the request of the applicant, can grant a full or partial waiver. For marketed drug and biological products, the rule became effective April 1, 1999.

Failure to comply can result in a drug being considered misbranded, an unapproved new drug, or an unlicensed biologic. In this case, the agency may seek an injunction, prosecution, or seizure to enforce sponsor commitments to conduct pediatric trials. The FDA has indicated that it does not intend to use seizure as a remedy on a routine basis, and only in a worst-case scenario will a com-

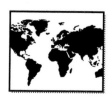

pany's failure to complete pediatric studies and submit the data from such studies according to the agreed timetable result in a drug product being considered misbranded. Similarly, although the agency could withdraw or deny a product's approval based on a sponsor's failure to conduct pediatric studies, it does not intend to do so, except possibly in "rare circumstances." Such circumstances might arise when a product's predominant use is in pediatric patients rather than adults, and when there are life-threatening risks associated with its use in the absence of pediatric dosing and safety information on the label.

The FDA plans to use publicity to encourage compliance by: (1) bringing appropriate cases to the attention of a panel of pediatric experts; (2) utilizing other forms of publicity to give consumers information about the status of required studies (i.e., FDAMA contains provisions for the disclosure of information on the status of postmarketing studies); and (3) considering the use of prominent warnings about the absence of data on pediatric use in particular cases.

Incorporating FDAMA and the Pediatric Rule into a Drug Development Plan

The FDA repeatedly emphasizes that the 1998 rule is currently being implemented to supplement FDAMA because antibiotics, biologics, and drugs without exclusivity or patent life generally will not qualify for FDAMA's pediatric exclusivity incentives. The agency also frequently notes that the focus and scope of the FDAMA incentive and the pediatric rule are different. Written requests for studies under FDAMA will cover an active moiety and possibly multiple indications and formulations, while the rule requires an assessment only for the drug product and indications contained in the application submitted for review (or for marketed drugs specified by the FDA). In addition, the FDAMA program is focused mainly on marketed products, while the 1998 pediatric rule is intended primarily to ensure that new drugs and biological products provide adequate pediatric labeling for the approved indications at the time of, or soon after, approval.

Even though a pediatric study could be rejected under the rule and still meet the terms of a written request (or vice versa), the FDA points out that the pediatric exclusivity program and the 1998 rule will overlap significantly for the next few years. The agency has estimated that just under half of the estimated $80 million that industry will spend in complying with the rule will actually be spent voluntarily on FDAMA-related pediatric studies that will perform "double-duty" to fulfill the 1998 rule requirements (or about 40 of the 80 or so product applications that the FDA estimates will be required to comply annually). Thus, while the pediatric exclusivity program is in effect, those constructing drug development plans should consider not only which drugs must comply with the rule and when, but also what types of studies will be necessary and the ideal timing of such studies with an eye towards complying with the 1998 rule as well as applying for pediatric exclusivity.

Planning Considerations I: Which Drugs Must Comply With the 1998 Pediatric Rule and When?
Initially, the agency's attention regarding an enforcement queue for the 1998 rule seemed to focus on the FDAMA list. At that time, the FDA emphasized three points about the import of the FDAMA list for the 1998 rule: (1) products designated as (high) priority may be appropriate candidates for required studies under the rule; (2) the list is not necessarily an exhaustive list of drugs potentially subject to the rule; and (3) inclusion on the list does not mean that a drug's sponsor will necessarily

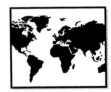

be required to submit a study. In its recent Draft Guidance for Industry on complying with the 1998 rule (November 2000), however, the agency steered away from discussing the FDAMA list in the context of the rule, most likely because it was planning to recommend, in the January 2001 report to Congress, that the FDAMA list be eliminated from the pediatric provision upon reauthorization. Nonetheless, the FDA has given some indications of how its prioritization scheme for enforcement of the 1998 rule will work. First, the agency has stated that it intends to exercise its authority to require studies with respect to marketed drugs and biologics that lack any remaining market exclusivity or patent life. Initially, the FDA will determine which marketed products "could pose significant risks to patients" (i.e., compelling circumstances). In making this determination, the agency will consider such factors as: (1) the severity of the illness; (2) the consequences of inadequate treatment; (3) the number of pediatric prescriptions; and (4) any available information on adverse events associated with the product. Since the FDA has stated that it expects to require studies for only two marketed drugs per year, drugs targeted early on must draw the agency's attention in some way (i.e., by being one of the ten drugs that the agency's proposed rule described as being the most widely prescribed drugs for pediatric outpatients despite inadequate labeling, or drugs and biologics recommended for study by the Pediatric Advisory Subcommittee).

Next, the FDA has stated that, after allowing manufacturers an adequate opportunity to voluntarily submit studies for already marketed drugs and biologics eligible for exclusivity, it will consider enforcing the rule for any remaining unstudied marketed drugs that the agency believes meet the "compelling circumstances" criteria. Finally, as discussed previously, the basic thrust of the 1998 rule is for new drugs or biological products. Upon a new drug's approval, the FDA's approval letter will discuss the following: (1) the need for pediatric studies; (2) the deferral date (if relevant); (3) the granting of a waiver (if relevant); and (4) the drug's potential for pediatric exclusivity. Thus, the FDA is now operating under the presumption that all new drugs and biologics will be tested in children, unless exemptions, waivers, or deferrals from the 1998 rule can be justified. In particular, many new drugs and biologics for serious and life-threatening illnesses will be considered to offer meaningful therapeutic benefit for pediatric populations—even if the products are not necessarily used in a substantial number of pediatric patients—at least until there are sufficient numbers of adequately labeled products available for such conditions.

Exemptions The formal language of the regulation makes only one category of products eligible for exemptions—new drugs, antibiotics, and biological products with an indication for which an orphan designation has been granted. The FDA notes in the preamble, however, that the automatic exemption does not apply to already-marketed drugs and biological products that meet "the compelling circumstances" threshold, which triggers the rule. The FDA further states that generic copies of approved drugs under section 505(j) do not fall under the rule, and that pediatric bioequivalence studies are not required for generic drugs.

While not considered an exemption per se, there is another significant category of drug usage that does not fall under the scope of the rule: The FDA does not require an applicant to conduct a pediatric assessment for an unapproved or unclaimed indication.

Waiver For new applications, the FDA may grant a full or partial waiver on its own initiative or at the request of an applicant. The agency will grant a full or partial waiver if it finds that there is a

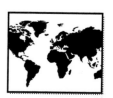

"reasonable basis" that one or more of the following grounds for a waiver exist: (a) studies are impossible or highly impractical; (b) evidence strongly suggests that the product would be ineffective or unsafe (this information would have to be included in a product's labeling); (c) reasonable attempts to produce a pediatric formulation have failed; or (d) there is no meaningful therapeutic benefit, the drug is not likely to be used in a substantial number of patients, and the absence of labeling would not pose a significant risk.

The FDA reviewing division responsible for a drug will make the waiver decision. To request a waiver from the appropriate reviewing division, the applicant must certify that one or more of the grounds for a waiver exist and supply supporting information and documentation. In other words, the burden is on the manufacturer to justify a waiver. The agency has emphasized that cost ordinarily will not be a factor in the waiver decision, that unsupported assertions will be rejected, that methods are available to conduct adequate studies in small populations, and that studies in small populations may have to be at least attempted before a waiver will be granted. Waiver discussions with the FDA should take place at the end-of-Phase 2 or pre-NDA/BLA meeting, or at least 60 days prior to an application's submission.

A manufacturer's first step in preparing a waiver request should be to check the FDA's list of diseases and conditions for which waivers are likely to be granted (see exhibit below for the list from the FDA's November 2000 Draft Guidance for Industry).

In its waiver request, an applicant seeking a waiver on the basis of this list should refer to the *Federal Register* notice in which the list appears or to any guidance that modifies the *Federal Register* notice (i.e., Regulations Requiring Pediatric Studies of Certain New and Marketed Drug and Biological Products, 63 *Fed. Reg.* 66,632, 66,648 (1998), or to the Draft Guidance when it becomes final). Modifications to this list, however, are anticipated in the future. Some changes are already being contemplated as products for the treatment, prevention, or diagnosis of listed diseases become available through gene therapy, diagnostic genetic testing, or chemoprevention.

The FDA's Waiver List

Alzheimer's disease	Age-related macular degeneration
Prostate cancer	Breast cancer
Non-germ cell ovarian cancer	Renal cell cancer
Hairy cell leukemia	Uterine cancer
Squamous cell cancers of the oropharynx	Pancreatic cancer
Basal cell and squamous cell cancer	Endometrial cancer
Osteoarthritis	Parkinson's disease
Amyotrophic lateral sclerosis	Arteriosclerosis
Infertility	Symptoms of menopause
Small cell and non-small cell lung cancer	

Source: FDA

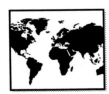

If formulation difficulties are to provide the basis for the waiver request, the burden is on the applicant to provide evidence that "experts" in formulation chemistry had encountered unusually difficult technical problems. In evaluating formulation issues, the FDA will also consider the potential importance of the product to pediatric patients. The agency will, at its discretion, subject the waiver request to the scrutiny of an advisory committee, which will consider whether reasonable attempts were made in a particular case. Although the FDA recognizes that the difficulty and cost of producing a formulation can vary "greatly" based on such factors as the compound's solubility and taste, the agency will have to rely on the manufacturer to supply "informative cost information." The FDA believes, however, that greater costs can be incurred when a product has "significant" patent or exclusivity life remaining. Even if a stable commercial formulation cannot be developed, the agency will consider, on a case-by-case basis, whether to accept labeling directions for producing extemporaneous pediatric formulations as an alternative.

Deferral The FDA may grant a deferral for a new application on its own initiative or at the request of an applicant. As it does for waivers, the FDA recommends that discussion regarding a deferral take place at the end-of-Phase 2 or pre-NDA/BLA meeting, or at least 60 days prior to an application's submission. To request a deferral, an applicant must: (1) certify the grounds for delaying pediatric studies; (2) describe the planned or ongoing studies; and (3) show that the studies are being or will be conducted with due diligence and at the earliest possible time.

If the agency determines that there is "adequate justification" for temporarily delaying the submission of assessments of pediatric safety and effectiveness, the drug product may be approved for use in adults subject to the requirement that the applicant submit the required assessments within a specified time. Adequate justification for deferral may exist if the pediatric studies cannot begin until some safety and/or effectiveness information has been collected on adults first, or when the need to await the completion of pediatric studies would delay the availability of the product for adults. For example, assessments for "me-too drugs" may be deferred until adequate safety and efficacy profiles have been established through extensive marketing in the adult population. In contrast, for drugs intended to treat life-threatening illnesses that lack adequate treatment, pediatric studies may begin as early as preliminary safety data become available in adults (i.e., after Phase 1).

Although the proposed rule discussed a two-year deferral period, this period was suggested as a maximum timeframe for a deferral. A decision regarding the amount of additional time allowed, like the decision to grant a deferral itself, will be made on a case-by-case basis. These decisions will depend on several factors, such as the need for the drug, when sufficient safety data become available, the nature and extent of the pediatric data that will be required to support pediatric labeling, and substantiated difficulties encountered in enrolling patients and in developing pediatric formulations. Deferral decisions will provide a specific date by which data submissions are required. Ordinarily, the FDA will expect that deferred pediatric studies will be initiated prior to a drug's approval for an adult indication, and that the results will be submitted no more than two years after the initial approval.

If the applicant fails to conduct the assessment within the specified time, the FDA reviewing division will first notify and meet with the applicant to discuss the reasons for this failure. When an applicant cannot provide a reasonable explanation for the delay and obtain a further deferral from the division, the division may pursue regulatory actions in consultation with the FDA's Office of the General

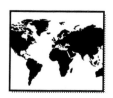

Counsel. If the study submitted with the application is not adequate, a further study will be necessary unless the review division waives or defers the requirement based on its desire to approve the application for adults.

FDAMA considerations may prove relevant to a manufacturer's plans for exemptions, waivers, or deferrals from the 1998 rule. For example, while an exemption for an orphan approved drug might be useful, there are three reasons why a company might want to investigate possible pediatric indications. First, any pediatric studies that a company undertakes may qualify for a six-month extension of its orphan exclusivity under FDAMA. Next, funding support for studies of pediatric orphan indications may be available through the FDA's orphan drug program. Finally, since even an orphan drug may become, at some point, subject to the pediatric rule if it meets the compelling circumstances criteria for marketed drugs, the sponsor may have to conduct pediatric studies ultimately, perhaps after the FDAMA incentive is no longer available.

The FDA has pointed out that a sponsor that submits an NDA for an indication not relevant to children and that receives a waiver from the 1998 pediatric rule for this indication would not be precluded from submitting a proposal under FDAMA to do pediatric studies of the drug for a different indication.

There is a similar potential for FDAMA interaction with the deferral decision. For example, consider a sponsor's options if it is developing an NME with uses in both the adult and pediatric population but is on target with only two of the three pediatric studies needed. The sponsor may want to submit an NDA, but seek a deferral for all pediatric studies until it can solicit an FDA written request, which would enable the company to submit the pediatric studies simultaneously to comply with the pediatric rule and to apply for FDAMA pediatric exclusivity.

Planning Considerations II: What Types of Studies Will Be Required For FDAMA and the Pediatric Rule?

As previously discussed, although FDAMA's scope is different from that of the 1998 pediatric rule, the types of studies and methodological issues involved will be similar. Additionally, because the FDA is committed under FDAMA to work toward the global harmonization of regulatory requirements, the agency's recommendations often refer to the guidelines developed by the International Conference on Harmonization (ICH), a joint regulatory/industry project designed to harmonize the regulatory requirements for developing and registering new medicinal products in Europe, Japan, and the United States. For both FDAMA and the 1998 rule, a company's determination of what types of studies will be needed should begin with an evaluation of animal toxicology, prior human experience, the relevance of adult efficacy data, and the ICH guidelines.

Age Group Considerations and Extrapolation Before determining what types of studies will be required, a company should take into account age group and extrapolation considerations.

The FDA has described three basic methods of providing evidence to support the safe and effective use of drugs in children: (1) evidence from adequate and well-controlled investigations of a specific pediatric indication different from the indication approved for adults; (2) evidence from adequate and

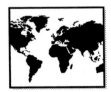

well-controlled investigations in children to support the same indication approved for adults; and (3) evidence from adequate and well-controlled adult studies in which the course of the disease and the effects of the drug, both beneficial and adverse, are sufficiently similar in the pediatric and adult populations to permit extrapolation of the adult efficacy data to pediatric patients. This last approach would likely involve the need for pharmacokinetic studies to permit appropriate dosing. There are two basic approaches for conducting pharmacokinetic studies: the standard pharmacokinetic approach and the population pharmacokinetic approach. The standard approach is, as the name implies, the approach typically employed, and involves the administration of either single or multiple doses of a drug to a relatively small (e.g., 6-12) group of subjects with relatively frequent blood and sometimes urine sample collection. The population PK approach is generally used in patients being given the drug therapeutically, and relies on infrequent (sparse) sampling of blood from a larger population.

Percent of Pediatric Studies by Age-Group for FDAMA and 1998 Rule

	Rule Studies*	FDAMA Studies**	1998 FDAMA list**
Neonate	5%	17%	21%
Infant	15%	26%	25%
Child	40%	30%	28%
Adolescent	40%	27%	26%

*Source: Tufts Center for the Study of Drug Development
** Source: Food and Drug Administration

In most cases, the FDA believes that pharmacokinetic (PK) data will be necessary in each age group to allow dosing adjustments, and that studies in more than one age group may be necessary, depending on the expected therapeutic benefit and use in each age group and on the degree to which data from one age group can be extrapolated to other age groups. When PK parameters have not been well correlated with activity in adults (e.g., topicals), a clinical study will most likely be necessary. Specific requirements for each study will be determined on a case-by-case basis, however. In general, the FDA states that specific drug studies in the relevant age category should be conducted whenever major differences, such as the formation of different metabolites, exist. The agency indicates that neonates, in particular, are likely to require age-specific studies.

Although the FDA and the American Academy of Pediatrics (AAP) maintain that the standard FDA age-groups (neonates: birth-1month; infants: 1month-2 years; children: 2-12 years; and adolescents: 12-16 years) provide acceptable guidelines, both organizations concede that the ranges should not be followed rigidly when it is reasonable to define subgroups by some other method, such as stage of development. If a sponsor conducts a study based on characteristics other than age, the company should support its categories with scientific, developmental, compliance, or ethical considerations. Most recently, the FDA has stated that age groups should be defined in a flexible manner, depending on the pharmacology of the drug or biological product, the manifestations of the disease in various age groups, and the ability to measure the response to therapy.

With regard to pre-term infants, neonates, and infants, the AAP emphasizes that the difficulties involved in studying drug effects in these groups do not outweigh the importance of studying them. The FDA acknowledges that studies in these groups may be waived, or at least deferred, until additional experience with the drug or biological product has been gained. There will be cases, however, in which the drug or biologic is an important advance and is expected to be used in these age groups. In such cases, studies will be required, unless the applicant obtains a partial waiver.

Diseases and Conditions for which Efficacy Trials were Requested by FDA for Pediatric Exclusivity Studies Under FDAMA

- Hypertension
- Depression
- Anesthesia/Sedation
- Pain
- Hepatitis C
- Complicated UTI
- Obesity
- Transplant rejection
- End stage renal disease
- Malaria
- GAD
- Allergic conjunctivitis
- Eye allergies
- Hepatitis B
- Asthma
- OCD
- HIV
- Influenza
- Seizures
- Atopic dermatitis
- Intraocular pressure
- Allergic rhinitis
- Cholesterol lowering
- Antibiotics
- Smoking cessation
- Migraines
- JRA
- Diabetes
- Anti-fungal
- Acne

Source: FDA

The ICH guidelines state that pre-term and term newborn infants may have unique manifestations of diseases, precluding the extrapolation of efficacy from older pediatric patients. Rarely is it possible to extrapolate efficacy from studies in adults or even older pediatric patients to the pre-term infant. Oral absorption of medicinal products may be less predictable in term newborn infants than in older pediatric patients. In children, it may be necessary to define age by Tanner stages. The extrapolation of efficacy data from older children to younger children may be necessary, especially when the assessment of outcome variables is particularly difficult in younger patients (e.g., forced expiratory volume (FEV1) below the age of 6 years).

Preclinical Studies Since the FDA has no standard requirements for the number or type of preclinical studies that must accompany an application for a pediatric indication, the agency may need to have the applicant conduct animal studies to provide adequate data. Each drug will be considered on a case-by-case basis.

The FDA believes that juvenile animal studies should be considered when the drug or biological product is for chronic use, when the product presents specific health concerns that require investigation (e.g., neurotoxicity), or when problems are associated with the drug class (e.g., bone/joint toxicity in the adult—human or animal).

To support pediatric exclusivity under FDAMA, toxicology studies in immature animals may be necessary even before determining if a written request should be issued and before conducting pediatric clinical studies.

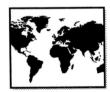

Clinical Studies When pediatric clinical studies are required, then an evaluation of their unique aspects must comprise the next stage of planning. Alternative endpoints are often necessary in pediatric clinical trials. For example, it may be impractical to measure the same clinical endpoints as used for adults in some cases (e.g., because it would require cooperation, verbal skills, or comprehension beyond the ken of the typical pediatric study participant). Suggested approaches for tailoring trial design to children involve modifying adult efficacy measures, devising new ones, or identifying and validating surrogate endpoints. Pediatric clinical studies will also have to accommodate school and caregiver schedules, and employ sampling schemes that will vary, in some cases, from those used in adult studies. The availability of appropriate facilities and specially trained staff are other considerations that the FDA has suggested should become a routine part of a sponsor's planning process for pediatric clinical studies.

The agency has noted that the type and amount of data required in any particular case will depend upon many factors (see the exhibits below). As for the number of pivotal clinical trials required, the FDA has further stated that two adequate and well-controlled clinical trials are not necessarily required to establish adequate evidence of a drug's safety and effectiveness. Under the agency's 1994 labeling regulation, for example, the FDA may approve a pediatric use for a drug on the basis of extrapolations from adult efficacy data that are supplemented with supporting pediatric data, such as pharmacokinetic, dosing, and safety information. If additional controlled trial data are needed to support a drug's effectiveness in a pediatric population, a single controlled trial generally should suffice. Safety studies are typically required when the drug has a narrow therapeutic index or when major safety problems have been identified from the adult data.

Types of Pediatric Studies for FDAMA and the 1998 Rule, by Percent

	Efficacy	PK	Safety	PK/PD	Other†
Rule*	23%	16%	21%	14%	26%
	Eff/Safety	PK/Safety	Safety	PK/PD	Other††
FDAMA ** (1999)	38%	28%	23%	9%	3%
FDAMA** (2001)	32%	31%	19%	9%	9%

Other†—Dosing and extrapolation studies
Other††—Prophylaxis, OTC use, and combination efficacy, safety and PK studies

*Source: Tufts Center for the Study of Drug Development
**Source: Food and Drug Administration

The ICH guidelines point out that a PK approach may not be sufficient for medicinal products for which blood levels are not known to correspond with efficacy, or for which there is concern that the concentration-response relationship may differ between adult and pediatric patients. When the compatibility of the disease course and/or outcome of therapy in the pediatric patient is expected to be similar but the appropriate blood levels are not clear, it may be possible to utilize measurements of a pharmacodynamic (PD) effect to confirm the expectations of effectiveness and to define the dose and concentration needed to attain that PD effect. Such studies would provide additional assurance that achieving a given pediatric exposure is likely to result in the desired therapeutic outcomes. This could circumvent the need for clinical efficacy studies. Aside from adult data, the necessary safety information would comprise repeat dose toxicology (may not be applicable for some biotechnology products) and reproductive toxicology and genotoxicology data.

Long-term Studies Long-term observational studies may be required when drugs could affect growth and development (e.g., steroids), CNS development (e.g., drugs affecting neurotransmitters, drugs given chronically during CNS/brain development, drugs with CNS toxicity), or the musculoskeletal system (e.g., quinolones). Other diseases and conditions that the FDA has suggested as likely to require long-term studies include chronic lung disease, asthma, inflammatory diseases, attention deficit disorder, depression, and psychoses. However, the FDA also has emphasized that, if early studies do not indicate a problem, then long-term studies will not be an impediment to marketing the product, and that post-marketing studies may be a tool to accomplish the twin goals of making needed products available while investigating long-term effects.

Formulations It is becoming increasingly clear that one of the FDA's main goals in the pediatric studies initiative is to promote the development of pediatric formulations. The development of age-appropriate formulations is technically challenging and time-consuming, and requires a number of steps, including the identification of problem drugs, the application of specialized formulation technology (e.g., tastemasking and transdermal enhancement), and the completion of dosing and pharmacokinetic studies. Taste is crucial for compliance, especially in children—an Ascent Pediatrics survey of 500 parents indicated that approximately 50% of children refuse to take their medication at some time and that, for 75% of the noncompliers, the reason related to a drug's taste.

Dosage form is another complicating factor in pediatric formulation, and significant variation occurs even between pediatric age groups. According to the Physician Drug & Diagnosis Audit conducted by Scott Levin in 1997, the percent of 6-year-olds taking their medicines as oral solids was 4 times less than in 16-year-olds. In addition, the selection of inert ingredients requires greater care, since children can have adverse reactions to preservatives, colorings, and flavoring agents routinely used in adult formulations.

The AAP emphasizes that the FDA must require appropriate formulations for each age group in which a drug will be used, taking into account the ease of administration and the ability to dose accurately. The agency believes that, for drugs and biologics that offer a meaningful therapeutic benefit, it is essential to ensure a drug's bioavailability and accurate dosing. The agency may require that an applicant develop a new formulation when one is needed for the targeted pediatric population.

The FDA recognizes that it may be necessary for a manufacturer to begin developing a pediatric formulation before initiating clinical trials—in some cases, as early as before Phase 1 studies are completed. In general, the agency believes that 25% of all new dosage forms developed would be initiated at the start of Phase 2 trials and 75% by the start of Phase 3 trials. By the FDA's own estimates, the financial impact of new formulation development is considerable: The agency has projected that, for

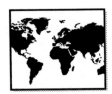

about 40% of drugs and biologicals studied each year under the rule, manufacturers would have to develop new dosage forms at an average cost of $1 million per formulation.

The ICH guidelines regard pediatric formulation needs as potentially expansive, despite the FDA's belief that a liquid formulation may serve all age groups in many cases. ICH suggests that several formulations, such as liquids, suspensions, and chewable tablets, may be needed or desirable for pediatric patients in different age groups. Different concentrations may be necessary, as well as alternative approaches, such as patches or suppositories. For injectables, the concentration must be appropriate for the doses administered, including doses for small premature infants or when fluid restrictions are relevant for very small patients. Since the development of pediatric formulations can be difficult and time consuming, it is important that this process be considered early in medicinal product development.

Planning Considerations III: When to Start Studies

Nothing in the pediatric rule requires concurrent testing of adults and children, or the testing of infants and neonates before older children (i.e., progressing up or down the age categories). For life-threatening diseases, the expectation is that pediatric trials will start after Phase 1. For less serious diseases, pediatric trials should begin no earlier than the point at which data from the initial well-controlled study in adults are available. Even for lower-priority drugs (e.g., "me-too drugs"), pediatric trials should not begin until after the FDA approves the drug or biological product in adults. In general, products with a narrow therapeutic index that do not fulfill an urgent need should be studied in pediatric patients later in drug development. The pediatric rule does not necessarily require separate studies in pediatric patients, since such patients may be included in the original trials conducted for the product.

The regulation indicates that a sponsor generally should forward, in advance of a submission for an end-of-Phase 2 meeting (at least one month in advance), a proposed timeline for protocol finalization, enrollment, study completion, data analysis, and the submission of pediatric studies. Alternatively, a sponsor may submit information to support a planned request for a waiver or deferral. For drugs and biologics for life-threatening diseases, the submission should be made in advance of the EOP1 meeting. If a pediatric drug development plan is not included in the background package for the EOP1 or EOP2 meeting, the reviewing division need not grant the meeting until the package is complete.

Alternatively, sponsors could submit information on the status of needed and ongoing pediatric studies in advance of the pre-NDA or pre-BLA meeting (i.e., not every sponsor elects to have an EOP1 or EOP2 meeting). While a formal request for a waiver or deferral is not required until the NDA/BLA submission, whenever the FDA receives such information, the agency will provide its best judgment "at that time" as to whether pediatric studies will be waived or deferred.

Planning Considerations IV: What Resources Are Available

Pediatric Research Organizations and Outsourcing Some pediatric research organizations predated the FDA's pediatric initiative. One of these is the network of Pediatric Pharmacology Research

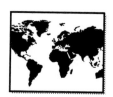

Units (PPRUs), which currently comprises 13 academic medical centers and children's hospitals in the United States. Collectively, these PPRUs, which are organized under the auspices of the NIH and have been operational since 1994, serve a population of 160,000 pediatric inpatients and nearly 3 million pediatric outpatients. Similarly, some additional children's hospitals and academic medical centers that were previously conducting pediatric research on an individual basis have established networks or other collaborations of their own. Moreover, the NIH and its Division of AIDS have created the Pediatric AIDS Clinical Trials Group to design and conduct pediatric HIV drug trials. In addition, a Pediatric Oncology Group has been established under the auspices of the National Cancer Institute.

There has also been an impressive marshaling of resources within the outsourcing sector in response to the FDAMA incentive and the perception that many pharmaceutical companies would find value in external pediatric research capacities and expertise.

Some organizations reshaped themselves in response to what they perceived as new industry needs and market opportunities. One form was the make-over of academic medical centers into academic research organizations (AROs). Another was the formation of site management organizations (SMOs) dedicated exclusively to pediatric research. Other outsourcing entities, including several CROs, supplemented existing resources and established discrete pediatric research units.

It is likely that the 1998 rule will further increase the pharmaceutical industry's demand for pediatric investigators. Generic drug sponsors, which do not routinely conduct clinical trials and which may face requirements for conducting pediatric studies for multisource drugs under the 1998 rule, may also have to look to the outsourcing industry to assist them in meeting their obligations.

Ethical Guidelines and the Pediatric Advisory Subcommittee Given the need for large numbers of pediatric patients within a relatively brief timeframe, ensuring the ethics of patient recruitment, informed consent procedures, trial design and conduct, and the use of appropriate facilities and adequately trained personnel has become especially challenging. This is one of the reasons that, although FDAMA mentioned consultation with pediatric experts only in passing and the 1998 rule referred to it even more obliquely, the FDA decided early on in the initiative to convene a panel with

Increase in Pediatric Studies Infrastructure After FDAMA

	1997	1999
Contract Research Organizations	32%	45%*
Site Management Organizations	30%	45%**
Clinical Research Centers	58	119***
Pediatric Pharmacology Research Units	7	13

*Source: CenterWatch Survey
** Source: Quintiles, Tufts CSDD Survey
*** CenterWatch Database

expertise in pediatric health. In April of 1999, the FDA held the first meeting of its Pediatric Advisory Subcommittee (officially the Pediatric Subcommittee of the Anti-Infective Drugs Advisory Committee). Currently, the Subcommittee comprises FDA and non-FDA clinicians, statisticians, and consumer representatives who are advising the agency on a range of issues related to the implementation of the 1998 rule:

- Providing an annual assessment of the rule's implementation
- Reviewing the agency's record of granting waivers and deferrals
- Discussing ethical issues raised by clinical trials in pediatric patients
- Reviewing the need for additional therapeutic options
- Recommending specific marketed drugs and biological products that should be studied in pediatric patients
- Monitoring the timeliness or progress of studies
- Reviewing trial design and data analysis

The Subcommittee is also addressing pediatric exclusivity, the interaction of the pediatric rule and exclusivity, and pediatric studies in general (e.g., matters of ethics). Ethical issues are discussed by the FDA's Pediatric Ethics Working Group, which held its first meeting in November 1999. The proceedings of these meetings are available online through the FDA's Pediatric Medicine Page web site (see Information Sources Checklist below).

The FDA's basic position statement on the ethical conduct of pediatric studies notes that pediatric clinical studies should adhere to the principles set forth by the Department of Health and Human Services (DHHS) as described in Subpart D-Additional Protections for Children Involved as Subjects in Research (45 CFR Subtitle A: 46.401-46.409). The APP's Committee on Drugs has also issued a document entitled, *Guidelines for the Ethical Conduct of Studies to Evaluate Drugs in Pediatric Populations* (see Information Sources Checklist below).

The ICH guidelines recommend minimizing the distress experienced by pediatric patients by providing: (1) protocols and investigations specifically designed for the pediatric population (i.e., not reworked adult protocols); (2) oversight by competent and experienced IRB/IECs (Independent Ethics Committee); (3) personnel knowledgeable and skilled in dealing with the pediatric population and its age-appropriate needs, including skills in performing pediatric procedures; (4) a physical setting with age-appropriate furniture, play equipment, activities, and food; and (5) a familiar environment for conducting the trials, such as hospitals or clinics at which pediatric patients normally receive care.

Information Sources

Since the pediatric studies initiative is constantly evolving and because many FDA decisions are being reached on a case-by-case basis after consultation with several different professional groups, access to up-to-date information is especially crucial. In addition, it is essential that sponsors communicate directly with the FDA when they have questions that appear to have been insufficiently addressed in currently available information sources.

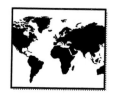

Information Sources Checklist

Contacting FDA Directly

PEDS Line: 301-594-PEDS (7337)
Office of Pediatric Drug Development and Program Initiatives (HFD-950): 301-594-7337
E-mail questions to CDER: pdit@cder.fda.gov
Human Subject Protection, CDER: 301-594-1026
Human Subject Protection, CBER: 301-827-6221

Websites

Http://www.fda.gov/cder/pediatric (FDA Pediatric Medicine Page)
Http://www.fda.gov/ (FDA Home Page)
Http://www.fda.gov/cder/pediatric/faqs.htm (FDA's Frequently Asked Questions on Pediatric Exclusivity (505A), The Pediatric "Rule," and Their Interaction)
Http://www.eudra.org/emea.html (International Conference on Harmonization [ICH] Guidelines including E3,E4,E6,& E8 and European Agency for the Evaluation of Medicinal Products [EMEA] Guidelines)
Http://helix.nih.gov:8001/ohsr/info/jinfo_10.phtml (NIH Information Sheet on Research in Children, or call NIH Office of Protection from Research Risks: 301-496-7041)
Http://helix.nih.gov:8001/ohsr/mpa/45cfr46.phtml (DHHS Regulations for Protection of Children as Research Subjects)
Http://www.aap.org/policy/00655.html (Guidelines for the Ethical Conduct of Studies to Evaluate Drugs in Pediatric Populations – RE9503)

Documents (available on-line from the FDA Pediatric Medicine Page)

The Pediatric Exclusivity Provision of FDAMA as codified: 21 U.S.C. 355a.
The 1998 FDA Pediatric Rule: 63 Fed. Reg. 66632 (December 2, 1998).
Guidance for Industry: Qualifying for Pediatric Exclusivity, CDER and CBER, September 1999.
CDER MAPP (Manual of Policies and Procedures) 6020.6: Review Management: Process for Handling Pediatric Exclusivity, October 1998
Guidance (Draft) for Industry: Recommendations for Complying with the Pediatric Rule, CDER and CBER, November 2000
Guidance (Draft) for Industry: General Considerations for Pediatric Pharmacokinetic Studies for Drugs and Biological Products, CDER and CBER, November 1998
Guidance for Industry: Pediatric Oncology Studies In Response to a Written Request, CDER and CBER, June 2000
Guidance for Industry: Providing Evidence of Clinical Effectiveness for Human Drug and Biological Products, CDER and CBER, May 1998
Guidance for Industry: The Content and Format for Pediatric Use Supplements, CDER and CBER, May 1996
Guidance for Industry: Format and Content of Clinical and Statistical Sections of New Drug Applications, CDER, July 1988
CDER Pediatric Drug Development Organization Chart
Sample Letter for Written Request for Pediatric Studies (basic template), August 1999
Sample Written Request for specific drug classes (oral hypertensives, antidepressants, HIV drugs, obsessive-compulsive disorder and oncology drugs), Aug/1999 – May/2000
Draft Guidance on Clinical Investigation of Medicinal Products in the Pediatric Population, 4/20/2000 (FDA publication of ICH Topic E-11: Clinical Investigation of Medicinal Products in the Pediatric Population (Draft), October 1999)

The Present

There is no doubt that FDAMA's pediatric provision has motivated the industry "to think pediatric." Already, close to 300 products have been the subjects of pediatric study proposals by nearly 60 different companies. Similarly, the 1998 rule also seems to be motivating the industry: The number of applications for new molecular entities (NMEs) accompanied by pediatric studies appears to be rising steadily (see exhibit below). The FDA has even noted that, of the NDAs submitted within the first six months of the rule's effective date, close to 60% had completed studies or had received waivers and documented deferrals.

Given the frenetic pace of the pediatric studies initiative, all of the affected parties—industry, researchers, regulators, and outsourcing companies—are scrambling to keep up. Such efforts will only intensify over the next few years as the "crunch times" for FDAMA and the 1998 rule begin to overlap. With over 400 studies in the works to support pediatric exclusivity and with an additional 40 or so products requiring pediatric studies under the pediatric rule each year, the number of pediatric drug studies already has tripled its pre-FDAMA level.

Although the pharmaceutical industry has been able to marshal resources to meet the demand so far, the FDA may be struggling under the increasing workload. Agency officials have conceded that the demands of the resource-intensive and deadline-driven pediatric studies initiative may have affected its capacity to deal with its traditional regulatory activities, such as reviewing standard NDAs. While industry has been prompted, through incentives, to devote additional resources to pediatric studies, the FDA actually has lost resources due to the exemption of pediatric supplements from user fees. The impact of the initiative on FDA personnel can be appreciated by considering the fact that, throughout most of the FDAMA implementation period, the FDA had 65 staffers spread over 12 pediatric oversight activities. This does not take into account the additional staffers involved at the CDER review division and CBER office levels. In the fall of 2001, in recognition of the "ever-increasing role

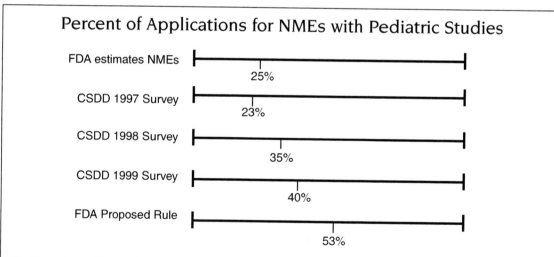

Percent of Applications for NMEs with Pediatric Studies

- FDA estimates NMEs: 25%
- CSDD 1997 Survey: 23%
- CSDD 1998 Survey: 35%
- CSDD 1999 Survey: 40%
- FDA Proposed Rule: 53%

The FDA estimated in 1997 that 25% of NDAs submitted for NMEs were accompanied by pediatric studies. Since then, the Tufts CSDD has been tracking the percent of NDAs for NMEs with pediatric studies through annual industry surveys. As illustrated above, the percent of applications with pediatric studies is now approaching the percent of NMEs estimated by the FDA to have potential uses in the pediatric population.

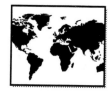

The Pediatric Studies Initiative

Chapter 16

that pediatric drug development" was playing in the agency's regulatory workload, the FDA established the Office of Pediatric Drug Development and Program Initiatives. In addition to pediatric issues, the new office is also responsible for pregnancy labeling and anti-bioterrorism efforts.

Another resource concern focuses on the dearth of pediatric patients. This was anticipated in therapeutic areas in which a large percentage of the pediatric patient population is already enrolled in studies (e.g., AIDS and cancer). So far, the few shortages that have been identified have occurred in less traditional pediatric research areas, including hypertension. In some cases, these problems were addressed by recruiting patients overseas. Despite such efforts, the pediatric studies initiative will put pediatric study participants at a premium.

According to the 1999 Tufts CSDD annual survey of NME sponsors, companies have enrolled an average of 247 patients per pediatric drug study in efforts to comply with the 1998 rule. If these numbers hold true for the approximately 80 drug and biological products that the FDA projected may be required to submit pediatric studies each year under the rule, about 20,000 pediatric patients will be needed annually (although the FDA estimates that half of these, or approximately 10,000 patients, would be studied to fulfill both the rule's requirements and to support pediatric exclusivity). In March 2000, the FDA announced that 131 of 274 studies for written requests issued under FDAMA had specified the numbers of patients for studies, and that those studies alone would require over 17,000 patients (and perhaps well over 30,000 for all 274 studies). Thus, over 40,000 children—and some say as many as 50,000—are participating or have participated in pediatric studies as a result of the initiative.

If the pediatric research infrastructure is capable of handling this increased level of activity over a longer term, it could have a very beneficial impact on children's health. For example, a 1996 study reported that over 70% of pediatric cancer patients were enrolled in clinical trials and that pediatric cancer has experienced a dramatic increase in cure rates over the last few years.

In the four years since the pediatric studies program was initiated, studies for 80 diseases and conditions in a dozen different therapeutic areas have been requested. Although only about two dozen drugs have been labeled to date under the pediatric exclusivity program, the level of research activity is an indicator of the program's public health promise.

There is, however, an additional and important element of the pediatric studies initiative—the economic incentive. As of year-end 2001, over 40 drugs had been awarded pediatric exclusivity—a reward is potentially worth hundreds of millions of dollars (see exhibit below).

In fact, impending incentive awards have even become key factors in merger negotiations, as reportedly was the case in the Astra-Zeneca merger (i.e., regarding Zeneca's blockbuster drug Zestril). Also, industry is taking notice of the sponsor's experience with the recently approved drug abacavir, for which pediatric studies were utilized to help support approval in adults.

The FDA examined a number of these considerations in a January 2001 report to Congress on all issues relevant to the pediatric exclusivity program. In particular, the FDA was directed to examine: (1) the program's effectiveness in improving information about important pediatric uses for approved drugs; (2) the adequacy of FDAMA's exclusivity incentive; (3) the program's economic impact on taxpayers and consumers, including lower-income patients; and (4) any suggestions for modifications that the HHS secretary deems appropriate.

The FDA's report and the testimony provided at congressional hearings held in the spring of 2001 convinced Congress to extend the pediatric provision of FDAMA until 2007. The pediatric exclusivity incentive will remain essentially the same in the reauthorized version of the law, although gaps in the program related to pediatric studies for off-patent drugs, expediting labeling changes, as well as facilitating implementation, enforcement and disseminating pediatric information are addressed in the reauthorized legislation.

Drugs with Sales Over $1 Billion Worldwide, for which FDA has Issued Written Requests for Pediatric Studies in the First Two Years of FDAMA

Drug (Generic Name)	Drug (Trade Name)	Manufacturer	Worldwide 1997 Sales (Millions)*	Patent Expiration*
Omeprazole	Losec	Astra-Zeneca	$2,816	2001
Fluoxetine	Prozac	Lilly	$2,559	2001
Enalapril	Vasotec	Merck	$2,510	2000
Omeprazole	Prilosec	Astra-Zeneca	$2,240	2001
Amlodipine	Norvasc	Pfizer	$2,217	2007
Loratadine	Claritin	Schering	$1,726	2012
Sertraline	Zoloft	Pfizer	$1,507	2005
Paroxetine	Paxil	SmithKline Beecham	$1,474	2005
Ciprofloxacin	Cipro	Bayer	$1,441	2004
Lavastatin	Mevacor	Merck	$1,100	2001
Sumatriptan	Imitrex	Glaxo Wellcome	$1,086	2006
Lisinopril	Zestril	Zeneca	$1,035	2001

* Source: Med Ad News, May 1998

Source: Tufts Center for the Study of Drug Development

The Future

The future is global. Why go global? For one reason, because that is where the potential research participants are in the short-term. Shortages of pediatric patients are likely to arise in the United States, especially in certain therapeutic areas (perhaps already a problem with cancer, AIDS and hypertension studies) and possibly for healthy pediatric study participants as well. Another reason is that off-label use of medicines in children is reportedly high in the United Kingdom, Japan, Australia, and likely the rest of the world. For this reason, there is a growing interest in the pediatric initiative overseas, with a number of countries having developed guidelines for pediatric research recently and some even considering voluntary or mandatory "incentive" programs. The growing movement toward regulatory harmonization and the internationalization of clinical research, together with the growth of multinational CROs, should facilitate the conduct of pediatric

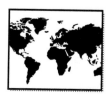

trials in multicountry settings, and should lay the groundwork for a global pediatric research infrastructure.

Another reason for the pharmaceutical industry to "go global" relates to patient needs in the long-term. The rest of the world is a mirror image of the United States as far as economic incentives for pediatric research are concerned. In the short-term, the economic incentives are strong in the United States, but weak overseas. In the long-term, it will be the reverse. Once the FDA's pediatric exclusivity program has played itself out, U.S. companies will still be conducting pediatric studies to fulfill regulatory requirements, but will have to search for pediatric market incentives elsewhere.

In the United States, the pediatric market is only 5% of the total market's dollar volume, even though it is growing at a rate 2% faster than pharmaceuticals overall and is estimated to be about $6 billion currently. While 10% to 15% of children in the United States are not covered by health insurance, there is a recent initiative to increase insurance coverage through the Children's Health Insurance Program (CHIP). Also, managed care organizations currently prefer the use of medicines for children over other treatment options.

Despite these positive trends, the actual economic impetus for the current boom in pediatric research in the United States is pediatric exclusivity, which can be worth a million dollars a day (i.e., for each additional day of exclusivity) to drug sponsors, but which is also a limited and temporary incentive. In fact, the decreasing proportion of children in our population over time, the comparatively short duration of use and low price of most pediatric medicines relative to adult medicines, as well as the increasing concerns about the overuse of antibiotics, psychotropics, and medicines in general in children do not portend favorably for a profitable long-term pediatric market in the United States. Large volume, large discount drug purchasers such as Medicaid (covers 16 million children, 23% of the total and 90% of pediatric AIDS patients) and the advent of disease management programs for chronic diseases in children (e.g., one 165,000-member HMO has a program for pediatric asthma that has reduced per-member, per-month costs by 12%) make the prospects for an economically self-sufficient pediatric drug market in the United States even less likely.

In contrast, long-term market dynamics may favor a sustainable pediatric market overseas, especially in developing countries. The demographics of such countries may support the development of a viable market for pediatric drugs in the near future based on volume alone. The under-18 population, which is about 25% of the total population in the United States and is likely to decrease, is approaching 50% in the developing world and is unlikely to decrease anytime soon. At the same time, the overall market for pharmaceuticals in the developing world is predicted to equal that of Europe (nearly $100 billion) by the year 2002. Additionally, the proportion of chronic diseases, such as depression and cardiovascular illness (generally requiring more cost-intensive therapeutic intervention), throughout the world is expected to rise from 55% in 1990 to 73% in 2020, with the most rapid increase expected in the developing world.

In the final analysis, statutory and regulatory incentives in the United States may help to build a global pediatric research infrastructure with enough economy of scale and performance to permit pediatric medicine development to come into its own as a sustainable sector of the drug and biological products industry. In this respect, it may be a harbinger of where research and development is head-ing as a whole. Pharmacogenomics, consumer empowerment, public policy pressures, incentive programs and competitive forces may compel the industry to subdivide R&D, marketing, and manufacturing units along subpopulation lines as well as by therapeutic areas. We may soon come to recognize the therapeutic orphan as the new face of drug development.

References

Milne, C.P., Pediatric research: coming of age in the new millennium, *Am J Therapeutics*, 1999; 6: 263-282.

Labson M.L., A legal and regulatory update on pediatric exclusivity and the pediatric rule. Presented at Barnett International workshop, "Pediatric Clinical Trials," Philadelphia, December 5-6, 2001.

Turner J., A regulatory perspective from the pharmaceutical industry for pediatric trials. Presented at Barnett International workshop, "Pediatric Clinical Trials," Philadelphia, December 5-6, 2001.